ADVANCES IN

Anesthesia

Editor-in-Chief
Laurence C. Torsher, MD
Assoicate Editors
Richard P. Dutton, MD
Francis V. Salinas, MD
Arna Banerjee, MD, MMHC, FCCM

ELSEVIER

An Imprint of Elsevier, Inc.

PHILADELPHIA LONDON TORONTO MONTREAL SYDNEY TOKYO

ADVANCES IN
Anesthesia

VOLUMES 1 THROUGH 35 (OUT OF PRINT)

VOLUME 36

VOLUME 37

VOLUME 38

Director, Continuity Publishing: Dolores Meloni
Editor: Joanna Collett
Developmental Editor: Karen Justine Solomon

Cover images courtesy of James P. Rathmell, MD, Brigham and Women's Hospital, Boston, MA

Reprints: For copies of 100 or more of articles in this publication, please contact the Commercial Reprints Department, Elsevier Inc., 360 Park Avenue South, New York, NY 10010-1710. Tel: 212-633-3874; Fax: 212-633-3820; E-mail: reprints@elsevier.com.

Editorial Office:
Elsevier
1600 John F. Kennedy Blvd,
Suite 1800
Philadelphia, PA 19103-2899

International Standard Serial Number: 0737-6146
International Standard Book Number-13: 978-0-323-89706-8

ADVANCES IN
Anesthesia

CONTRIBUTORS

RAVIE ABOZAID, MD, Assistant Professor, Department of Anesthesiology and Perioperative Medicine, University of Rochester School of Medicine & Dentistry, Rochester, New York

MEHMET K. AKTAS, MD, Associate Professor, Department of Medicine, Cardiology, University of Rochester School of Medicine & Dentistry, Rochester, New York

MOEED AZAM, MD, FASA, Board of Directors, Legislative Committee, Florida Society of Anesthesiologists, Orlando, Florida

ADITI BALAKRISHNA, MD, Assistant Professor of Anesthesiology, Vanderbilt University School of Medicine, Nashville, Tennessee

MONICA BHUTIANI, MD, MEd, Clinical Instructor, Department of Anesthesiology, Vanderbilt University Medical Center, Nashville, Tennessee

KAITLYN A. BRENNAN, DO, MPH, Assistant Professor of Anesthesiology and Critical Care Medicine, Department of Anesthesiology, Vanderbilt University Medical Center, Nashville, Tennessee

LUCILLE BRUNKER, MD, Assistant Professor of Anesthesiology, Vanderbilt University School of Medicine, Nashville, Tennessee

MAXIME CANNESSON, MD, PhD, Department of Anesthesiology and Perioperative Medicine, Professor and Chair, Ronal L. Katz Chair, David Geffen School of Medicine at UCLA, Ronald Reagan UCLA Medical Center, Los Angeles, California

VALERIA CARCAMO-CAVAZOS, MD, Department of Anesthesiology and Perioperative Medicine, Assistant Clinical Professor, Regional Anesthesiology and Acute Pain Management (RAAPM) Fellowship Associate Program Director, David Geffen School of Medicine at UCLA, Ronald Reagan UCLA Medical Center, Los Angeles, California

FRANCIS M. CHANG, MD, Assistant Professor, Department of Anesthesiology and Perioperative Medicine, University of Rochester School of Medicine & Dentistry, Rochester, New York

ADAORA M. CHIMA, MBBS, MPH, Department of Anesthesiology, Cincinnati Children's Hospital Medical Center, Cincinnati, Ohio

HUGO S. CLIFFORD, MD, Assistant Professor, Department of Anesthesiology and Perioperative Medicine, University of Rochster School of Medicine and Dentistry, Rochester, New York

JENNIFER E. DOMINGUEZ, MD, MHS, Department of Anesthesiology, Division of Women's Anesthesia, Duke University School of Medicine, Durham, North Carolina

RICHARD P. DUTTON, MD, MBA, FASA, Adjunct Professor, Department of Anesthesiology, Texas A&M College of Medicine, Baylor University Medical Center, Dallas, Texas

YANG GU, MD, Assistant Professor, Department of Anesthesiology and Perioperative Medicine, University of Rochester School of Medicine & Dentistry, Rochester, New York

ASHRAF S. HABIB, MBBCh, MSc, MHSc, FRCA, Department of Anesthesiology, Division of Women's Anesthesia, Duke University School of Medicine, Durham, North Carolina

WILLIAM R. HARTMAN, MD, PhD, Department of Anesthesiology, Office of Clinical Research, University of Wisconsin-Madison, Madison, Wisconsin

CHRISTOPHER G. HUGHES, MD, MS, FCCM, Professor of Anesthesiology, Vanderbilt University School of Medicine, Nashville, Tennessee

STEPHANIE JONES, MD, Postdoctoral Clinical Fellow in Anesthesiology Critical Care, Columbia University Irving Medical Center, New York, New York

MEREDITH A. KINGETER, MD, Assistant Professor of Anesthesiology, Cardiothoracic Division, Assistant Program Director, Anesthesia Residency

ALLAN M. KLOMPAS, MB, BCh, BAO, Assistant Professor of Anesthesiology, Department of Anesthesiology and Perioperative Medicine, Mayo Clinic College of Medicine, Rochester, Minnesota

HEATHER L. LANDER, MD, Assistant Professor, Department of Anesthesiology and Perioperative Medicine, University of Rochester School of Medicine & Dentistry, Rochester, New York

BRANDON F. LEBOW, MD, Assistant Professor, Department of Anesthesiology and Perioperative Medicine, University of Rochester School of Medicine & Dentistry, Rochester, New York

TODD J. LIU, MD, Department of Anesthesiology and Critical Care Medicine, Memorial Sloan Kettering Cancer Center, Department of Anesthesiology, Weill Cornell Medicine, New York, New York

YING HUI LOW, MD, FASE, FASA, Staff Physician, Department of Anesthesiology, Massachusetts General Hospital, Boston, Massachusetts

MOHAMED A. MAHMOUD, MD, Department of Anesthesiology, Cincinnati Children's Hospital Medical Center, Cincinnati, Ohio

MATTHEW D. McEVOY, MD, Professor of Anesthesiology and Surgery, Vice-Chair of Perioperative Medicine, Medical Director, VUMC Enhanced Recovery Programs, Program Director, Perioperative Medicine Fellowship Medical Director, Hi-RiSE Preoperative Optimization Clinic Director, Perioperative Consult Service, Department of Anesthesiology, Vanderbilt University Medical Center, Nashville, Tennessee

TERESA A. MULAIKAL, MD, FASE, Associate Professor of Anesthesiology and Critical Care Medicine, Division of Cardiothoracic and Critical Care, Columbia University Irving Medical Center, New York, New York

SURYAKUMAR NARAYANASAMY, MBBS, MD, Department of Anesthesiology, Cincinnati Children's Hospital Medical Center, Cincinnati, Ohio

KUNAL PANDA, MD, Assistant Professor, Department of Anesthesiology and Perioperative Medicine, University of Rochester School of Medicine & Dentistry, Rochester, New York

JUAN G. RIPOLL, MD, Fellow, Department of Anesthesiology and Perioperative Medicine, Mayo Clinic College of Medicine, Rochester, Minnesota

KAYLYN SACHSE, MD, Assistant Professor, Department of Anesthesiology, Vanderbilt University Medical Center, Nashville, Tennessee

FRANCIS V. SALINAS, MD, FASA, Staff Anesthesiologist-Swedish Medical Center, Seattle and Issaquah, Medical Director of Anesthesia Services and Interventional Platform-Swedish Issaquah Hospital, Issaquah, Washington

BRETT A. SIMON, MD, PhD, Department of Anesthesiology, Weill Cornell Medicine, Department of Anesthesiology and Critical Care Medicine, Memorial Sloan Kettering Cancer Center, New York, New York

BRADFORD B. SMITH, MD, Assistant Professor, Department of Anesthesiology and Perioperative Medicine, Mayo Clinic College of Medicine, Phoenix, Arizona

MARK M. SMITH, MD, Associate Professor, Department of Anesthesiology and Perioperative Medicine, Mayo Clinic College of Medicine, Rochester, Minnesota

YASMINE TAMEZE, MD, Staff Physician, Department of Anesthesiology, Massachusetts General Hospital, Boston, Massachusetts

CAMERON R. TAYLOR, MD, Department of Anesthesiology, Division of Women's Anesthesia, Duke University School of Medicine, Durham, North Carolina

HANAE K. TOKITA, MD, Department of Anesthesiology, Weill Cornell Medicine, Department of Anesthesiology and Critical Care Medicine, Memorial Sloan Kettering Cancer Center, New York, New York

JULIE A. WYROBEK, MD, Assistant Professor, Department of Anesthesiology and Perioperative Medicine, University of Rochester School of Medicine & Dentistry, Rochester, New York

MARY YURASHEVICH, MD, MPH, Department of Anesthesiology, Division of Women's Anesthesia, Duke University School of Medicine, Durham, North Carolina

SHERIF ZAAFRAN, MD, FASA, Board of Directors, Texas Society of Anesthesiologists, Chair, Texas Medical Board, Houston, Texas

ADVANCES IN
Anesthesia

CONTENTS

VOLUME 40 • 2022

A shortage of inpatient beds and nurses during the coronavirus disease 2019 pandemic has lent priority to safe same-day discharge after surgery. The minimally invasive nature of robotic surgery has allowed an increasing number of procedures to be done on an outpatient basis. Anesthetic management should be designed to complement the technical advantages of robotic surgery in facilitating early discharge.

Ambulatory surgery centers (ASC) serve an important role for hospital systems of increasing operating capacity and offloading patient volume. When seeking to perform more complex cancer surgeries at an ASC, a systematic approach with care pathways can yield success by facilitating quick recovery for patients and reducing complication rates. End-to-end patient engagement is a key component of patient-centered care at the Josie Robertson Surgery Center and begins the moment the decision to have surgery is made and extends to the postdischarge period to track recovery. Engagement includes comprehensive education, standardization of processes, and setting clear expectations for recovery and discharge.

Severe acute respiratory syndrome coronavirus 2 (SARS-CoV-2) emerged in late 2019. To date, this coronavirus is responsible for greater than 90 million cases in the United States and more than 1 million confirmed deaths. When this virus came to the United States, testing was unorganized, no effective treatments were known, and no vaccines had been discovered. A plan to correct these deficiencies through cooperative science and efficient clinical trials was implemented to combat this novel virus. This plan developed efficient and inexpensive tests, highly effective medicines to treat and prevent disease progression, and vaccines to immunize the population.

Over two-thirds of the world's population do not have access to safe surgical and anesthetic care. Barriers to care include a lack of specialty trained personnel and unavailability of essential operating room resources. Aid efforts with the greatest impact focus on forming partnerships between high- and low-income communities, with the goal of creating self-sustaining programs run by local communities. Together these partnerships can work to build local capacity and expand the trained workforce by educating local providers.

Vasoplegic syndrome occurs relatively frequently in cardiac surgery, liver transplant, major noncardiac surgery, in post-return of spontaneous circulation situations, and in pateints with sepsis. It is paramount for the anesthesiologist to understand both the pathophysiology of vasoplegia and the different treatment strategies available for rescuing a patient from life-threatening hypotension.

Direct oral anticoagulants (DOACs) have rapidly emerged as popular alternatives to warfarin in the setting of nonvalvular atrial fibrillation, prevention and treatment of venous thromboembolism, and secondary prevention of arterial thrombosis. It is now estimated that more patients in the United States take DOACs than warfarin for approved indications. Studies to date have shown that these drugs are similarly efficacious with perhaps a lower bleeding risk than warfarin. The purpose of this review is to provide insight into the currently available DOACs and discuss the management and reversal strategies for patients in the perioperative period.

Dexmedetomidine's unique sedative properties have led to its widespread use. Dexmedetomidine has a beneficial pharmacologic profile including analgesic sparing effects, anxiolysis, sympatholysis, organ-protective effects against ischemic and hypoxic injury, and sedation which parallels natural sleep. An understanding of predictable side effects,

effects of age-related physiologic changes, and pharmacokinetic and pharmacodynamic effects of dexmedetomidine is crucial to maximize its safe administration in adults and children. This review focuses on the growing body of literature examining advances in applications of dexmedetomidine in children and adults.

The number of electrophysiology (EP) procedures being performed has dramatically increased in recent years. This escalation necessitates a full understanding by the general anesthesiologist as to the risks, specific considerations, and comorbidities that accompany these now common procedures. Procedures reviewed in this article include atrial fibrillation and flutter ablation, supraventricular tachycardia ablation, ventricular tachycardia ablation, electrical cardioversion, pacemaker insertion, implantable cardioverter-defibrillator (ICD) insertion, and ICD lead extraction. General anesthetic considerations as well as procedure-specific concerns are discussed. Knowledge of these procedures will add to the anesthesiologist's armamentarium in safely caring for patients in the EP laboratory.

Appropriate perioperative pain control is essential to aid in patients' recovery after surgery; however, acute postsurgical pain remains poorly treated and there continues to be an overreliance on opiates. Perioperative pain control starts in the operating room, and opiate-free anesthesia (OFA), where no opiates are used intraoperatively, has been proposed as a feasible strategy to further minimize opiates in the perioperative period. In this article, we address the potential benefits and shortcomings of OFA, while exploring tools available to accomplish multimodal anesthesia and ideally OFA, and the evidence behind the techniques proposed.

higher risk of maternal and fetal complications. Anesthesia also poses higher risks for obese parturients and may be more technically challenging due to body habitus. Safe anesthesia practice for these patients must take into consideration the unique challenges associated with the combination of pregnancy and obesity.

Electroconvulsive therapy (ECT) is a medical treatment most often used in patients with severe major depression that has not responded to other treatments. ECT is also indicated for patients with other severe psychiatric conditions, including bipolar disorder, schizophrenia, schizoaffective disorders, catatonia, and neuroleptic malignant syndrome. Contemporary "modified ECT" involves inducing general anesthesia with neuromuscular blockade before inducing the therapeutic seizure. The goal of this review is to combine an evidence-based update with the experience of the author's institution to provide a practical approach to anesthetic care for the patient undergoing ECT.

Advocating for anesthesiology is a professional responsibility. We need to make the public aware of the role we play in assuring their safety and comfort; and we must also ensure that payment models are fair and commensurate with the quality of our work.

Advances in Anesthesia 40 (2022) xxiii–xxv

ADVANCES IN ANESTHESIA

PREFACE

Anesthesiology in 2022: Ever in Demand and Ever Evolving

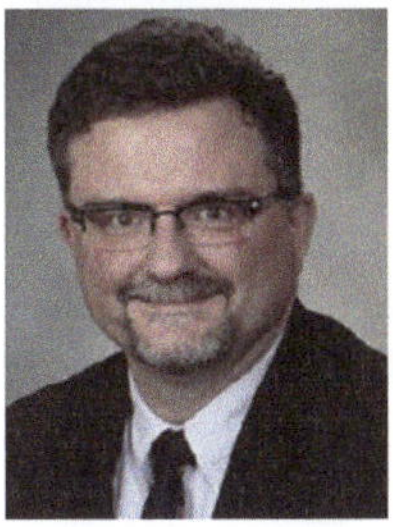
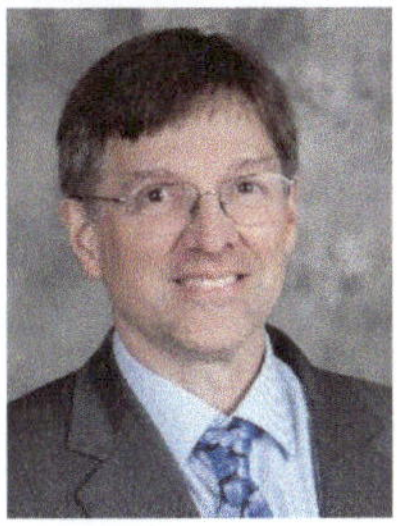
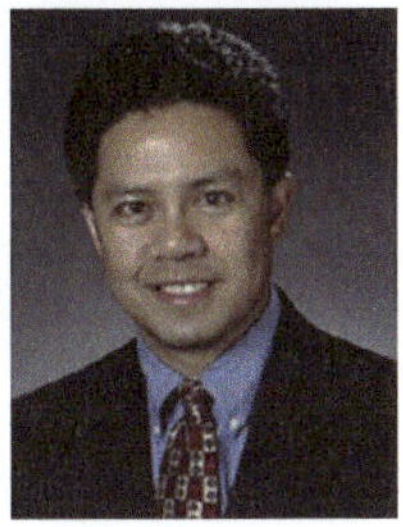
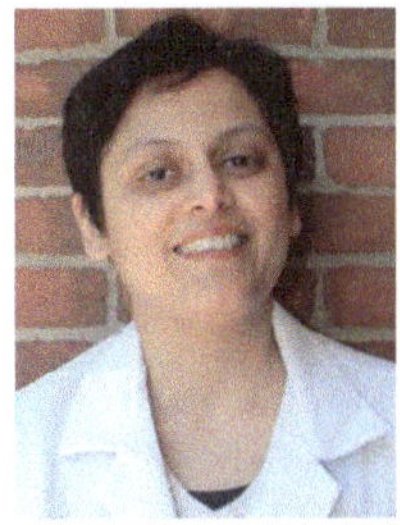

Laurence C. Torsher, MD

Richard P. Dutton, MD, MBA

Francis V. Salinas, MD

Arna Banerjee, MD, MMHC, FCCM

Editors

Welcome to the 2022 *Advances in Anesthesia*! This year's issue has 14 articles from all corners of our profession. As we do every year, the Editors have sought to find active and contentious topics to address, and we have invited the best experts we could find to discuss each topic. It's a truism in anesthesia practice management that we don't sit around and talk about everything that's going well. As a profession, we have always been future oriented: what is the next threat? What has to change? And where are we headed next? This year's collection of articles covers future-oriented anesthesia practice ranging from the clinically esoteric to the rough and tumble of health care professionalism in the modern era.

In the first category, we have solicited reviews on robotic surgery, electroconvulsive therapy, and cardiac electrophysiology procedures. We have a new and updated review of anesthesia for obese obstetric patients, and a first summary of best practice for those with COVID-19. We review new anesthesia technology for intraoperative ventilation and current uses of dexmedetomidine. And for those interested in the cutting edge of translational resuscitation, we offer a pair of articles on management of vasoplegia and coagulation: two sides of the same basic science understanding of surgical inflammation, now beginning to influence evidence-based clinical management.

https://doi.org/10.1016/j.aan.2022.08.001
0737-6146/22/© 2022 Published by Elsevier Inc.

We live in a challenging time for health care professionals, with both internal and external challenges to our daily existence. Articles on aspects of modern anesthesia practice include a review of advocacy and current political issues, guidance on opioid prescribing, an illustration of how anesthesiologists can influence end-of-life care, and a very specific example (the Josey Robertson Surgical Hospital in New York City) of how a perioperative process can be built from the ground up to promote a positive patient experience. While many of our professional articles are focused on US anesthesia practice, we have also included an important review of how anesthesiologists anywhere can contribute to positive patient outcomes in low- and middle-income countries.

Demand for anesthesia services has never been higher, with close to half our work today outside of the traditional OR environment. More than ever, our profession needs innovative solutions for both clinical work and professional development; we hope this issue of *Advances in Anesthesia* will help you find both.

Laurence C. Torsher, MD
Department of Anesthesiology
Mayo Clinic Rochester
Rochester, MN 55905, USA

E-mail address: torsher.laurence@mayo.edu

Richard P. Dutton, MD, MBA
US Anesthesia Partners
12222 Merit Drive
Dallas, TX 75225, USA

Department of Anesthesiology
Texas A&M College of Medicine
Bryan, TX 77807, USA

E-mail address: Richard.dutton@usap.com

Francis V. Salinas, MD
US Anesthesia Partners–Washington
1229 Madison Street, Suite 1440
Seattle, WA 98104, USA

Swedish Medical Center
Seattle, WA 98104, USA

Department of Anesthesiology and Pain Medicine
University of Washington
Seattle, WA 98195, USA

E-mail address: fvsalinasmd@gmail.com

Arna Banerjee, MD, MMHC, FCCM
Vanderbilt University School of Medicine
Nashville, TN 37232, USA

E-mail address: arna.banerjee@vumc.org

Advances in Anesthesia 40 (2022) 1–14

ADVANCES IN ANESTHESIA

End of Life: What Is the Anesthesiologist's Role?

Stephanie Jones, MD[a], Teresa A. Mulaikal, MD[b,*]

[a]Columbia University Irving Medical Center, Division of Critical Care Medicine, 622 W. 168th St, New York, NY 10032, USA; [b]Division of Cardiothoracic and Critical Care, Columbia University Medical Center, 622 W. 168th St., PH 5 Stem 133, New York, NY 10032, USA

Keywords

• Anesthesiologist • End of life • Palliative care • Advance care planning • Death • Ethics • COVID-19 • Mechanical circulatory support

Key points

- Anesthesiologists are central in the hub of contemporary medicine and have multiple opportunities to elevate the quality of care patients receive at the end of life.
- Effective communication and empathy are evidence-based interventions that can improve patient and family satisfaction scores and decrease costs associated with an over-medicalized death.
- More training should be incorporated into anesthesiology residencies to enhance the understanding of how best to improve end-of-life care.

BACKGROUND

Advance care planning (ACP) is a vital component of contemporary medicine that has been garnering attention and gaining momentum since the patient Self-Determination act of 1990. It ensures that any adult, regardless of the present state of competence, has the right to participate in decisions pertaining to surgical and medical care through living wills and designation of surrogate decision makers. These advanced decisions are federally mandated to be respected and honored. While ACP has always been important, its role is even more crucial in the era of COVID-19 when providers encounter major strains on our health care systems due to shortages in supplies as well as medical personnel. Patients who previously had no terminal diagnoses may

*Corresponding author. *E-mail address:* tam36@cumc.columbia.edu

https://doi.org/10.1016/j.aan.2022.07.007
0737-6146/22/

unexpectedly find themselves in hospitals and intensive care units being faced with these decisions far sooner than they had anticipated. Despite increasing efforts to have patients document their wishes in advance, there are no compelling studies proving this improves goal-concordance or quality of end of life [1]. There is, however, an emerging trend to shift the understanding of ACP from advancing *planning* to ongoing *processing* with the support of the patient's medical team and caregivers [2]. What is the anesthesiologist's role at the end of life? As perioperative physicians, we interface with our patients at all phases of peri-procedural care, as well as in intensive-care units, palliative care teams, and acute and chronic pain treatment teams. We have extensive opportunities to alleviate suffering, improve the quality of life and death, and help guide our patients and their loved ones to navigate the most vulnerable and difficult time of life. This article examines the role of the anesthesiologist in the care of patients at the end of life.

DEFINITIONS

As we navigate goals of care discussions with our patients and their family, it is important to ensure the terms and vocabulary we use are consistent and universally understood. Terms such as do-not-resuscitate and do-not-intubate are among the delineated terms, but since the initial policies on DNR orders were made in the 1970s, significant advancements have occurred in medicine to include mechanical support therapies, electrical therapies, and advanced respiratory support measures. At their inception, laws surrounding orders of DNR were aimed at providing patients with autonomy to refuse attempts at life-sustaining resuscitation, which previously had been considered the default when patients experienced cardiopulmonary arrest [3]. Major developments in the bioethical community evolved during this era, and the emerging consensus contained within the report of the 1983 President's Commission was that competent patients had the autonomy to refuse life-sustaining treatment through advance directives, or surrogate decision makers for patients lacking capacity [3]. An important distinction when discussing goals of care with families is that DNR orders are not tantamount to "do not treat" practices [4]. Patients with terminal diagnoses such as heart failure or cancer may wish to refuse attempts at life-sustaining resuscitation, but still opt for life-prolonging therapies such as dialysis, mechanical heart support, or electrical pacemakers. As the medical experts guiding these conversations, it is important to present these options as recommendations when medically appropriate, and not to offer patients a list of choices, some of which may be nonbeneficial and even harmful. The American Heart Association reports that roughly only 15%, or 1 in 6 patients, who have CPR in the hospital will survive to discharge [5]. This number is even lower for patients in the ICU and patients with cancer and should be referenced when talking with patients and their families about the reality of their illnesses.

Often the progression of code status following hospital admissions for the critically ill evolves from full code to DNR to capped care to comfort care and eventually the withdrawal of life-sustaining therapy. This progression highlights the ambiguity that lies in the middle stages of withholding therapies to withdrawing therapies. Multiple studies have shown that ACP does not correlate with goal-concordant care or improve patient satisfaction scores [1]. This is likely because what we theoretically plan for in times of health is not always what we choose in times of critical illness when death is imminent. What does correlate with patient and family satisfaction, however, is an ongoing conversation with a medical provider they perceive as empathetic and invested in their care. Navigating the middle ground between full-code and withdrawal of treatment can be especially challenging for physicians as we balance bioethical principles of patient autonomy, nonmaleficence, and physician integrity. Patient demands for nonindicated therapies, partial DNR orders, and arbitrary involvement in choosing the cap of vasopressor doses challenge physician judgment and our ability to provide care that is indicated and avoid medical futility. Studies have demonstrated that when the family wishes for heroic medical care conflict with physician recommendations for withdrawal of life-sustaining therapy in instances of futility, time-limited trials of intensive care can help decrease the overall intensity and duration of nonbeneficial medical therapy [6].

While most professional societies have consensus statements surrounding do-not-resuscitate orders, no such consensus exists for partial DNR orders or definitions of capped care. Even the term comfort care is ambiguous since what one patient may choose for comfort may differ from the next. As we navigate these challenging conversations, it is helpful to reframe the concept of advance care "planning" to "processing" while we guide our patients and their families through these difficult times. Involving our palliative care colleagues, bioethics committees, and institutional leaders should also occur, particularly when our medical recommendations are not concordant with patients' and their surrogates' wishes.

SETTINGS

Preoperative

Anesthesiologists have an integral role in caring for dying patient. We are the center hub of a complex medical environment, in both in-patient and outpatient settings (Fig. 1). Having claimed our role as leaders of the perioperative surgical home, we have demonstrated an organizational system that helps improve patient recovery outcomes and decrease hospital utilization [7]. What if we were able to use that same integrated model to help improve the family satisfaction scores and quality of life for our dying patients? Beginning with the preoperative consultation in the office or in the holding area on the day of surgery, anesthesiologists have an opportunity to participate in goals of care conversations, normalizing this as an integrated part of whole-person care and taking steps to destigmatize it as a conversation spared for the actively dying. Less than 50% of older adults have engaged in ACP and only 10% to 20% have discussed those wishes with clinicians [8]. In one study using a standardized patient actor, just over half of anesthesiologists included preoperative

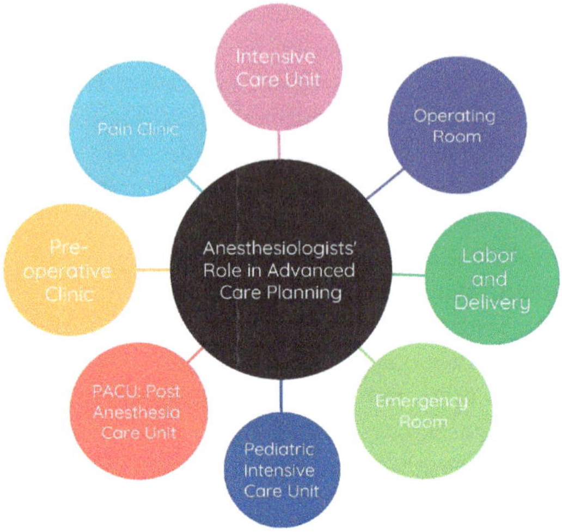

Fig. 1. Anesthesiologists' role in ACP.

discussions about resuscitation with a patient who had a documented do-not-resuscitate order [9]. Given a significant number of patients will encounter an anesthesiologist in one of the various spokes on the medical system wheel (see Fig. 1), we have an opportunity and obligation to improve the rates and quality of ACP for all patients.

Intraoperative

Care of the patient with a do-not-resuscitate order often brings up ethical concerns with anesthesiologists in the operating room (OR) setting [10]. The origin of cardiopulmonary resuscitation came from closed-chest compressions in the OR [11], and the duty of the anesthesiologist in the OR is ongoing resuscitation. Is caring for a patient who explicitly wishes to not be resuscitated at odds with our fundamental duty? Despite the American Society of Anesthesiologists recommending against the automatic rescinding of DNR orders when undergoing surgery [12], a 2013 study from Mayo Clinic found that 30% of physicians and 18% of anesthesiologists believed DNR orders should be automatically suspended when undergoing surgery [13]. The perception among patients is even more concerning with the study finding that 57% of patients believed that DNR orders were automatically suspended in the OR. Institutional policies which automatically rescind advance directives and orders not to resuscitate in the periprocedural period fail to accommodate a patient's right to self-determination. The ASA recommends that anesthesiologists participate in goals of care discussions preoperatively to better understand the patient's goals and values. Many operations and procedures are palliative in nature, including fixing pathologic fractures, tracheostomies, laparotomies for bowel obstructions, and many more. Patients with a terminal illness may elect to undergo surgery to improve the quality of their remaining life, and it is important that we support their right to self-determination, providing their requests are not medically futile. When patients with existing orders to limit resuscitative efforts present for anesthetic care, anesthesiologists should engage in conversation to clarify these orders and explain the requisite resuscitative efforts used when undergoing anesthesia. The ASA recommends providing one of the 3 alternatives for satisfactory outcomes: (1) full attempt at resuscitation; (2) limited attempt at resuscitation defined with regard to specific procedures; and (3) limited attempt at resuscitation defined with regard to the patient's goals and values (Fig. 2) [12]. Arriving at one of these conclusions requires a thoughtful and empathetic conversation with our patients, their surrogate decision makers, and the surgeons and other providers on their care team. Accurate documentation should occur, particularly when modifying or clarifying existing patient directives, including at which point in the postoperative/postprocedural course the prior directives should go back into effect. While it may be impossible to demarcate the exact moment when this occurs, care should be taken to accurately understand and document the guiding values and wishes of our patients and their families. In some circumstances, the anesthesiologist may be unwilling to abide by a patient's wishes to qualify for a do-not-resuscitate order when undergoing anesthesia. It is important to not abandon patients under our care, but in these circumstances, an alternative physician should be sought to provide care concordant with the patient's wishes.

Intensive care unit

End-of-life considerations are perhaps nowhere more relevant than in intensive care units whereby we care for our most critically ill, many of whom will not survive to discharge. Anesthesiologists in this setting have an obligation to the dying patient not only when functioning as the anesthesiologist-intensivist, but also when acting as a consultant for pain and symptom management. Given the inevitability of death, surprisingly few patients have advance directives when admitted to the intensive care unit. One proven way to improve ICU satisfaction scores is to require the review of a bundled procedural consent on admission that reviews the most common invasive procedures encountered in intensive care [14]. This prompts early goals of care conversation with the physician, and compassionate communication is one of the most valuable interventions we have to offer [15,16]. By addressing goals of care on admission to the ICU, the intensivist can normalize the conversation around end-of-life and acknowledge that goals of care are an integral part of every daily plan.

The integration of palliative care teams into the ICU is a critical part of improving the quality of life for critically ill patients and their families [17]. In 2014, the World Health Organization stated that it was an imperative "ethical duty of health care professionals" to incorporate palliative care in the treatment of serious illnesses [18]. The growth of this specialty over the past 3 decades and the integration of palliative care teams in the ICU has significantly improved multiple facets of care including patient quality of life [19],

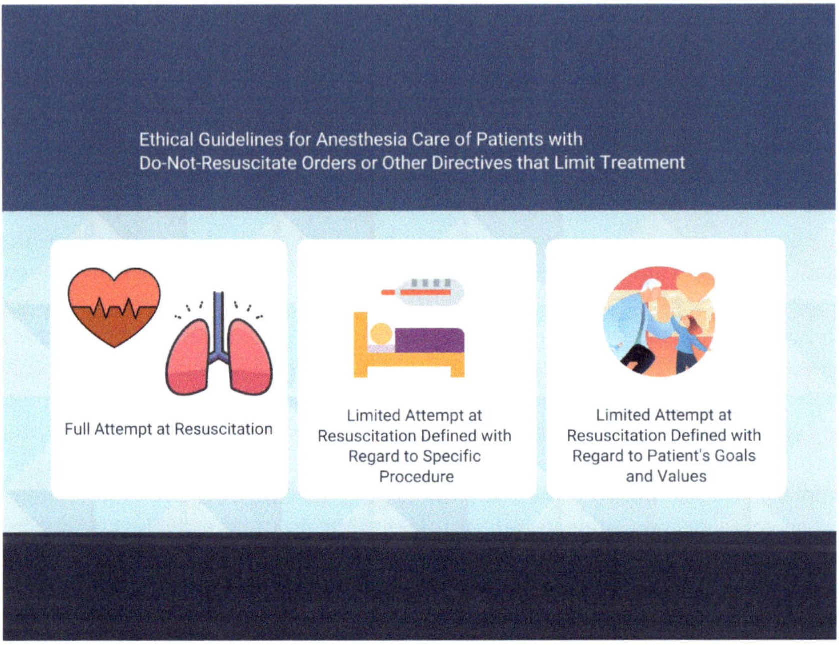

Fig. 2. ASA Ethical Guidelines. (*Data from* Ethics, A.S.o.A.C.o., Ethical Guidelines for the Anesthesia Care of Patients with Do-Not-Resuscitate Orders or *Other* Directives That Limit Treatment, in Ethics Committee. 2018: Schaumburg, IL.)

higher satisfaction among patients and caregivers [20], and reduced costs associated with end-of-life care [21]. Despite what some may falsely perceive, specialty palliative care interventions do not increase mortality [22]. Anesthesiologists are adept at components of primary palliative care such as symptom management, addressing code status, and discussing patients' goals and values and should incorporate these into regular practice patterns. When these primary needs cannot be met by the anesthesiologist-led team caring for the patient, the involvement of a specialty palliative care team is recommended. This multidisciplinary team includes advanced practice providers, nurses, chaplains, social workers who have undergone advanced training, and physicians who have completed an additional 1-year palliative medicine fellowship. Specialty teams can be particularly helpful for managing patients with unclear goals of care, uncertain prognoses, refractory pain symptoms, and for navigating complex communication dynamics with patients and families [23]. Involving specialty palliative care teams can help alleviate provider burnout, as well as the significant spiritual and emotional distress of patients, families, and caregivers [23].

The advent of mechanical circulatory support in the ICU has allowed the prolongation of life beyond what has ever before been possible for patients with advanced cardiopulmonary disease. Durable ventricular assist devices serve as both destination therapy and a bridge to transplantation for patients with advanced stages of heart failure. Within the ICU, patients are now able to undergo prolonged life support on venoarterial or venovenous extracorporeal membrane oxygenation (ECMO). This form of life support can only serve as a bridge to a more durable form of support, such as recovery, transplantation, or durable assist devices. Given how resource-intensive and elaborate this support is, there are significant ethical dilemmas relating to initiating and withdrawing this therapy. Data collected between 2002 and 2012 in the extracorporeal life support organization (ELSO) registry showed a mortality of 58.6% for all patients placed on VA-ECMO [24]. As anesthesiologists caring for these patients in the ICU, it is important to counsel patients and their surrogates on the limitations and risks of this salvage therapy, as well as the potential benefits [25]. In some cases, a potential benefit of ECMO is allowing patients to be extubated and alert enough to participate in goals of care discussions when they may have otherwise been too sedated to effectively communicate. Inevitably, circumstances may arise in which recovery is no longer possible and contraindications to destination therapies or transplantation have arisen. ECMO then becomes a "bridge to no recovery." [26] This presents significant ethical and emotional challenges for all parties, particularly in the era of COVID-19 when the rapid deterioration of previously healthy patients may prompt physicians to consider ECMO as rescue therapy when there is no viable destination. Our obligation to respect patient autonomy must be continually balanced with our obligation to do no harm. This balancing act is increasingly challenging when considering the myriad possibilities for risk and benefit with advanced mechanical support.

While our primary obligation will always be to our patients, we must also acknowledge that our care extends to their community units. The experience of having a loved one admitted to the ICU has always been stressful, but this has been made even worse in an era of limited visitation privileges, prolonged ICU stays, and disrupted physical contact due to personal protective equipment. Families who have loved ones admitted to the ICU report posttraumatic stress responses characterized by anxiety, depression, and grief [27]. If the death of their loved one occurs while in the ICU, they are at risk of developing prolonged grief which can become a debilitating condition that threatens mental, physical, and emotional well-being and consumes additional health care resources [28].

We can help mitigate this burden of stress, grief, and anxiety by implementing structured communication and support strategies with our patients' loved ones. Multiple studies have been conducted to quantify what interventions help reduce these burdens. A prospective, randomized controlled trial conducted in France studied the effects of physician-initiated and nurse-aided support strategies for families with a loved one dying in the ICU. The strategy used one the of strongest tools of medical care, effective communication, and focused on the 3 following areas: attentive listening, recognition of nonverbal communication, and empathy. When this strategy was used, the number of relatives reporting prolonged grief symptoms was significantly reduced compared with relatives randomized to standard care (21% vs 15%; $P = 0.035$) [29]. A qualitative study using focus groups used the feedback of patients and their families to attempt to define "high-quality palliative care in the intensive care unit." [16] The findings again illustrate the importance of structured, compassionate communication as a central component of high-quality medical care. Shared-decision making among all stakeholders–physicians, nurses, patients, and family members–is another strategy that has demonstrated improvement in the satisfaction of all parties [30]. With communication, compassion, and inclusive teaming, we can significantly improve the care we extend to dying patients and their loved ones.

HEALTH CARE DISPARITIES

There are a growing number of reports that highlight disparity in medical care provided to different ethnic and minority groups. Black and Hispanic patients, as well as patients with limited health literacy, are less likely to have a documented advance care plan compared with white patients, even after adjusting for clinical and demographic factors [31,32]. Members of the LGBTQIA community as well as incarcerated patients experience disparities in rates of ACP planning as well [33,34]. Black families who experience the death of a loved one in the hospital are more likely than families of white decedents to report absent or problematic communication with physicians, as well as express concerns with the level of support offered to their family [35].

In addition to disparities in the documentation of patients' wishes for times of critical illness, disparities exist among gender and ethnic divides regarding aggressive care received at the end of life. Women are more likely than men to have documentation of DNR status, a finding that supports existing data that show women receive less aggressive treatment of myocardial infarction, transplantation, renal dialysis, and end-of-life care [3,36–38]. Gender bias may also influence the way we treat the pain and suffering of our dying patients [39]. Women's pain is more likely to be attributed to psychological rather than organic reasons [40], and may explain why they receive less analgesia than men [41]. Despite the fact that US women spend an estimated 50% more of their lives caregiving than men [42], they are more likely to die in hospitals and nursing homes out of concern for not wanting to burden other family members when they themselves require care [43]. End-of-life care is best realized when treating and recognizing the individual as autonomous, unique, and worthy of compassionate, dignified care. As anesthesiologists caring for a diversity of patients, awareness of these disparities and inequities can help us strive to provide equally excellent care to all dying patients, regardless of gender or ethnic background.

ETHICS

As we navigate complex issues around end-of-life with our patients in the clinic, intensive-care units, and periprocedural settings, we will inevitably encounter situations whereby conflicts arise relating to principles of autonomy, beneficence, nonmaleficence, and distributive justice. We are taught to respect patient autonomy and to provide care that is concordant with their preferences and goals, but what if their requests are discordant with our own integrity as physicians? What do we do when patient autonomy conflicts with our right of conscience? Dr. Robert Orr argues that it is important to distinguish between cases of negative versus positive autonomy [44]. The right of a patient to refuse indicated and offered medical treatment (negative autonomy) is well established, and the guiding ethical principle behind allowing patients to choose DNR status [45]. However, the right of a patient to demand nonindicated treatments (positive autonomy) that conflict with a physician's conscience is not a right of self-determination. We have all taken an oath to do no harm (nonmaleficence) and both national society organizations and local institutional guidelines should support this practice. For example, the American Thoracic Society, American Association of Critical Care Nurses, American College of Chest Physicians, European Society of Intensive Care Medicine, and Society of Critical Care published a joint policy statement about the limits of "potentially inappropriate treatment in the intensive care unit" [46]. These are treatments that have some chance of accomplishing the effect sought by the patient or surrogate but clinicians feel has competing ethical considerations. These situations are often complex medically and socially and should not be shouldered by the individual anesthesiologist alone. To avoid burnout and excessive moral distress, when ethical conflicts arise institutional support and guidance from internal ethics committees and administrators should be sought to help guide decision making.

How do these national organizations define medical futility? The American Thoracic Society states a "life-sustaining intervention is futile if reasoning and experience indicate that the interventions would be highly unlikely to result in meaningful survival for the patient." The Society for Critical Care Medicine defines futile treatment as therapy that cannot accomplish its intended goal or has "no beneficial physiologic effect." [46] In approaching these complex conversations, it is important to understand why a family or patient may request futile therapy. Often religious values or a belief in miracles guides their decision making. Physician distrust or anger may also be a factor, especially if the medical team is not unified in their recommendations or prognostication. Finally, denial or guilt can be a very powerful emotion at the end of life [47]. The approach to a family or patient requesting futile therapy should be an interdisciplinary one involving bioethicists, palliative care teams, anesthesiologists, and the primary care team. Initially, it may be best to withhold therapy that is not indicated rather than withdraw therapy patients are already receiving. For example, the decision to not offer ongoing blood transfusions or escalations in vasopressors when that treatment is futile in changing the outcome is separate from the decision to withdraw existing forms of life-sustaining therapy such as dialysis, mechanical cardiopulmonary support, or mechanical ventilation. While patients and families come to terms with the reality of their illness, it may be important to withhold further escalations in care while giving families time to agree to recommendations to withdraw life-sustaining therapy. During this period, avoid confrontation, agree on unanimous medical recommendations before family meetings, seek to understand underlying values, and give families time and space to agree to recommendations for withdrawal of therapies and comfort care.

When patients and their surrogates insist on continuing life-sustaining therapy despite medical recommendations against doing so, what is our legal obligation despite major ethical concerns? The Texas Advanced Directives Act does legally protect physicians who withhold or withdraw medically futile cases after certain procedures are followed [48]. However, most states have not upheld unilateral physician decision making. There is no federal mandate universally protecting physicians who withhold or withdraw medically futile therapy, even during "crisis standards of care." [49,50] The lack of societal consensus on this issue, even at the height of the COVID-19 pandemic, illustrates the importance of defining this ambiguous landscape for the future of medicine.

MORAL RESILIENCE AND HEALTH CARE PROVIDER SUPPORT

The impact of ethical challenges involved in providing care that seems to prolong the dying process rather than improve quality of life has a tremendous toll on health care providers. Moral distress can occur when providers feel their care is inconsistent with their professional or personal values [51,52]. The advent of sophisticated technology such as mechanical circulatory support including extracorporeal membrane oxygenation and ventricular assist devices presents unique concerns. Technology exists to prolong life without the requisite legal and societal landscape to support providers, patients, and families. In a recent single-center study of moral distress in the intensive care unit setting, clinician burnout and moral distress were higher in providers caring for those receiving mechanical circulatory support than those caring for patients without it; and nurses reported higher levels of moral distress than physicians or advanced practice providers [53]. In this study, interventions such as palliative care consultations, ethics consultations, and debriefings were found to be most likely to reduce moral distress and thereby promote moral resilience [53]. Another recent study that investigated moral distress as a consequence of the pandemic identified the following factors as likely to promote resilience: greater support from employers and coworkers and regulated sleep patterns [54]. Younger providers with pre-existing mental health conditions were at highest risk for distress [54]. In this era of health care whereby providers are one of the most limited resources, we have a responsibility to ourselves and the other members of our team to support one another and create the space to process the grief we all experience while caring for our most vulnerable patients.

SUMMARY

As anesthesiologists, we are well-equipped with knowledge on how to save lives. The official mantras of the American Society of Anesthesiologists have emphasized this role throughout the years: "Anesthesiologists: Physicians providing the *lifeline* of modern medicine." The succinct motto "vigilance" shines a light on our job to stay alert, intervene early, and save lives "when seconds count." While the importance of this vigilant role in saving a life is central to our job, that unilateral focus neglects to define our role in the compassionate care of dying patients. We are a lifeline for the living, but we are undeniably equipped to ease the suffering of dying patients and their loved ones. Death is the natural conclusion to life. We cannot focus on one without acknowledging the other [55].

In the presence of incurable illness, our position in the central hub of contemporary medicine should shift focus to ameliorating the inevitable loss, stress, and sadness that accompany overmedicalized death. High-income earning countries spend a disproportionate amount of health care funds caring for dying patients. Up to 11% of annual health expenditure for the whole population is spent to care for the less than 1% who will die that year [55]. This significant expenditure may result in small increases in quantity with significant sacrifices in quality. Before the COVID-19 pandemic, up to 40% of Americans spent a portion of their final 6 months of life in an ICU [56]. From 2000 to 2019, the number of years lived *in the absence of good health* increased from 8.6 to 10 years [57]. We sacrificed quality for quantity.

In our earnestness to do no harm and remain vigilant, may we take the lead to improve the experience of our patients and their loved ones during the end of life. This can start by encouraging discussions about our patients' values and ACP wherever we encounter them: in the clinic, on the day of surgery, and on admission to the intensive care unit. We should use our vigilance to watch out for instances when systemic racism and unconscious bias lead to marginalized patient populations receiving inferior care when they are most vulnerable. We should never hesitate to use our advanced armamentarium to alleviate the pain and suffering that may accompany death, but we should also be wary of perpetuating harm to our patients by offering false hope or tying up their final weeks in the hospital instead of at home if that is where they wish to die. We cannot control nature and the inevitable conclusion that accompanies the life we strive to protect. We can, however, elevate the value placed on death free of pain, loneliness, and anxiety and full of compassion for those left behind after the loss. Our leadership as anesthesiologists in the perioperative realm is as critical during the final weeks of life as it is during complex resuscitations and procedures. Each of us, regardless of our exact subspecialty and scope of practice, can make a meaningful impact on our patients, their families, and the care they receive from us, both in life and in death.

CLINICS CARE POINTS

- Advanced care planning (ACP) ensures that patients have the right to participate in decisions pertaining to their medical care through living wills and surrogate decision makers.

- Anesthesiologists have a unique role in perioperative advanced care planning (ACP). Their role extends from the pain and preoperative clinic, to the operating room, and the intensive care unit. We can lead interdisciplinary teams in clarifying goals of care and navigating ethical challenges at the end of life.
- There are documented disparities in medical care provided to ethnic and minority groups, including in advanced care planning. Awareness of these gaps allows us to serve our patients more equitably.

Disclosure

Neither author has any financial interests to disclose.

References

[1] McMahan RD, Tellez I, Sudore RL. Deconstructing the Complexities of Advance Care Planning Outcomes: What Do We Know and Where Do We Go? A Scoping Review. J Am Geriatr Soc 2021;69(1):234–44.
[2] Sudore RL, Lum DL, You JJ, et al. Defining Advance Care Planning for Adults: A Consensus Definition From a Multidisciplinary Delphi Panel. J Pain Symptom Manage 2017;53(5):821–32.e1.
[3] Burns JP, Edwards J, Johnson J, et al. Do-not-resuscitate order after 25 years. Crit Care Med 2003;31(5):1543–50.
[4] Smith CB, Bunch O'Neill L. Do not resuscitate does not mean do not treat: how palliative care and other modalities can help facilitate communication about goals of care in advanced illness. Mt Sinai J Med 2008;75(5):460–5.
[5] Morrison LJ, Neumar RW, Zimmerman JL, et al. Strategies for improving survival after in-hospital cardiac arrest in the United States: 2013 consensus recommendations: a consensus statement from the American Heart Association. Circulation 2013;127(14):1538–63.
[6] Chang DW, Neville TH, Parrish J, et al. Evaluation of Time-Limited Trials Among Critically Ill Patients With Advanced Medical Illnesses and Reduction of Nonbeneficial ICU Treatments. JAMA Intern Med 2021;181(6):786–94.
[7] Cline KM, Clement V, Rock-Klotz J, et al. Improving the cost, quality, and safety of perioperative care: A systematic review of the literature on implementation of the perioperative surgical home. J Clin Anesth 2020;63:109760.
[8] Morrison RS, Meier DE, Arnold RM. What's Wrong With Advance Care Planning? JAMA 2021;326(16):1575–6.
[9] Waisel DB, Simon R, Truog RD, et al. Anesthesiologist management of perioperative do-not-resuscitate orders: a simulation-based experiment. Simul Healthc 2009;4(2):70–6.
[10] Nurok M, Green DST, Chisholm MF, et al. Anesthesiologists' familiarity with the ASA and ACS guidelines on Advance Directives in the perioperative setting. J Clin Anesth 2014;26(3):174–6.
[11] Kouwenhoven WB, Jude JR, Knickerbocker GG. Closed-chest cardiac massage. JAMA 1960;173:1064–7.
[12] Ethical guidelines for the anesthesia care of patients with do-not-resuscitate orders or other directives that limit treatment. IL: American Society of Anesthesiologists: Schaumburg; 2018.
[13] Burkle CM, Swetz KM, Armstrong MH, et al. Patient and doctor attitudes and beliefs concerning perioperative do not resuscitate orders: anesthesiologists' growing compliance with patient autonomy and self determination guidelines. BMC Anesthesiol 2013;13:2.
[14] Dhillon A, Tardini F, Bittner E, et al. Benefit of using a "bundled" consent for intensive care unit procedures as part of an early family meeting. J Crit Care 2014;29(6):919–22.

[15] Nelson JE, Tardini F, Bittner E, et al. Improving comfort and communication in the ICU: a practical new tool for palliative care performance measurement and feedback. Qual Saf Health Care 2006;15(4):264–71.
[16] Nelson JE, Puntillo KA, Pronovost PJ, et al. In their own words: patients and families define high-quality palliative care in the intensive care unit. Crit Care Med 2010;38(3):808–18.
[17] Epstein AS, Morrison RS. Palliative oncology: identity, progress, and the path ahead. Ann Oncol 2012;23(Suppl 3):43–8.
[18] World Health O. Strengthening of palliative care as a component of integrated treatment throughout the life course. J Pain Palliat Care Pharmacother 2014;28(2):130–4.
[19] Haun MW, Estel S, Rucker G, et al. Early palliative care for adults with advanced cancer. Cochrane Database Syst Rev 2017;6:CD011129.
[20] Casarett D, Shreve S, Luhrs C, et al. Measuring families' perceptions of care across a health care system: preliminary experience with the Family Assessment of Treatment at End of Life Short form (FATE-S). J Pain Symptom Manage 2010;40(6):801–9.
[21] May P, Normand C, Cassel JB, et al. Economics of Palliative Care for Hospitalized Adults With Serious Illness: A Meta-analysis. JAMA Intern Med 2018;178(6):820–9.
[22] Aslakson R, Cheng J, Vollenweider D, et al. Evidence-based palliative care in the intensive care unit: a systematic review of interventions. J Palliat Med 2014;17(2):219–35.
[23] Crooms RC, Gelfman LP. Palliative Care and End-of-Life Considerations for the Frail Patient. Anesth Analg 2020;130(6):1504–15.
[24] Smith M, Vukomanovic A, Brodie D, et al. Duration of veno-arterial extracorporeal life support (VA ECMO) and outcome: an analysis of the Extracorporeal Life Support Organization (ELSO) registry. Crit Care 2017;21(1):45.
[25] Abrams DC, Prager K, Blinderman CD, et al. Ethical dilemmas encountered with the use of extracorporeal membrane oxygenation in adults. Chest 2014;145(4):876–82.
[26] Mulaikal TA, Nakagawa S, Prager KM. Extracorporeal Membrane Oxygenation Bridge to No Recovery. Circulation 2019;139(4):428–30.
[27] Azoulay E, Pochard F, Kentish-Barnes N, et al. Risk of post-traumatic stress symptoms in family members of intensive care unit patients. Am J Respir Crit Care Med 2005;171(9): 987–94.
[28] Kentish-Barnes N, Chaize M, Seegers V, et al. Complicated grief after death of a relative in the intensive care unit. Eur Respir J 2015;45(5):1341–52.
[29] Kentish-Barnes N, Chevret S, Valade S, et al. A three-step support strategy for relatives of patients dying in the intensive care unit: a cluster randomised trial. Lancet 2022;399(10325):656–64.
[30] Wubben N, van den Boogard M, van der Hoeven JG, et al. Shared decision-making in the ICU from the perspective of physicians, nurses and patients: a qualitative interview study. BMJ Open 2021;11(8):e050134.
[31] Smith AK, McCarthy EP, Paulk E, et al. Racial and ethnic differences in advance care planning among patients with cancer: impact of terminal illness acknowledgment, religiousness, and treatment preferences. J Clin Oncol 2008;26(25):4131–7.
[32] Rao JK, Anderson LA, Lin FC, et al. Completion of advance directives among U.S. consumers. Am J Prev Med 2014;46(1):65–70.
[33] Hughes M, Cartwright C. Lesbian, gay, bisexual and transgender people's attitudes to end-of-life decision-making and advance care planning. Australas J Ageing 2015;34(Suppl 2): 39–43.
[34] Ekaireb R, Ahalt C, Sudore R, et al. We Take Care of Patients, but We Don't Advocate for Them": Advance Care Planning in Prison or Jail. J Am Geriatr Soc 2018;66(12):2382–8.
[35] Welch LC, Teno JM, Mor V. End-of-life care in black and white: race matters for medical care of dying patients and their families. J Am Geriatr Soc 2005;53(7):1145–53.
[36] Gan SC, Beaver SK, Houck PM, et al. Treatment of acute myocardial infarction and 30-day mortality among women and men. N Engl J Med 2000;343(1):8–15.

[37] Miesfeldt S, Murray K, Lucas L, et al. Association of age, gender, and race with intensity of end-of-life care for Medicare beneficiaries with cancer. J Palliat Med 2012;15(5):548–54.
[38] Sharma RK, Prigerson HG, Penedo FJ, et al. Male-female patient differences in the association between end-of-life discussions and receipt of intensive care near death. Cancer 2015;121(16):2814–20.
[39] Gott M, Morgan T, Williams L. Gender and palliative care: a call to arms. Palliat Care Soc Pract 2020;14:2632352420957997.
[40] Schafer G, Prkachin KM, Kaseweter KA, et al. Health care providers' judgments in chronic pain: the influence of gender and trustworthiness. Pain 2016;157(8):1618–25.
[41] Michael GE, Sporer KA, Youngblood GM. Women are less likely than men to receive prehospital analgesia for isolated extremity injuries. Am J Emerg Med 2007;25(8):901–6.
[42] Caregiver statistics: demographics. Family caregiver alliance, National Center on Caregiving. 2016. https://www.caregiver.org/caregiver-statistics-demographics. [Accessed 24 March 2022].
[43] Gott M, Frey R, Wiles J, et al. End of life care preferences among people of advanced age: LiLACS NZ. BMC Palliat Care 2017;16(1):76.
[44] Orr RD. Autonomy, conscience, and professional obligation. Virtual Mentor 2013;15(3): 244–8.
[45] Bouvia v Superior Court. Cal Rptr 297 (Cal. Ct. App 1986.
[46] Bosslet GT, Pope TM, Rubenfeld GD, et al. An Official ATS/AACN/ACCP/ESICM/SCCM Policy Statement: Responding to Requests for Potentially Inappropriate Treatments in Intensive Care Units. Am J Respir Crit Care Med 2015;191(11):1318–30.
[47] Prager K. When physicians and surrogates disagree about futility. Virtual Mentor 2013;15(12):1022–6.
[48] Texas Advance Directive Act. Procedure If Not Effectuating a Directive or Treatment Decision. In: Texas Health and Safety code - health & Safety § 166.046. USA: Texas Health and Safety Code; 1999.
[49] Fischkoff K, Neuberg G, Dastidar J, et al. Clinical Ethics Consultations during the COVID-19 Pandemic Surge at a New York City Medical Center. J Clin Ethics 2020;31(3):212–8.
[50] Fins JJ, Prager KM. The COVID-19 crisis and clinical ethics in new york city. J Clin Ethics 2020;31(3):228–32.
[51] Dodek PM, Wong H, Norena M, et al. Moral distress in intensive care unit professionals is associated with profession, age, and years of experience. J Crit Care 2016;31(1):178–82.
[52] Johnson-Coyle L, Opgenorth D, Bellows M, et al. Moral distress and burnout among cardiovascular surgery intensive care unit healthcare professionals: A prospective cross-sectional survey. Can J Crit Care Nurs 2016;27(4):27–36.
[53] Emple A, Fonseca L, Nakagawa S, et al. Moral Distress in Clinicians Caring for Critically Ill Patients Who Require Mechanical Circulatory Support. Am J Crit Care 2021;30(5): 356–62.
[54] Spilg EG, Rushton CH, Phillips JL, et al. The new frontline: exploring the links between moral distress, moral resilience and mental health in healthcare workers during the COVID-19 pandemic. BMC Psychiatry 2022;22(1):19.
[55] Sallnow L, Smith R, Ahmedzai SH, et al. Report of the Lancet Commission on the Value of Death: bringing death back into life. Lancet 2022;399(10327):837–84.
[56] Bekelman JE, Halpern SD, Blankart CR, et al. Comparison of Site of Death, Health Care Utilization, and Hospital Expenditures for Patients Dying With Cancer in 7 Developed Countries. JAMA 2016;315(3):272–83.
[57] Collaborators GBDD. Global age-sex-specific fertility, mortality, healthy life expectancy (HALE), and population estimates in 204 countries and territories, 1950-2019: a comprehensive demographic analysis for the Global Burden of Disease Study 2019. Lancet 2020;396(10258):1160–203.

Advances in Anesthesia 40 (2022) 15–32
ADVANCES IN ANESTHESIA

Outpatient Robotic surgery: Considerations for the Anesthesiologist

Yasmine Tameze, MD*, Ying Hui Low, MD
Department of Anesthesiology, Massachusetts General Hospital, 55 Fruit Street, Boston, MA 02114, USA

Keywords

• Robotic surgery • Outpatient/ambulatory surgery • Urologic surgery • Gynecologic surgery • Same-day discharge surgery

Key points

- Robot-assisted surgical techniques are being used in an expanding number of procedures.
- Generally good outcomes, or outcomes comparable with inpatient surgery, have been reported.
- Known challenges and intraoperative management considerations include extremes of Trendelenburg positioning, CO_2 insufflation, and having limited access to the patient after robot docking.
- Risk factors associated with failure to achieve same-day discharge in robotic surgery include patient age, preexisting lung disease, occurrence of intraoperative complications, and surgery end time.
- Awareness of risk factors is key to selecting patients for robotic surgery for same-day discharge.

INTRODUCTION: NATURE OF THE PROBLEM

Robotic surgery was initially developed in the 1990s as a military project that would allow for a remote surgeon to operate on wounded soldiers on a battlefield [1]. Since then, robotic surgery has gained popularity across a broad range of common surgical procedures: from general and colorectal surgery to urogynecologic procedures and mitral valve repairs [1]. In the field of general surgery, the use of robotic surgery accounted for only 1.8% of all procedures in

*Corresponding author. *E-mail address:* ytameze@partners.org

https://doi.org/10.1016/j.aan.2022.06.001

2012, and this increased to 15.1% by 2018 [2]. Robotic surgery is attractive for several reasons: like laparoscopic surgery, it offers smaller incisions, a lower risk of infection, a shorter hospital stay, and a shorter convalescence than its open counterpart [3]. In addition, unlike laparoscopic surgery, robotic surgery has the advantage of increasing surgical dexterity due to the increased degrees of freedom of the instruments. The increased dexterity allows for more precise dissection during the operation [4].

For the anesthesiologist, robotic surgery comes with the following challenges: steep Trendelenburg or reverse Trendelenburg to provide the best field of view for the surgeon, longer duration of pneumoperitoneum especially during the initial part of an operator's learning curve, and limited access to the patient after robot docking [3,5–8].

Despite the high initial costs of robotic surgery, the hope is that it will ultimately reduce health care costs by decreasing complications and reducing inpatient length of stay after surgery, thereby reducing hospital resource utilization and reducing risks of nosocomial infections [2,9], a benefit that has been highlighted by the recent coronavirus disease 2019 pandemic. The quick recovery associated with the minimally invasive nature of robotic surgery can allow for early discharge from the hospital, making it an attractive option for patients looking to reduce their time spent in health care facilities.

This article describes the role and challenges of anesthesia in promoting same-day discharge after robotic surgery: the indications, procedures, common complications, and management of postoperative care.

INDICATIONS/CONTRAINDICATIONS OF AMBULATORY ROBOTIC SURGERY

To date, outpatient robotic surgery has been described for an expanding list of procedures as shown in Table 1. Some procedures, such as colectomies,

Table 1
Robotic surgeries that have been described in the ambulatory setting

General Surgery	Head and Neck	Gynecologic	Urologic	Orthopedic
• Ventral hernia repair • Inguinal hernia repair • Cholecystectomy • Bariatric surgery	• Transoral tumor removal • Facelifts • Thyroidectomy	• Hysterectomy • Salpingo-oophorectomy • Tubal ligation • Sacrocolpopexy	• Prostatectomy • Adrenalectomy • Nephrectomy (including partial and living donors) In pediatrics: • Pyeloplasty • Extravesical ureteral implant • Ureteroureterostomy	• Total knee arthroplasty • Total hip arthroplasty

bariatric surgeries, and nephrectomies (including partial and living-related donor resections), have not hitherto been described in the peer review literature but are well established in select practices. In essence, the indications for ambulatory robot-assisted surgery will likely continue to grow rapidly with different institutions developing experience in various surgical procedures, and this is a list that is expected to evolve over time.

Commonly performed ambulatory robotic surgical procedures

General surgery: cholecystectomy [4], hernia repair [10], colectomy, bariatric surgery.

Head and neck surgery: facelift, thyroidectomy [11].

Gynecology: hysterectomy ± bilateral salpingo-oophorectomy, staging for endometrial or cervical cancer [12–16], salpingo-oophorectomy [13], tubal ligation [17], and sacrocolpopexy [18].

Urology: radical prostatectomy [19], nephrectomy (including partial and living-related donor resections) [20], pyeloplasty, adrenalectomy [21].

Pediatric surgery: Robotic outpatient pediatric surgery is mainly reported in urology in procedures such as pyeloplasty or extravesical ureteral reimplantation, but other procedures such as ureteroureterostomy and nephrectomy/heminephrectomy have been done as outpatients as well [22].

Orthopedic surgery: Orthopedic surgery such as total knee and hip arthroplasty: although not specifically described as outpatient procedures, successful discharge within 24 hours has been reported [23] and may move progressively toward quicker discharges.

Relative contraindications to robotic surgery

Although there are not any absolute contraindications to robotic surgery, one must review the suitability of the surgical goals and the ability of the patient to tolerate the hemodynamic changes associated with the pneumoperitoneum or extremes in positioning. As surgeons and anesthesia providers become more experienced and familiar with robot-assisted methods, however, the list of contraindications will also likely grow and dwindle over time.

Surgical factors that make robot-assisted surgery a poor choice will vary depending on the type of surgery. Relative contraindications to robot-assisted ventral hernia repairs, for instance, include strangulated or acutely incarcerated hernias, cirrhosis or ascites, prior open abdominal surgery, recurrent or complex ventral hernias, and redundant skin and soft tissue, although the degree to which each of these poses a contraindication to surgery will vary depending on surgical experience [24]. For colectomies and urologic and gynecologic procedures, these include a high likelihood of needing an open procedure, for instance, a laparotomy for tumor debulking or extensive adhesions [25].

Poor candidates for robotic surgery generally include patients who may not tolerate insufflation or extremes of positioning well, and this will vary based on surgical location. Certain cardiopulmonary conditions such as severe pulmonary hypertension, or congenital heart disease including single-ventricle physiology or intra/extracardiac shunts, may not tolerate a pneumoperitoneum well

[26,27]. The presence of ascites may result in challenging port placement. In colectomies and gynecologic and urologic surgery, for instance, severe obesity or respiratory pathology such as chronic obstructive pulmonary disease (COPD) may lead to inadequate ventilation or oxygenation; the same considerations are less of a problem with bariatric surgery because of the reverse Trendelenburg positioning. However, this may result in decreased venous blood return and lead to hypotension that may be poorly tolerated in patients with severe carotid stenosis or cardiac disease [26,27]. Again, the extent to which these factors pose a limit to the use of a robotic approach depends on the severity of disease and surgical and anesthetic experience. Modifying, for instance, the speed of abdominal insufflation, or a shorter duration of Trendelenberg positioning with a faster surgeon, may enable surgery to proceed despite the aforementioned comorbidities.

Technique/procedure

Companies such as Medtronic, Johnson & Johnson, Stryker, Zimmer Biomet, Smith and Nephew, and NuVasive are currently manufacturing surgical robots. At present, Intuitive Surgical, which makes the da Vinci robot system, has the largest market share. For the purpose of describing the robot-assisted technique here, the authors refer to the da Vinci system.

The da Vinci robot surgical system consists of 3 major components (https://www.intuitive.com/en-us/products-and-services/da-vinci/systems) (Fig. 1).

- A console for the operating surgeon: where the surgeon sits to view the operating field and control the robot's arms
- A patient-side cart with 4 interactive robotic arms; also known as the surgical cart: instruments have 7 degrees of freedom

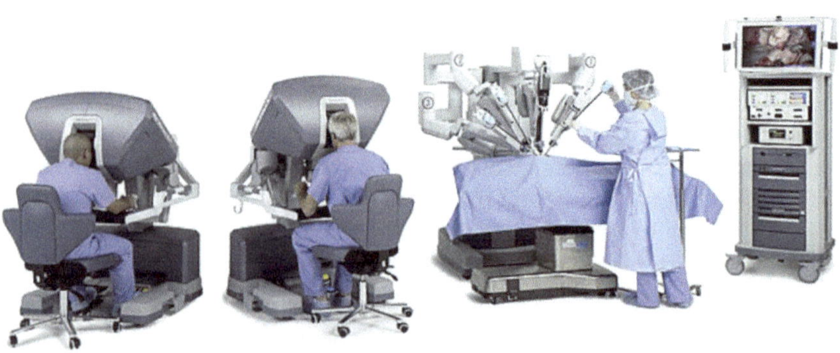

Fig. 1. The da Vinci robot surgical system consists of 1 or 2 surgical consoles, a patient cart, and a vision cart. (*From* Pietrabissa A, et al. Cirugia robótica: controversias actuales y expectativas futuras.Cir Esp. 2013;91:67–71.)

- A vision cart including optical devices for the robotic camera (optical 3D vision tower): a viewscreen as well as computer equipment needed to integrate the optical channels and provide stereoscopic vision

Challenges for the anesthesiologist

As robotic surgery continues to gain popularity, the anesthesiologist is faced with challenges related to patient positioning and limited access to the patient after docking [28] (Tables 2 and 3), and pneumoperitoneum (Table 4).

- Patient positioning and limited access to patient (see Tables 2 and 3):

Robotic surgery depends on establishing and maintaining the best possible field of view for the surgeon, which is partly achieved by insufflation of carbon dioxide to create a pneumoperitoneum and partly by positioning the patient in such a way that noninvolved organs move away from the surgical site. For bariatric surgery, cholecystectomy, and other upper abdominal procedures this means elevating the head and lowering the feet (extreme reverse Trendelenburg position). For prostatectomy, hysterectomy, and other lower abdominal surgeries this means the opposite: for much of the procedure the patient will be head down (see Fig. 1). A steep Trendelenberg is defined as a 30° to 40° head down position, and most operating room tables can achieve a maximum of a 45° tilt; for gynecologic surgery some investigators have reported that an average Trendelenburg angle of 28° was sufficient for surgical visualization [29]. For colectomy, nephrectomy, and other midabdominal operations the bed may remain in a neutral position or the position may be changed from one extreme to the other throughout the operation. Extremes of lateral tilt to the right or left may also occur and may vary over the course of the surgical dissection.

Proper patient positioning should allow for safe docking of the robot and adequate access to the robot arms and ports for the surgical assistant [3,30]. Although each case is different, the footprint of the robot, the desired bed position, the anticipated length of the procedure, and the body habitus of the patient should all be taken into account when docking the robot. It is sometimes useful to move the patient and bed through the full range of possible positions before making the surgical incision, to determine the safe limits of the procedure and likely intraoperative pressure points; this is especially true when dealing with unusual circumstances such as a patient with high body mass index scheduled for bariatric surgery in extreme reverse Trendelenburg position.

The robotic surgical equipment is heavy and bulky and can inadvertently place excess pressure on various parts of the body depending on the position of the surgery. For instance, when the surgery is in Trendelenburg position, it is important to monitor the face of the patient to avoid injury from the robot arms and to ensure that the height of surgical tables is adjusted to avoid impact with the patient when going into Trendelenburg or reverse Trendelenburg position (for instance, stands above the patient's feet and steep head down positions) (Fig. 2). Furthermore, given the limited access to the patient and

Table 2
Patient positioning: summary of challenges and management considerations

Consideration	Consequence	Management
Heavy and bulky robot	Can contact the head of the patient if not positioned correctly	Make sure that the face of the patient is visible during surgery
Arms are tucked by the sides of patient	No access to arms once the robot is docked	• Ensure IV is working well after arms tucked • Consider second IV after induction • Invasive lines only in high-risk patients
Steep Trendelenburg: physiologic consequences	• Downward/cephalad movement of the diaphragm by abdominal contents in conjunction with pneumoperitoneum • ⇓Pulmonary compliance • ⇓Functional residual capacity • ⇓Tidal volumes • ⇑Peak and plateau airway pressures • Exacerbates V/Q mismatch • ⇓Vital capacity • ⇑ Intracranial pressure • ⇑ Cerebral blood flow • ⇑ Intraocular pressure	Careful preoperative assessment regarding ability of patient to tolerate positioning such as patients with • severe underlying lung disease (ie, COPD) • severe obesity • glaucoma
Steep Trendelenburg: physical consequences	• Displacement of the ETT → mainstem intubation • Reflux of stomach acid • Upper airway, periorbital, and brain edema • Postoperative corneal abrasion and vision loss • Trunk shifting during positioning • High venous pressures in ear lobe	• Ensure face visibility • Consider orogastric tube for long surgeries • Ensure ETT is well secured • Limit the amount of CO_2 insufflation to decrease upper extremity venous congestion • Goal-directed fluid management • Ensure proper eye protection to avoid corneal abrasions • Ensure pressure points are padded • Most adjuncts (such as shoulder braces) have been associated with neuropathic injury • Placement of the pulse oximeter on the finger

Abbreviations: ETT, endotracheal tube; IV, intravenous; V/Q, ventilation perfusion ratio.

Table 3
Limited access to patient: summary of challenges and management considerations

Consideration	Consequence	Management
Robot is over the chest and abdomen of the patient	If airway or cardiovascular events happen intraoperatively might delay intervention	• Ensure proper communication among team members • Consider simulation exercises
	Peripheral nerve and soft tissue injuries	Ensure proper pressure point padding

Table 4
Pneumoperitoneum: summary of challenges and management considerations

Consideration	Consequence	Management
Long continuous insufflation with cold gas	Hypothermia	Ensure that the patient has a warming air blanket before docking
	Venous air embolism	• Removal of pneumoperitoneum • Undock robot • Hyperventilation with oxygen • Place the patient on left lateral decubitus • Leave the patient in Trendelenburg position • Consider aspirating with central venous catheter
	• Subcutaneous emphysema • Pneumothorax, pneumomediastinum, pneumopericardium	• Vigilance
Pneumoperitoneum: physiologic consequences	• Fluid shifts and changes in venous return/preload and afterload may lead to hemodynamic compromise • ⇑ LV filling pressures • ⇓Cardiac output • ⇑SVR and MAP • ⇓Renal, splanchnic, and portal flow→ • ⇑Renin-angiotensin system → ⇑ vasopressin	• Careful patient selection • ⇓Urine output, goal-directed fluid therapy
	Hypercarbia and respiratory acidosis	Consider pressure-controlled ventilation

Abbreviations: LV, left ventricular; MAP, mean arterial pressure; SVR, systemic vascular resistance

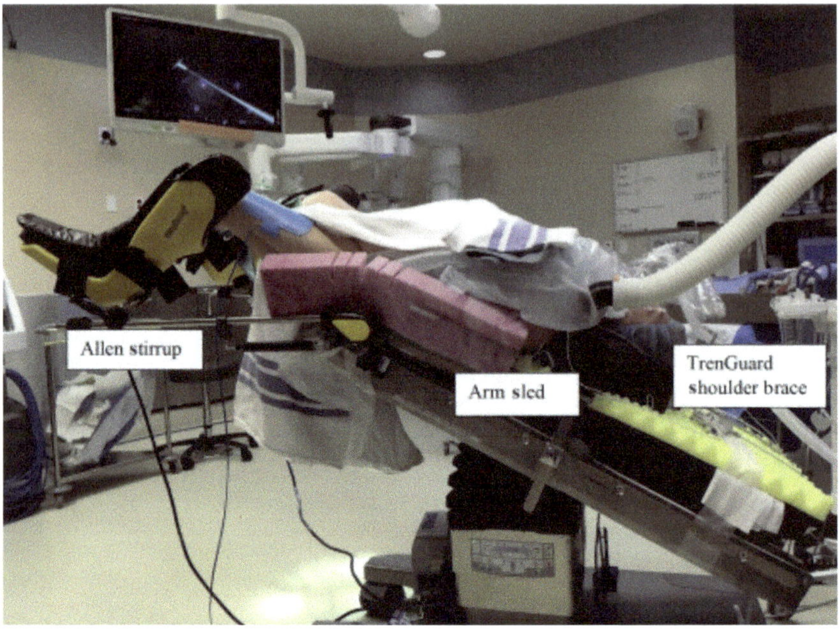

Fig. 2. Steep Trendelenberg positioning. Surgical tables are often placed over the patient's head (or legs) and have to be adjusted to ensure they do not cause any injury to patients. (*From* Lim PC, Kang E. How to prepare the patient for robotic surgery: before and during the operation. Best Pract Res Clin Obstet Gynaecol 2017 Nov;45:32-47.)

different spatial consideration of the operating room, the pressure points must be adequately padded before draping and docking the robot. A patient's arms are often tucked by the side to facilitate robot docking, which means venous or arterial access cannot be easily monitored, for instance, for leaks or infiltration, and new access sites are not easily obtained once the robot is positioned (Fig. 3). The limited access to the patient also increases the risk of peripheral nerve and soft tissue injuries [31] and occult blood loss and can present challenges during emergent situations [3,28] (Fig. 4). Given the complexity of the room setup, it is crucial to have good communication between the team members.

To improve visualization for pelvic and lower abdominal surgeries, the patient is often required to be in a steep Trendelenburg with or without exaggerated lithotomy position [3,8,32]. Upper abdominal surgery requires a reverse Trendelenburg position with the robot docked above the head of the patient (Fig. 4). This position requires the head of the bed to be rotated away from the anesthesia machine further increasing the risk of injury to head and neck [28]. The physiologic effect seen in this position is mainly a consequence of venous pooling, which can lead to resistant hypotension [33]. Prolonged reverse Trendelenburg positioning, along with increased abdominal pressures from insufflation, has also been associated with a higher deep vein thrombosis

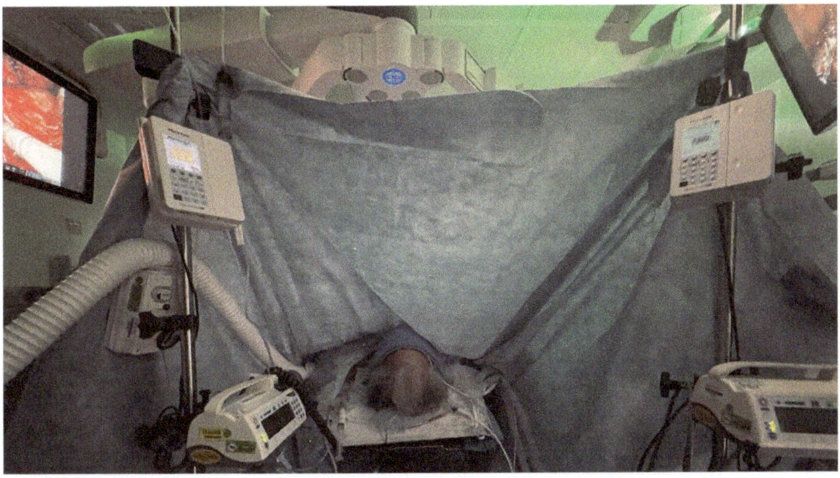

Fig. 3. Limited access to patient's head and airway.

(DVT) risk due to venous pooling in the legs, and attention should be paid to proper DVT prophylaxis.

The physiologic consequences associated with steep Trendelenburg position include downward movement of the diaphragm by abdominal contents. Together with the increased abdominal pressure from pneumoperitoneum, this leads to a decrease in pulmonary compliance and subsequently tidal volumes, a decrease in functional residual capacity and vital capacity, increase

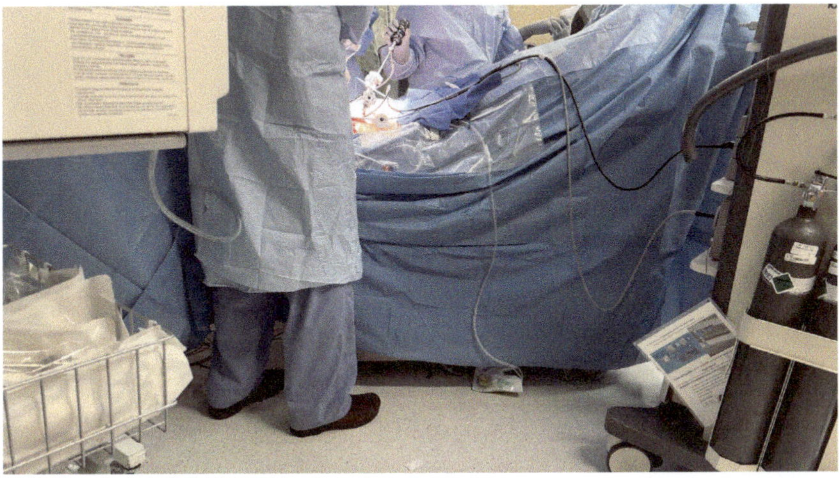

Fig. 4. Limited access to patients. Arms are tucked, venous/arterial access sites cannot be easily monitored for integrity, increases the risk of peripheral nerve, soft tissue injuries and occult blood loss, thus creating a challenge during emergencies.

in peak and plateau airway pressures, and exacerbation of ventilation perfusion ratio mismatch [32]. Some studies have found that pressure-controlled ventilation will allow for lower peak airway and plateau pressures as well as greater pulmonary compliance [5].

Steep Trendelenburg positioning and pneumoperitoneum can also lead to an increase in intracranial pressure, cerebral blood flow, and intraocular pressure [6]. Some investigators have reported erroneous pulse oximeter readings resulting from high venous pressures in the ear lobe induced by Trendelenburg positioning, and suggest that if possible, the pulse oximeter should be placed on a finger instead [7]. Prolonged time spent in steep Trendelenburg may also lead to upper airway, periorbital, and brain edema [8]. The cephalad movement of the diaphragm can lead to the displacement of the endotracheal tube and subsequent mainstem intubation. If not well secured in the bed, the patient may shift position during the course of the surgery, creating a risk for friction burns to the skin, nerve injury to the extremities, and even fall from the operating room table [34].

Pneumoperitoneum

Pneumoperitoneum for robotic surgery has similar consequences to that of laparoscopic surgery (see Table 4). However, especially during the early parts of a surgical team's learning curve, the patient is exposed to these consequences for longer periods given the longer duration of the cases. For instance, the risk of hypothermia is increased secondary to insufflation with cold gas (CO_2) for a prolonged period [34,35].

Fluid shifts, changes in venous return (preload), and afterload may lead to hemodynamic compromise in patients with preexisting cardiopulmonary disease. Factors that contribute to a decrease in cardiac output include [34]:

- Decrease in renal, splanchnic, and portal flow
- Increased systemic vascular resistance
- Increased mean arterial pressure: both from direct compression and from an increase in renin-angiotensin system activation that ultimately results in increased circulating vasopressin levels [34]

Prolonged carbon dioxide (CO_2) insufflation may result in postoperative hypercarbia and respiratory acidosis especially in patients with COPD in whom the efficiency of CO_2 elimination is decreased [32].

Finally, consequences such as venous air embolisms [36], subcutaneous emphysema [37], pneumothorax, pneumomediastinum, and pneumopericardium are rare but may result in hemodynamic collapse [38,39]. Providers should remain vigilant for any of these potential complications and should have plans in place to deal with each.

Management goals

Preoperative assessment

In addition to the standard preoperative assessment, providers should have a good understanding of the ability of the patient to tolerate consequences related to steep Trendelenburg positioning and pneumoperitoneum. For instance, patients with underlying lung disease or morbid obesity might be difficult to ventilate and therefore poor candidates for outpatient robotic surgery [3,8]. Special attention should be paid to patients with a history of glaucoma who are scheduled for lower abdominal procedures, given the potential increase in intraocular pressure [5]. Patients with congenital heart disease or significant cardiovascular disease may not tolerate changes in preload or afterload caused by extreme positioning and pneumoperitoneum [6,8].

Intraoperative

In addition to proper patient selection, intraoperative anesthetic management for planned outpatients must ensure timely emergence and recovery in the Post Anesthesia Care Unit (PACU) [10,12,13,18,23].

Once a standard induction is achieved and the airway is secured, obtaining additional intravenous access is often useful because access to patient's arms will be extremely limited once the robot is docked [3,6,8]. An invasive arterial line may be helpful as well, if suggested by comorbidities or the potential for fluid volume shifts; direct arterial pressure monitoring may also be helpful in larger patients where a noninvasive cuff may not fit or work well. Subsequently providers should also pay attention to ensuring that all access sites are working after the arms have been tucked and the robot docked. Similarly, it is important to ensure proper padding of pressure points (ie, elbow, axilla, back, and shoulders) given the limited access to the patient during the case. Transitioning to Trendelenburg position can lead to the patient shifting down the table: several adjuncts such as shoulder braces, leg suspension, and iliac support have been associated with neuropathic injury and therefore are not recommended [40,41]. Placing the patient on an antiskid material (egg-crate pink foam) has shown minimal shift of the patient without evidence of skin or neurologic injuries [42] (Fig. 5).

Given the known physiologic changes associated with Trendelenburg and pneumoperitoneum, plans should be made to achieve adequate ventilation and for judicious fluid administration. Trendelenburg positioning alone and in combination with pneumoperitoneum can lead to hypercarbia, or the need for high airway pressures, which may run the risk of barotrauma and subsequent lung injury [32,37]. Some investigators have reported that in patients in whom ventilation or oxygenation is challenging, a pressure-controlled ventilation mode might allow for larger tidal volumes and lower peak and plateau pressures [37]. Muscle relaxation is typically maintained throughout the case to facilitate pneumoperitoneum and avoid the catastrophic consequences associated with patient movement while the robot is docked [3].

A carefully designed fluid strategy balancing hemodynamic goals individual to the patient and minimizing facial and airway edema is important. If the patient can tolerate it, a restrictive fluid management strategy may allow for reduction of edema and, in some urologic procedures, improve surgical visualization by reducing urine output [43].

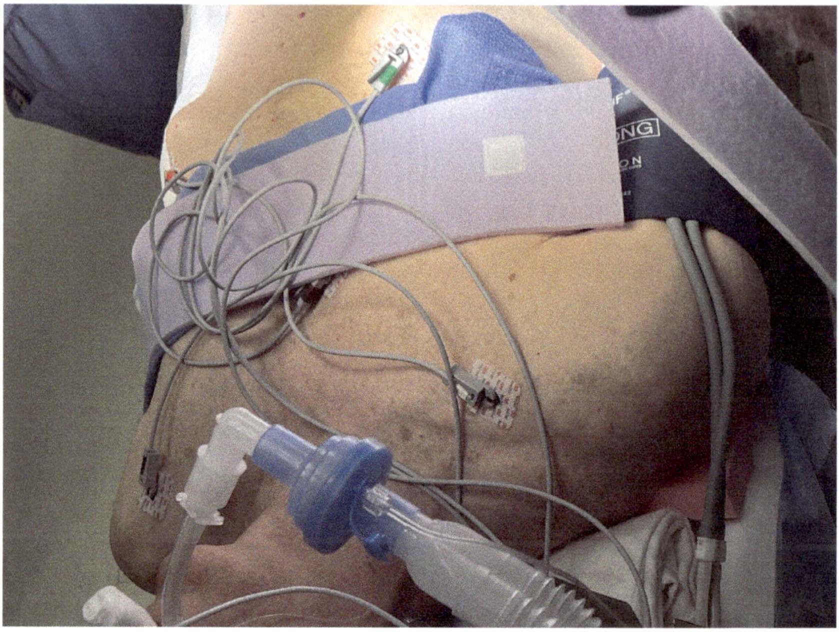

Fig. 5. Pink foam to minimize patient skidding during steep Trendelenberg, reverse Trendelenberg, or lateral tilts.

Pain management should complement the gains offered by robotic surgery by thus allowing for safe and expedient discharge. A multimodal approach to analgesia, including regional blocks where appropriate, can help minimize postoperative opioid use, nausea and vomiting, and ileus, and forms a key part of any ambulatory surgery [44]. Although epidural analgesia may promote quicker return of bowel function by minimizing narcotics, its use should be balanced by the fact that dosing the epidural in the Trendelenburg position might lead to a high block [45]. In addition, epidural-associated hemodynamic changes might contribute to greater fluid loading. Furthermore, the patient will not be eligible for discharge home until all block-related muscle weakness has resolved.

Ultrasound-guided transversus abdominis plane or quadratus lumborum blockade may be performed after induction or placed under laparoscopic guidance by the surgical team to provide postoperative analgesia. This approach is a common adjunct for pain relief after robotic surgery, especially in cases wherein a larger incision will be needed for hand assist or specimen removal, such as in the case of nephrectomies [46,47]. This approach might be favorable to decrease the length of stay in the hospital postoperatively. [48], and has been reported by some groups to decrease opioid requirement and the time to ambulation and bowel function recovery [47,48], and even decrease the development of chronic pain [46].

Postoperative
In most ambulatory patients, the use of standard postanesthesia discharge criteria such as the Post Anesthetic Discharge Scoring System (PADSS) [49] is commonly implemented. The PADSS discharge criteria includes ensuring that vital signs are within 20% of preoperative baseline, that the patient ambulates with a steady gait, and that there is good control of nausea/vomiting, pain, and surgical bleeding. Criteria should be developed and systematically applied for both patients going home on the day of surgery and "23-hour" patients scheduled to leave the next morning.

Because the ability to select patients for rapid discharge is not perfect, and cannot account for intraoperative surprises, any facility performing outpatient robotic procedures must have an established relationship with an inpatient facility, and an organized protocol for transferring care when needed.

OUTCOMES

Most published studies evaluating the feasibility of outpatient robotic procedures have been done in the urology and gynecologic fields. Most of the studies have observed low rates of complications and readmissions, although the longest follow-up period of available studies is 6 weeks postoperatively [12,14]. Several groups have tried to identify factors that contribute to successful discharge and patient outcomes. In a study of patients undergoing robotic hysterectomies, older age, preoperative lung disease, and later surgical end time were risk factors for requiring a prolonged hospital stay [16]. Another study in robotic hysterectomies found that the need for abdominal hysterectomy, older age, Medicare insurance, ethnicity, higher number of comorbidities, and concomitant procedures were associated with the need for inpatient stay [15].

CURRENT CONTROVERSIES/FUTURE CONSIDERATIONS

Successful outpatient robotic surgery depends on the following key factors: appropriate patient selection and identification of risks to patients (Table 5), good surgical technique, and skilled anesthetic management.

At present, there are only limited studies describing readmission rates or short-term safety outcomes after outpatient robotic surgery. Further data about which patients have consistently good or poor outcomes after outpatient robotic surgery and what types of procedures are most appropriate might be useful. There is conflicting data on whether the use of robot-assisted techniques in outpatient surgery increases or decreases costs [13,16,50]; facility fees for outpatient procedures are lower than for inpatient ones, but the costs for the robot and associated disposables may outweigh this benefit.

Future studies are needed to better characterize the risk-benefit ratios of ambulatory robotic surgery in different patient populations, and to better capture the economic or financial costs of expanding the various indications for outpatient robotic surgery.

Table 5
Risks to patients undergoing abdominal or pelvic robotic surgery and management goals

Cardiovascular	• Decreased venous return with pneumoperitoneum • Decreased mesenteric perfusion with pneumoperitoneum Reverse Trendelenburg: • Decreased venous return • Hypotension • Increased DVT risk	• Consider preoperative consult for patients with congenital or other significant heart disease • Slow insufflation in patients who are more preload dependent Optimal volume status • in steep Trendelenberg, avoid too much crystalloid • in reverse Trendelenberg, ensure adequate volume repletion Maintain adequate MAP with pressors as needed Adequate DVT prophylaxis
Respiratory	Trendelenburg positioning: • Hypercapnia (decreased ventilation from FRC, ERV; CO_2 insufflation) • Hypoxemia (atelectasis and decreased ventilation)	• Use lowest peritoneal insufflation pressure needed to provide surgical visualization • Pressure-controlled ventilation, optimize PEEP and other ventilation settings to achieve adequate ventilation
Airway	Trendelenburg positioning: • Airway edema • Subcutaneous emphysema	• Check proper ETT positioning after being placed in steep Trendelenburg/reverse • Consider performing cuff leak test before extubation • Judicious fluid administration, consider using goal-directed fluid administration, to decrease edema risk.
Nervous system	Trendelenburg: • Raised ICP • Raised IOP • Visual changes/loss Reverse Trendelenburg: • Hypotension • Decreased cerebral perfusion	• Check that there is no equipment causing external pressure on eyes, head/neck • Maintain adequate MAP for cerebral and ocular perfusion • Consider neurologic consult for patients at risk for increased ICP or IOP

Positioning	• Nerve injuries • Compartment syndrome • Limited access to airway, extremities	Team effort: • Obtain adequate arterial and venous access before positioning • Adequate padding of all pressure points • Decrease sliding/skidding risk: antiskid bedding and cross-torso straps • Use smallest degree and shortest duration of Trendelenburg/reverse Trendelenburg positioning required for surgical success

Abbreviations: ERV, expiratory reserve volume; FRC, functional residual capacity; ICP, itracranial pressure; IOP, intraoccular pressure ; MAP, mean arterial pressure; PEEP, positive end expiratory pressure.

SUMMARY

Patient selection, surgical technique, and prudent perioperative anesthetic management are important to reduce surgical duration and the risk of complications. More robust data are required to support the use of ambulatory robotic surgery in various surgical and patient populations.

CLINICS CARE POINTS

- Careful patient selection is an important factor insuring safe discharge after ambulatory surgery.
- Steep trendelenberg position used in pelvic and urologic surgery leads to physiological changes which may or may not be tolerated by every patient.
- As the lenght of the surgery decreases, there should be less risks of severe positional injuries seen with prolonged procedure.

DISCLOSURE

The authors have nothing to disclose.

References

[1] George EI, Brand TC, LaPorta A, et al. Origins of robotic surgery: from skepticism to standard of care. JSLS 2018;22(4).
[2] Sheetz KH, Claflin J, Dimick JB. Trends in the adoption of robotic surgery for common surgical procedures. JAMA Netw Open 2020;3(1):e1918911.
[3] Lee JR. Anesthetic considerations for robotic surgery. Korean J Anesthesiol 2014;66(1): 3–11.

[4] Newman RM, Umer A, Bozzuto BJ, et al. Surgical value of elective minimally invasive gallbladder removal: a cost analysis of traditional 4-port vs single-incision and robotically assisted cholecystectomy. J Am Coll Surg 2016;222(3):303–8.
[5] Oğurlu M, Küçük M, Bilgin F, et al. Pressure-controlled vs volume-controlled ventilation during laparoscopic gynecologic surgery. J Minim Invasive Gynecol 2010;17(3):295–300.
[6] Molloy BL. Implications for postoperative visual loss: steep trendelenburg position and effects on intraocular pressure. Aana j 2011;79(2):115–21.
[7] Ludbrook G, Sutherland P. Erroneous pulse oximetry readings during robotic prostatectomy. Anaesth Intensive Care 2007;35(1):144–5.
[8] Phong SV, Koh LK. Anaesthesia for robotic-assisted radical prostatectomy: considerations for laparoscopy in the Trendelenburg position. Anaesth Intensive Care 2007;35(2):281–5.
[9] Lanfranco AR, Castellanos AE, Desai JP, et al. Robotic surgery: a current perspective. Ann Surg 2004;239(1):14–21.
[10] Escobar Dominguez JE, Ramos MG, Seetharamaiah R, et al. Feasibility of robotic inguinal hernia repair, a single-institution experience. Surg Endosc 2016;30(9):4042–8.
[11] Terris DJ, Singer MC, Seybt MW. Robotic facelift thyroidectomy: II. Clinical feasibility and safety. Laryngoscope 2011;121(8):1636–41.
[12] Penner KR, Fleming ND, Barlavi L, et al. Same-day discharge is feasible and safe in patients undergoing minimally invasive staging for gynecologic malignancies. Am J Obstet Gynecol 2015;212(2):186–8.
[13] Rivard C, Casserly K, Anderson M, et al. Factors influencing same-day hospital discharge and risk factors for readmission after robotic surgery in the gynecologic oncology patient population. J Minim Invasive Gynecol 2015;22(2):219–26.
[14] Nahas S, Feigenberg T, Park S. Feasibility and safety of same-day discharge after minimally invasive hysterectomy in gynecologic oncology: A systematic review of the literature. Gynecol Oncol 2016;143(2):439–42.
[15] Borahay MA, Patel PR, Kilic CH, et al. Outpatient robotic hysterectomy: clinical outcomes and financial analysis of initial experience. Int J Med Robot 2014;10(2):244–50.
[16] Cappuccio S, Li Y, Song C, et al. The shift from inpatient to outpatient hysterectomy for endometrial cancer in the United States: trends, enabling factors, cost, and safety. Int J Gynecol Cancer 2021;31(5):686–93.
[17] Rodgers AK, Goldberg JM, Hammel JP, et al. Tubal anastomosis by robotic compared with outpatient minilaparotomy. Obstet Gynecol 2007;109(6):1375–80.
[18] Kisby CK, Polin MR, Visco AG, et al. Same-day discharge after robotic-assisted sacrocolpopexy. Female Pelvic Med Reconstr Surg 2019;25(5):337–41.
[19] Wilson CA, Aminsharifi A, Sawczyn G, et al. Outpatient extraperitoneal single-port robotic radical prostatectomy. Urology 2020;144:142–6.
[20] Bernhard JC, Robert G, Ricard S, et al. Day-case robotic-assisted partial nephrectomy: feasibility and preliminary results of a prospective evaluation (UroCCR-25 AMBU-REIN study). World J Urol 2022;40(6):1351–7.
[21] Abaza R, Murphy C, Bsatee A, et al. Single-port robotic surgery allows same-day discharge in majority of cases. Urology 2021;148:159–65.
[22] Neheman A, Kord E, VanderBrink BA, et al. Outpatient robotic surgery in pediatric urology: assessment of feasibility and short-term safety. J Urol 2022;207(4):894–900.
[23] Sephton BM, De la Cruz N, Shearman A, et al. Achieving discharge within 24 h of robotic unicompartmental knee arthroplasty may be possible with appropriate patient selection and a multi-disciplinary team approach. J Orthop 2020;19:223–8.
[24] Loor M, Liang M. Robotic ventral hernia repair. In: Chen W, editor. Uptodate. 2022 Waltham, MA. www.uptodate.com/contents/robotic-ventral-hernia-repair; 2022 (Accessed July 2022).
[25] Schmitt JJ, Occhino JA, Weaver AL, et al. Vaginal versus robotic hysterectomy for commonly cited relative contraindications to vaginal hysterectomy. J Minim Invasive Gynecol 2017;24(7):1158–69.

[26] Aceto P, Beretta L, Cariello C, et al. Joint consensus on anesthesia in urologic and gynecologic robotic surgery: specific issues in management from a task force of the SIAARTI, SIGO, and SIU. Minerva Anestesiol 2019;85(8):871–85.
[27] Corcione A, Angelini P, Bencini L, et al. Joint consensus on abdominal robotic surgery and anesthesia from a task force of the SIAARTI and SIC. Minerva Anestesiol 2018;84(10):1189–208.
[28] Pathirana S, Kam P. Anaesthetic issues in robotic-assisted minimally invasive surgery. Anaesth Intensive Care 2018;46(1):25–35.
[29] Gould C, Cull T, Wu YX, et al. Blinded measure of Trendelenburg angle in pelvic robotic surgery. J Minim Invasive Gynecol 2012;19(4):465–8.
[30] Jara RD, Guerrón AD, Portenier D. Complications of robotic surgery. Surg Clin North Am 2020;100(2):461–8.
[31] Bjøro B, Mykkeltveit I, Rustøen T, et al. Intraoperative peripheral nerve injury related to lithotomy positioning with steep Trendelenburg in patients undergoing robotic-assisted laparoscopic surgery - A systematic review. J Adv Nurs 2020;76(2):490–503.
[32] Carry PY, Gallet D, François Y, et al. Respiratory mechanics during laparoscopic cholecystectomy: the effects of the abdominal wall lift. Anesth Analg 1998;87(6):1393–7.
[33] Knight DJ, Mahajan RP. Patient positioning in anaesthesia. Continuing Educ Anaesth Crit Care Pain 2004;4(5):160–3.
[34] Hsu RL, Kaye AD, Urman RD. Anesthetic challenges in robotic-assisted urologic surgery. Rev Urol 2013;15(4):178–84.
[35] Dean M, Ramsay R, Heriot A, et al. Warmed, humidified CO(2) insufflation benefits intraoperative core temperature during laparoscopic surgery: A meta-analysis. Asian J Endosc Surg 2017;10(2):128–36.
[36] Hong JY, Kim JY, Choi YD, et al. Incidence of venous gas embolism during robotic-assisted laparoscopic radical prostatectomy is lower than that during radical retropubic prostatectomy. Br J Anaesth 2010;105(6):777–81.
[37] Miller RD, Eriksson LI, Fleisher LA, et al. Miller's anesthesia, 1647. Philadelphia: Elsevier Churchill Livingstone; 2005.
[38] Kim A, Geynisman-Tan J, Lewicky-Gaupp C. Pneumothorax after laparoscopic robotic-assisted supracervical hysterectomy and sacrocolpopexy. Female Pelvic Med Reconstr Surg 2017;23(3):e22–4.
[39] Huang TJ, Ahmed A, D'Souza D, et al. Delayed diagnosis of contralateral tension pneumothorax during robotic lung wedge resection. J Clin Anesth 2018;45:30–1.
[40] Barnett JC, Hurd WW, Rogers RM Jr, et al. Laparoscopic positioning and nerve injuries. J Minim Invasive Gynecol 2007;14(5):664–72 [Quiz: 673].
[41] Irvin W, Andersen W, Taylor P, et al. Minimizing the risk of neurologic injury in gynecologic surgery. Obstet Gynecol 2004;103(2):374–82.
[42] Klauschie J, Wechter ME, Jacob K, et al. Use of anti-skid material and patient-positioning to prevent patient shifting during robotic-assisted gynecologic procedures. J Minim Invasive Gynecol 2010;17(4):504–7.
[43] Danic MJ, Chow M, Alexander G, et al. Anesthesia considerations for robotic-assisted laparoscopic prostatectomy: a review of 1,500 cases. J Robot Surg 2007;1(2):119–23.
[44] Richebé P, Brulotte V, Raft J. Pharmacological strategies in multimodal analgesia for adults scheduled for ambulatory surgery. Curr Opin Anaesthesiol 2019;32(6):720–6.
[45] Irvine M, Patil V. Anaesthesia for robot-assisted laparoscopic surgery. Continuing Educ Anaesth Crit Care Pain 2009;9(4):125–9.
[46] Covotta M, Claroni C, Costantini M, et al. The effects of ultrasound-guided transversus abdominis plane block on acute and chronic postsurgical pain after robotic partial nephrectomy: a prospective randomized clinical trial. Pain Med 2020;21(2):378–86.
[47] Rogers T, Bhat KRS, Moschovas M, et al. Use of transversus abdominis plane block to decrease pain scores and narcotic use following robot-assisted laparoscopic prostatectomy. J Robot Surg 2021;15(1):81–6.

[48] Damadi AA, Lax EA, Smithson L, et al. Comparison of therapeutic benefit of bupivacaine hcl transversus abdominis plane (TAP) block as part of an enhanced recovery pathway versus traditional oral and intravenous pain control after minimally invasive colorectal surgery: a prospective, randomized, double-blind trial. Am Surg 2019;85(12):1363–8.
[49] Barash PGCB. Clinical anesthesia. 7th edition. Philadelphia: Lippincott Williams & Wilkins; 2013.
[50] Schwaitzberg SD. Financial modeling of current surgical robotic system in outpatient laparoscopic cholecystectomy: how should we think about the expense? Surg Endosc 2016;30(5):2082–5.

Advances in Anesthesia 40 (2022) 33–44
ADVANCES IN ANESTHESIA

An Enhanced Ambulatory Surgery Experience for Patients with Cancer Through End-to-End Patient Engagement

Todd J. Liu, MD[a,*], Hanae K. Tokita, MD[b,c], Brett A. Simon, MD, PhD[b,c]

[a]Department of Anesthesiology and Critical Care Medicine, Memorial Sloan Kettering Cancer Center, 1275 York Avenue, M-309, New York, NY 10065, USA; [b]Department of Anesthesiology, Weill Cornell Medicine, New York, NY, USA; [c]Department of Anesthesiology and Critical Care Medicine, Memorial Sloan Kettering Cancer Center, 1133 York Avenue, New York, NY 10065, USA

Keywords

• Ambulatory surgery center • Anesthesia • Patient engagement
• Enhanced recovery after surgery (ERAS) • Recovery tracker

Key points

- Josie Robertson Surgery Center is an ambulatory surgical center for patients with cancer at Memorial Sloan Kettering Cancer Center and was designed for patient-centered care including end-to-end patient engagement and standardized clinical pathways.
- Electronic symptom tracking during recovery through a patient portal (up to 10 days after discharge from ambulatory surgery) has high participation rates, may reduce readmissions, increase patient satisfaction, and expedite appropriate triage if complications occur.
- Real-time location system is a useful tool for patient engagement through automated communication of patient progress and may promote efficiency in an ambulatory surgery center.

BACKGROUND/INTRODUCTION

When faced with projected shortages of operating room capacity and tightening inpatient bed availability, the Memorial Sloan Kettering Cancer Center (MSK) opted to build a freestanding ambulatory surgery center (ASC) with

*Corresponding author. 1275 York Avenue; C-309, New York, NY 10065. *E-mail address:* liut@mskcc.org

https://doi.org/10.1016/j.aan.2022.07.001
0737-6146/22/

2 unique requirements. First, the center would need to accommodate more complex cancer surgeries than were typically done in the outpatient setting, and second, patient engagement and the patient and family experience were to be central to every aspect of the design and operation of the facility. In 2016, this vision was realized with the opening of the Josie Robertson Surgery Center (JRSC) on the Upper East Side of New York [1]. This article will review the organization and operation of JRSC, with a focus on how patients are engaged in their care throughout their surgical journey from the time the decision to have surgery is made through their follow-up clinic visit.

CASE MIX AND PATIENT POPULATION

One of the early challenges for MSK in building an ambulatory surgical center for patients with cancer was that the case complexity that needed to be offloaded from the main hospital would be significantly higher than at typical ASCs. As a hospital-associated outpatient department (as opposed to an independent ASC [2]), regulations permitted a single overnight stay for appropriate procedures. Thus, the facility itself was designed to comfortably handle the needs of overnight patients and their caregivers. Crucial to the early development process for JRSC was creating a multidisciplinary task force to identify case types and patients appropriate for a short stay that would be suitable for this unique ASC. The task force divided cases appropriate for the ASC into 2 types: conventional outpatient (OP) procedures and "ambulatory extended recovery" procedures (AXR). OPs would undergo simpler procedures and be discharged on the same day following a short recovery, whereas AXR patients would plan for discharge after an overnight stay. Before the opening of the JRSC, proposed AXR procedures were piloted at the main inpatient hospital to optimize management and prove feasibility, working out and refining processes for successful overnight discharge of patients. This helped facilitate a smooth transition and aided in the development of standardized care pathways. From the beginning, the JRSC case mix has been diverse but some of the most common AXR procedures done there include the following:

- Mastectomy with or without immediate tissue expander reconstruction
- Robotic prostatectomy
- Robotic total/partial nephrectomy
- Thyroidectomy
- Robotic hysterectomy and pelvic procedures
- Axillary lymphatic reconstruction

All surgical patients at MSK undergo preoperative evaluation before the day of surgery. Specific preoperative screening criteria were initially developed for JRSC with several exclusion criteria identified including body mass index (BMI) greater than 45, end-stage renal disease/dialysis, ASA score greater than 3, implanted cardiac devices (defibrillators and pacemakers), need for blood salvage/Jehovah's witness, severe obstructive sleep apnea, and high risk of alcohol withdrawal. As experience grew at JRSC, these "exclusions" were liberalized to "flags for individualized evaluation" because it was shown that patient outcomes were often not impacted. For example, studies of outcomes at JRSC demonstrated that appropriately selected patients with BMI greater than 50 [3] or obstructive sleep apnea [4] could still be safely managed at the ambulatory center. Cases that are flagged in advance are reviewed by an anesthesiologist for triage to the appropriate location based on case complexity, patient comorbidity, and clinical judgment.

LAYOUT AND FACILITIES

JRSC is located 6 city blocks south from the main MSK Memorial Hospital and has approximately 180,000 ft^2 of space over 15 floors. There are 12 operating rooms, 4 of which are equipped for robotic surgery. The center has 28 private patient rooms with bathrooms for postoperative recovery and an 18-room unit for preoperative care that can be flexed into postoperative recovery rooms for OPs as needed. Rooms are simply furnished and use extralarge stretchers with thicker mattresses rather than beds. The patient floors have ample natural light, inviting wide hallways to encourage postoperative ambulation, and a central "oasis" featuring a self-serve pantry for snacks and drinks and living room-type seating areas. Furthermore, on the JRSC premises are a large patient/caregiver waiting lounge with attached café, a staff cafeteria with outdoor space, and multiple staff workrooms and collaboration spaces. The on-site pharmacy provides all medications during the stay as well as discharge medications for the patient's convenience. A surgical pathology laboratory is also located on-site to facilitate immediate evaluation of surgical specimens. Although only procedures that are not expected to require transfusion are scheduled, 4 units of O-negative emergency blood are always available in a blood refrigerator managed and monitored by the hospital central blood bank to ensure inventory does not expire. In the event that additional blood products are needed emergently, an emergency massive transfusion protocol was setup to mirror the protocol on the main campus via a dedicated courier traveling to blood bank. The building has no critical machinery in the basement in case of flooding. Infrastructure includes 2 backup diesel generators as well as independent chillers and steam generators–a lesson learned from other hospitals in New York City after Hurricane Sandy. A real-time location system (RTLS, Midmark Corp.) is hard-wired into the ceilings and stairwells (details in later discussion).

CARE PATHWAYS

Core to the strategy for providing consistent, patient-centered, and continuously improving care at JRSC is using standardized pathways and, equally importantly, creating standardized, structured documentation, particularly for nursing assessments and pathway milestones. Enhanced recovery after surgery (ERAS) pathways has been widely used in inpatient care to standardize perioperative patient management, reduce complications, and shorten recovery time [5]. By standardizing operations around perioperative care at JRSC, not only do patients benefit but it also facilitates examination and improvement of the processes themselves. For example, monitoring of standardized outcomes such as postoperative nausea and vomiting (PONV), pain, time to first ambulation, and opioid consumption provides a basis for evaluating and steadily improving these pathways, even in the face of external factors such as drug shortages or changes in surgical practice [6]. A comparison of AXR cases occurring at JRSC versus the main hospital demonstrated that cases performed at JRSC had a significantly better pathway completion rate compared with JRSC-eligible cases performed at the main hospital (98.3% vs 86.4%, $P<.001$) [7]. JRSC's design and philosophy lends itself well to research projects focused on the development of evidence-based care pathways.

At JRSC, care standardization is broadly implemented across the surgical journey and includes preoperative (patient evaluation, testing, and preparation, patient education), intraoperative (surgical instrument kits, draping and set-up, anesthetic management guidelines, surgical site infection, venous thromboembolism (VTE) and urinary catheter management, nursing documentation), postoperative (symptom assessments and treatment, early ambulation, patient and family education, milestone based pathway advancement, discharge criteria), and postdischarge (analgesic management, follow-up phone calls, electronic symptom reporting) components. From its conception, JRSC leadership had a focus on hiring a dedicated staff who were well-educated regarding these standardized care pathways. Building a highly qualified and effective team committed to a process-focused approach to patient care was critical for the success at JRSC. Every week, a multidisciplinary meeting oversees and reviews the clinical operations at JRSC. These meetings have representatives from nearly all departments from nonclinical employees (eg, plant operations and security) to clinical staff (eg, pharmacists, nurses, midlevel providers, and physicians). The bottom–up engagement of the complete JRSC workforce ensures excellent patient care, positive patient experiences, and effective process improvement.

When the COVID pandemic began, inpatient beds and OR access were severely restricted at the main hospital and the rest of New York City. As a result, the overnight stay restriction was temporarily lifted and JRSC was able to accommodate large procedures such as colectomies, distal pancreatectomies, and small liver resections that required multinight stays. Despite this increase in case complexity, no major complications or deviations from the standard of care occurred during this time period. Once the crisis of inpatient bed/OR access improved, JRSC returned to its usual, pre-pandemic operations. However, it does suggest that perhaps more complex care pathways could be carefully attempted at JRSC in the future on a more routine basis.

Patient engagement

Preoperative engagement

Perioperative engagement begins well before a patient arrives at a surgical center. Patient engagement is enhanced the more that care can be given on the patient's own terms, particularly by providing patients and their caregivers the information they need at the time they both need it and when they are able to absorb it. Once the decision is made to have surgery, patients are given standardized written, procedure-specific educational materials that are reviewed with the surgeon's office practice nurse and can also be stored in a personal digital library on the patient portal for later access. At the preoperative clinic, trained nurse practitioners evaluate the patient and provide additional materials, such as to describe regional blocks if appropriate. Patients are risk assessed for PONV, the presence of cardiac devices, alcohol withdrawal, and so forth and, if excess risk is determined, standard protocols are activated. All preoperative educational materials are designed to clearly define expectations and goals for the surgical experience and mirror what information will be given at JRSC (Fig. 1). A good example of the innovation of preoperative processes at JRSC occurred during a recent routine presurgical visit at a satellite location when the nurse practitioner became concerned about a history of difficult airway for a patient. She was able to call and conference with an anesthesiologist who obtained an in-depth history, performed a remote physical examination of the patient's airway, and generated an effective perioperative plan before the day of surgery. As the day of surgery approaches, videos describing what to expect on site are provided, so there is a familiarity to both the physical surroundings and care processes for the patient once they arrive.

Engagement during the surgical visit

All paperwork and insurance verification are completed before arrival, so that the patient only needs to check in on the morning of surgery. On registration, each patient and their caregiver are provided with RTLS badges that identify their location throughout the visit. Similar RTLS badges are worn by all staff and placed on important equipment. This RTLS technology is interfaced to the electronic medical record and communication systems so as to enhance processes and workflows in a transparent and patient-centered way. For example, there is no public paging in the waiting area. Instead, the unit assistant finds where the patient or family is sitting from the RTLS monitor and can walk over to them to directly give a message or indicate that it is time to go up to the preoperative area, rather than announcing overhead. This helps create a serene atmosphere, especially for those anxiously waiting for important information. In the patient rooms, when staff members enter the room, their name and role are prominently displayed on the television monitor through the technology of the RTLS system (Fig. 2). This feature helps empower the patient and caregiver with timely information that lets them know with whom they are speaking, automatically and in an unobtrusive manner. When a nurse call button is pressed and the staff respond, the call alert is automatically inactivated on their entering the room, allowing them to go directly to the aid of the patient. In the waiting area, caregivers can see real-time updates on the patient's location through coded identifiers (only known to caregivers) on status boards (Fig. 3). Postoperatively, a check box on the nurse's electronic flow sheet

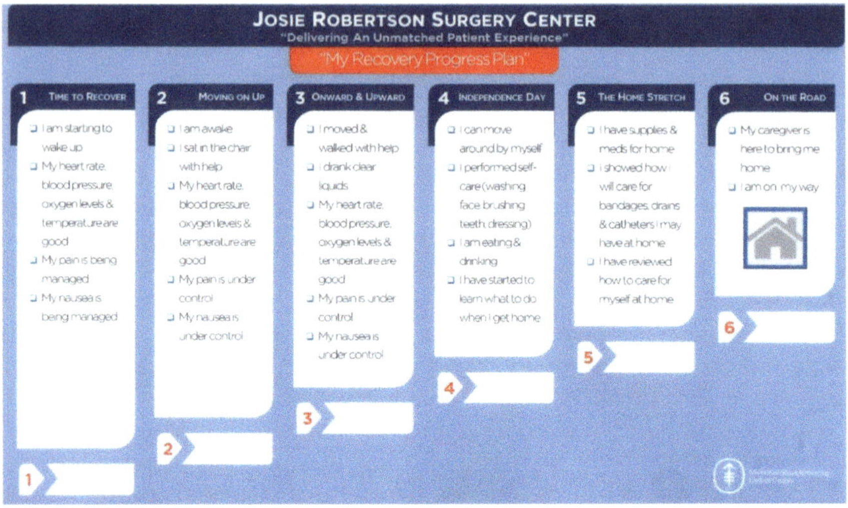

Fig. 1. "My Recovery Progress Plan" Worksheet—Before their surgery visit, patients receive a roadmap to their recovery with expected milestones and progressive steps toward discharge.

automatically indicates when the patient is "ready for visitors" on the status board, so the caregiver does not need to repeatedly ask but can approach the unit assistant for help when it is time to go see the patient.

RTLS is used to automate documentation and communication in other ways as well. For example, when the patient leaves the preoperative area to go to the OR and their badge is detected on the OR floor, this location event triggers the following: (1) the preop room status changes to red on the floor plan monitor to

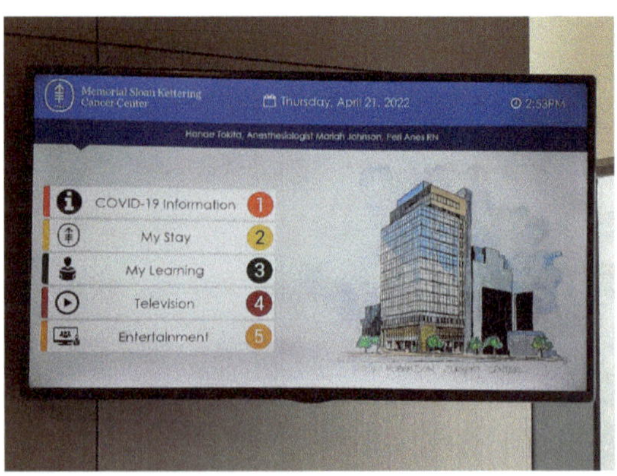

Fig. 2. Example interactive display of "Welcome Screen" in a patient's room displaying the name/role for providers currently in room through RTLS badge technology.

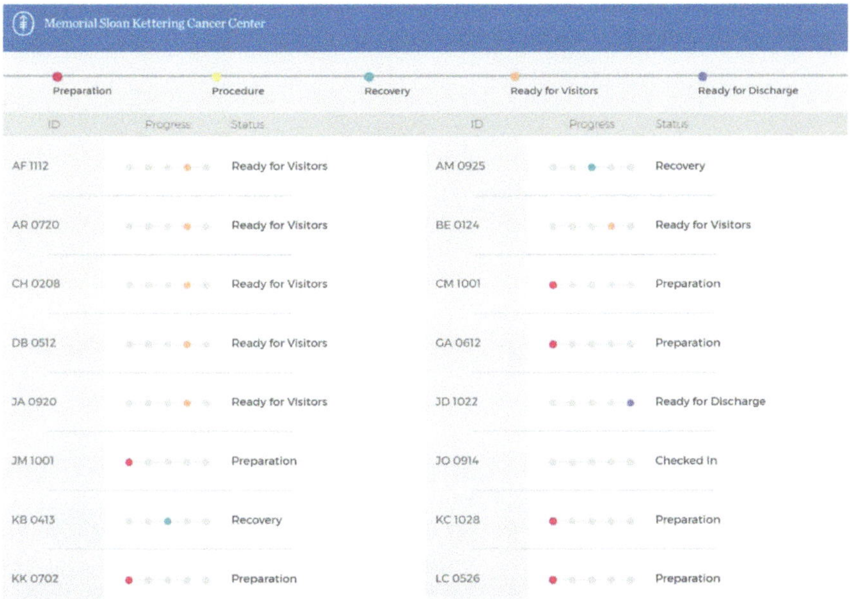

Fig. 3. Example of status board in waiting area to display patient progression through their stay with coded identifiers.

signal to the environmental services team to come clean it and (2) a page goes out to the attending anesthesiologist to inform them that the patient is about to arrive in the OR (Fig. 4). On arrival of the patient into the OR, the RTLS automatically records the "patient in room" time into the medical record, allowing the staff to focus on the patient rather than documentation or paging. Similar automated events occur at the end of surgery and on transfer to the postop room. Precise time-date location stamps for patients and staff provide clean data for operational analysis of wait times and turn over times. Anesthesiologists using the RTLS technology at JRSC are significantly more efficient in completing their preoperative workflow than at the main hospital where RTLS is not used [8]. The RTLS badge is also used to identify when a surgeon has arrived in the building so their first case can proceed, contributing to enhanced OR efficiency.

During the COVID-19 pandemic, the RTLS had an unanticipated use for contact tracing purposes. When a patient or staff member was diagnosed with COVID, their badge location from the last few days could be compared against other individuals. All individuals noted to be in the same room for the 15 minutes (as defined by the CDC COVID-19 exposure time period) were then contacted for appropriate quarantine management. Although not well studied, this methodology allowed for efficient and seemingly effective contact tracing when compared with traditional methods [9]. Many staff found this

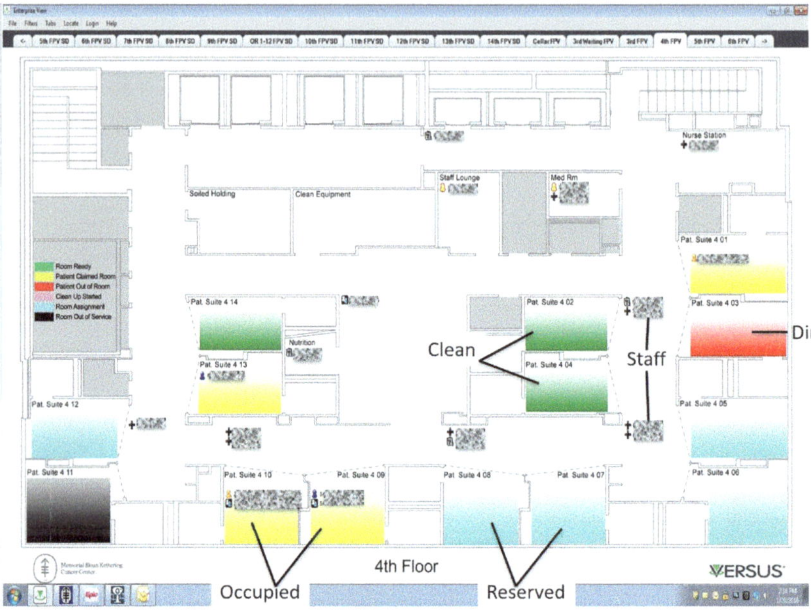

Fig. 4. Example of clinical floor plan of postoperative unit with real-time location information and color coding to optimize workflow efficiency.

very reassuring as compared with other locations without RTLS technology. RTLS is also useful for tracking the location of high-value, mobile equipment. Knowing exactly where a fiberoptic or laryngoscope is located may expedite urgent management and prevent misplaced equipment.

Developing ERAS protocols for the various AXR procedures at JRSC was critical to standardized perioperative methodology [6]. Provider education and engagement, including compliance audits, has been fundamental for successful deployment and ongoing improvement of ERAS protocols. Furthermore, reviewing postoperative pathways with patients and their caregivers, including setting clear expectations for progress, enhances the ability of patients to actively participate in their recovery (see Fig. 1). Continuously monitoring patient ambulation after surgery using the RTLS system and feeding back their progress to them is another way in which "gamification" of recovery helps engage and motivate patients. By prominently displaying walking distance traveled and passed recovery milestones, the clinical staff can quickly assess a patient's recovery and what next step may be necessary, focusing their attention on those patients not making their pathway benchmarks.

The morning after surgery, many surgeons use the telemedicine capability built into every recovery room to check in with their patients before discharge. This is greatly appreciated and highly satisfying to patients while very convenient for the surgeons, who may have responsibilities that prohibit a visit to JRSC. Reducing any barriers between communication between patients and the care team helps keep all parties engaged and informed. The practice also promotes timely discharge because patients are not held to wait for the surgical team to visit.

Postdischarge engagement

Postdischarge engagement is probably the most overlooked opportunity to ensure a successful ambulatory surgery experience for patients, particularly when patients are recovering from increasingly complex surgeries at home. Supporting patients after discharge begins with clear and comprehensive discharge education from the nursing team, including concise and easy to follow written instructions. Whenever possible, a caregiver is included in the discharge teaching. At JRSC, discharge medications, including analgesics and antibiotics as indicated, are provided by the on-site pharmacy so the patient does not need to stop on the way home or take a separate trip to obtain needed medications. This is intended to improve both patient satisfaction and medication compliance. All patients receive phone calls from JRSC nurses and the surgical office practice nurses on the day after discharge to check on their progress, answer any questions, and reinforce discharge instructions.

A unique feature of postdischarge support for JRSC patients is the recovery tracker (RT), an electronic patient-reported outcome (PRO) symptom monitoring system with automated clinical alerts for concerning responses [1,10]. AXR patients receive daily email reminders to complete 10 days of symptom questionnaires through the secure MyMSK Patient Portal. This brief survey contains 14 questions, adapted from the validated National Cancer Institute Patient-Reported Outcomes version of the Common Terminology Criteria for Adverse Events PRO-CTCAE [11] covering 12 common symptoms such as pain, fatigue, nausea, vomiting, shortness of breath, and wound condition. If patient responses exceed preset thresholds, "yellow alerts" (for moderate symptoms) or "red alerts" (for severe or concerning symptoms) are sent to the surgeon's office team by secure message. During business hours, patients are contacted for follow-up after the alerts. For "red alerts" patients are also instructed to immediately call the office or, if it is after hours, the on-call coverage so urgent problems are managed in a timely manner. A similar but simpler survey is also sent to patients after the smaller OP procedures, asking 5 symptom questions for 5 days.

The RT has been highly successful. Since initial rollout in 2016, more than 120,000 surveys have been returned by 21,000 patients, with an average of 5 of the 10 surveys offered completed, very high patient acceptance (participation rates of 86%, with 72% of patients returning 4 or more surveys) and patient satisfaction. A retrospective analysis of the impact of the RT on MSK urgent care center (UCC) visits and readmissions within 30 days of surgery before and after implementation showed that the RT reduced potentially avoidable UCC visits (ie, UCC visits that did not result in readmission) by 22%. Postimplementation, if a patient completed a single RT survey, their risk of a potentially avoidable UCC visit was reduced by 44% [10]. There were no differences in UCC visits resulting in readmission or readmissions overall, suggesting that RT did not create a false sense of security and delay treatment of important complications. These successes have led to the expansion of similar PRO systems at MSK to support patients after inpatient surgeries, radiation treatment, and acute hospitalizations for medical oncology [12].

The RT is a flexible, evolving platform. Specific questions, based on patient characteristics (ie, age, gender), procedure, surgeon, or even prior responses can be delivered to particular patients at specific times as needed, such as questions about vaginal bleeding directed only to hysterectomy patients. Pilot or test questions can be rapidly evaluated, including randomizing a subgroup of patients to different versions of questions. For example, after a quality improvement project in which hundreds of patients were called postoperatively to determine how many opioid pain pills they actually consumed, we significantly reduced the number of opioid pills prescribed on discharge [13]. We then added standard questions to RT asking patients how many opioid and nonopioid pain pills they had taken, with the question delivered first on postoperative day 7 and repeated daily until answered. These data are now used to further improve and monitor the opioid reduction program and were the primary outcome data for a prospective clinical trial evaluating the elimination of opioid prescriptions after breast lumpectomy [14]. Another enhancement to the PRO program was allowing patients to upload photographs for surgical review when they reported wound problems on the survey. This technology allows for timely and remote visual evaluation of surgical wounds through established telemedicine techniques.

Recognizing that patients expect to have health changes after surgery but may not know whether the symptoms they are experiencing are expected or indicate a brewing problem, a randomized clinical trial [15] supported by the Patient-Centered Outcomes Research Institute was performed comparing the standard RT "Team Monitoring," with alerts and nursing follow-up, to the use of "Enhanced Feedback," in which a customized, formatted report is immediately displayed after symptom reporting, which gave context and interpretation of the patients responses [15]. Results of this 2700 patient study indicated that the use of Enhanced Feedback reports resulted in the same reduction of potentially avoidable urgent care visits as the traditional Team Monitoring but with the added benefit of reduced patient anxiety, reduced nursing workload, and very high patient satisfaction [16]. As a result, enhanced feedback is now standard on all the RT-related PRO systems at MSK.

The standardized ERAS approach is maintained in the postoperative period as well. Standardization allows examination of outcomes on a systems level rather than on an individual level. This makes possible the identification of potential areas of improvement for the system. For example, JRSC performed a quality initiative to assess opioid usage after robotic/laparoscopic hysterectomy, radical prostatectomy, partial nephrectomy, or total mastectomy with or without reconstruction [13]. It was discovered that the standard prescriptions offered a median of 20 pills or 140 oral morphine milliequivalents

(MME) but the median consumption was 2 pills or 10 MME. The standardized prescriptions were lowered to 7 to 10 pills with no change in reported pain scores and a reduction of more than 28,000 opioid pills distributed in a single year. Among lumpectomy and sentinel lymph node biopsy patients, modification of discharge prescriptions from opioids to nonsteroidal anti-inflammatories and acetaminophen resulted in a 78% absolute reduction in opioid prescriptions, a 2% pain management failure rate, and no change in pain scores [14].

SUMMARY

The use of ambulatory surgical centers has become an increasingly popular option for health-care systems to increase operating room capacity while offloading inpatient volumes. JRSC exemplifies how, despite the increasing case complexity and patient comorbidities that may occur when pursuing this type of growth, a focus on end-to-end patient engagement and standardized pathways can insure a successful program. Engagement must extend beyond the patient and include their caregivers as well as clinical staff involved in a patient's surgical journey. Engagement must be comprehensive, starting the moment a patient consents to a surgery and extending until they are fully recovered at home. As an indication of the success of this approach, JRSC won Press Ganey "Guardian of Excellence in Patient Experience" awards for the last 3 years running (2019, 2020, 2021), based on continuous performance in the top 5 percentile on the CMS OAS-CAHPS (Outpatient and Ambulatory Surgery Consumer Assessment of Healthcare Providers and Systems) survey. As surgical procedures increasingly move to the ambulatory setting, targeting effective patient engagement and data-driven continuous improvement reaps benefits of increased efficiency, improved outcomes, as well as an optimized patient experience.

CLINICS CARE POINTS

- End-to-end patient engagement throughout the perioperative journey from surgical consent to postdischarge recovery is fundamental to excellent patient-centered ambulatory surgery care.
- Josie Robertson Surgery Center demonstrates how ambulatory surgical centers can successfully perform more complex cancer surgeries by using a systematic approach with care pathways with reduced complications and quick recoveries.
- The patient portal is a powerful tool to track recovery progress after discharge to reduce readmissions and facilitate appropriate triage.
- Ambulatory surgical centers can leverage technology such as real-time location system to enhance efficiency and focus care.

Disclosure

There are no commercial or financial conflicts of interests or relevant funding sources for the authors.

References

[1] Tokita H, Twersky R, Laudone V, et al. Complex Cancer Surgery in the Outpatient Setting: The Josie Robertson Surgery Center. Anesth Analg 2020;131(3):699–707.
[2] Vetter TR, Joshi GP. Ambulatory Extended Recovery: Coming to an Operating Theater Near You. Anesth Analg 2020;131(3):695–8.
[3] Vertosick EA, Assel M, Tokita HK, et al. Suitability of outpatient or ambulatory extended recovery cancer surgeries for obese patients. J Clin Anesth 2019;58:111–6.
[4] Szeto B, Vertosick EA, Ruiz K, et al. Outcomes and Safety Among Patients With Obstructive Sleep Apnea Undergoing Cancer Surgery Procedures in a Freestanding Ambulatory Surgical Facility. Anesth Analg 2019;129(2):360–8.
[5] Ljungqvist O, Scott M, Fearon KC. Enhanced Recovery After Surgery: A Review. JAMA Surg 2017;152(3):292–8.
[6] Afonso AM, McCormick PJ, Assel MJ, et al. Enhanced Recovery Programs in an Ambulatory Surgical Oncology Center. Anesth Analg 2021;133(6):1391–401.
[7] Laudone VP, Durany R, Ehdaie B, et al. Performing complex cancer surgery in the ambulatory setting. J Clin Oncol 2017;35(8_suppl):106.
[8] Yeoh C, Tan KS, Mascarenhas J, et al. Effects of Different Communication Tools on the Efficiency of Anesthesiologists in the Perioperative Setting. J Anesth Clin Res 2017;8(12):794.
[9] Ho HJ, Zhang ZX, Huang Z, et al. Use of a Real-Time Locating System for Contact Tracing of Health Care Workers During the COVID-19 Pandemic at an Infectious Disease Center in Singapore: Validation Study. J Med Internet Res 2020;22(5):e19437.
[10] Simon BA, Assel MJ, Tin AL, et al. Association Between Electronic Patient Symptom Reporting With Alerts and Potentially Avoidable Urgent Care Visits After Ambulatory Cancer Surgery. JAMA Surg 2021;156(8):740–6.
[11] National Cancer Institute Division of Cancer Control and Population Science. Patient-Reported Outcomes version of the Common Terminology Criteria for Adverse Events (PRO-CTCAETM). National Cancer Institute. 2022. Available at: https://healthcaredelivery.cancer.gov/pro-ctcae. Accessed April 3, 2019.
[12] Daly B, Nicholas K, Flynn J, et al. Analysis of a Remote Monitoring Program for Symptoms Among Adults With Cancer Receiving Antineoplastic Therapy. JAMA Netw Open 2022;5(3):e221078.
[13] Fearon NJ, Benfante N, Assel M, et al. Standardizing Opioid Prescriptions to Patients After Ambulatory Oncologic Surgery Reduces Overprescription. Jt Comm J Qual Patient Saf 2020;46(7):410–6.
[14] Moo TA, Pawloski KR, Sevilimedu V, et al. Changing the Default: A Prospective Study of Reducing Discharge Opioid Prescription after Lumpectomy and Sentinel Node Biopsy. Ann Surg Oncol 2020;27(12):4637–42.
[15] Stabile C, Temple LK, Ancker JS, et al. Ambulatory cancer care electronic symptom self-reporting (ACCESS) for surgical patients: a randomised controlled trial protocol. BMJ Open 2019;9(9):e030863.
[16] Pusic AL, Temple LK, Carter J, et al. A Randomized Controlled Trial Evaluating Electronic Outpatient Symptom Monitoring After Ambulatory Cancer Surgery. Ann Surg 2021;274(3):441–8.

ELSEVIER
MOSBY

Advances in Anesthesia 40 (2022) 45–62

ADVANCES IN ANESTHESIA

An Executed Plan to Combat COVID-19 in the United States

William R. Hartman, MD, PhD

Department of Anesthesiology, Office of Clinical Research, University of Wisconsin-Madison, Madison, WI, USA

Keywords

• COVID-19 • SARS-CoV-2 • Pandemic • COVID screening • Convalescent plasma • Monoclonal antibodies • Antivirals • Vaccine

Severe acute respiratory syndrome coronavirus 2 (SARS-CoV-2) is a highly transmissible coronavirus that emerged in late 2019 [1]. High SARS-CoV-2 transmissibility has led to a worldwide pandemic of acute respiratory disease, devastating populations by overwhelming health systems and causing many deaths. To date, this coronavirus is responsible for greater than 90 million cases in the United States and more than 1 million confirmed deaths [2].

As a coronavirus, SARS-CoV-2 belongs to a group of diverse viruses infecting many different animals including domesticated cattle and sheep, as well as avian mammals including bats [3]. New coronaviruses often lead to upper respiratory infections when they infect humans, infections that more recently have caused a wide clinical spectrum from mild-to-severe disease and death. Before the advent of these coronaviruses, these viruses were not thought to be pathogenic in humans, in fact, before 2002, most coronaviruses were believed to be quite mild and caused little or no disease in humans. SARS-CoV-2, a novel coronavirus responsible for COVID-19, is related to other pathogenic coronaviruses including SARS-CoV and MERS-CoV [3]. Although these other coronaviruses sparked a worldwide concern early due to rapid transmissibility and initial fatalities, both SARS-CoV and MERS-CoV were relatively quickly contained preventing a worldwide pandemic situation seen with SARS-CoV-2.

SARS-CoV-2 arose from Wuhan, China at the end of 2019 and, although attempts at containment were initiated, quickly spread to every country in the world [4]. The virus has proven to be highly contagious among humans, and with the timing of its emergence during the lunar New Year, travel of

E-mail address: Wrhartman@wisc.edu

https://doi.org/10.1016/j.aan.2022.07.002
0737-6146/22/

families to and from Wuhan made containment logistically difficult [5]. SARS-CoV-2 has caused to the largest viral pandemic in our lifetime and is a true threat to worldwide public health.

The emergence of SARS-CoV-2 in the United States, as in other countries, was met with great angst. The hospitals and health-care systems were quickly overwhelmed, and no treatments were known. People were dying and there was little that could be done other than supportive care. The SARS-CoV-2 pandemic highlighted the need for and importance of clinical trials to identify diagnostics, therapeutics, and vaccines that would combat this virus, as well as novel methods to get these therapies produced and trialed quickly but safely.

This review is written from the perspective of an anesthesiologist/clinical trialist who helped execute a plan at a large midwestern university to bring old and novel therapies for trial to help treat suffering people and to bring vaccines to trial with a goal of preventing severe disease and slowing viral transmission. To understand how and why this plan was needed, a firm understanding of the virus itself, as well as its impact on society are also very important.

VIRAL EMERGENCE AND EFFECTS ON SOCIETY

Emergence

Before 2002, coronaviruses were thought to not cause serious infections in humans. In fact, coronaviruses were better studied in mammals other than humans as human pathogenic coronaviruses were not seen. The emergence of SARS-CoV in a southern China animal market altered that theory. Pathogenic in humans, SARS-CoV caused respiratory illness in more than 8000 people and caused 774 deaths worldwide [6,7]. Still another coronavirus, MERS-CoV, emerged in 2012. This virus was responsible for Middle East respiratory syndrome and led to respiratory infections in approximately 2428 individuals and killing 838 [8]. SARS-CoV and MERS-CoV had bat origins before jumping to new mammalian hosts. SARS-CoV invaded the Himalayan civet. In the Middle East, MERS-CoV jumped to the dromedary camel in the Middle East. Both of these coronaviruses subsequently infected humans, with deadly consequences [9,10]. SARS-CoV-2 may have also originated in bats as bats have a similar coronavirus relative, a coronavirus known as RaTG13 [11]. SARS-CoV-2 and RaTG13 have similar S-proteins with about 98% amino acid sequence homology, only dramatically differing in the sequence of the S-gene coding for the spike protein [11]. Following initial SARS-CoV-2 cases that dated to December 8, 2019, in Wuhan, the World Health Organization (WHO) was notified of a pneumonia outbreak of unidentified cause by the Wuhan Municipal Health Organization [12]. By mid-January, 2020, Chinese scientists had identified the pathogen as a betacoronavirus with a single-stranded RNA genome. By January 12, 2020, the complete viral RNA genome sequence was made publicly available via the GISAID database [12,13]. On January 30, the WHO declared SARS-CoV-2 a public health emergency with international potential. Unable to contain the virus in China, and with a large international travel population, the highly transmissible virus was determined to be a threat in all countries. According to Johns Hopkins University, by August, 2020, 216 countries and regions from all 6 continents had reported more than 20 million cases of SARS-CoV-2 (now called COVID-19), overwhelming local health resources and leading to high mortality [14].

COVID-19 IN THE COMMUNITY

COVID-19 has had a tremendous impact on all communities in the United States but a disproportionate effect on communities of color. The COVID-19 pandemic has highlighted several health inequities within our health system. For instance, non-Hispanic Black or African American people and Hispanic people are both more than twice as likely to be hospitalized due to COVID-19 than non-Hispanic white people [14,15]. Further, non-Hispanic Native Americans or Alaska Native people are 3.1 times more likely to be hospitalized due to COVID-19 than non-Hispanic white people. Racial and socioeconomic factors play a role in these inequities. These factors likely contribute to these inequities including, comorbid conditions, access to health care, location, and type of housing. Historically, Black, Hispanic, Native American, and Asian American people are at higher risk of developing comorbid conditions including diabetes mellitus, reactive airway disease, and hypertension. These comorbid conditions may predispose a person to developing severe disease from COVID-19 [15,16]. It is thought that type of work can also predispose a person to developing COVID-19 as having a job that is considered essential, which cannot be performed remotely, or involves public interaction, can increase one's exposure to symptomatic and asymptomatic individuals and thus increase the risk of contracting COVID-19 [17]. People in racial and ethnic diversity groups might be more likely to live in multigenerational homes [18], crowded conditions, and densely populated urban areas. Living under the same roof or in groups can make the viral mitigating factor of social distancing difficult. Some diverse populations might also have higher rates of uninsured people causing disparities in health-care access [18]. Finally, stresses of racism itself can lead to early aging in diverse groups and could contribute to the development of severe disease from COVID-19 [19].

Within our communities, COVID-19 disproportionately affects people living in nursing homes. Often, this population has a high number of elderly, frail adults who are more likely to have a multitude of comorbid conditions [20]. An inability to properly social distance, a lack of adequate ventilation at the beginning of the pandemic, and the higher likelihood of this population having a multitude of chronic conditions all contributed to the waves of COVID-related deaths we saw in nursing homes at different times during the pandemic. Without question, the nursing home population suffered tremendous death counts because of swift transmission of COVID-19 within this environment and an inability to adequately institute viral mitigating methods, especially early in the pandemic.

COVID-19 and pregnancy

Although COVID-19 was deadly in the community, it was also thought that SARS-CoV-2 might also influence growing populations. Pregnant people infected with the SARS-CoV-2 could be asymptomatic or symptomatic. COVID-19 symptomatic pregnant people were found to be at increased risk for developing severe sequelae of COVID-19 compared with nonpregnant reproductive-aged women [21]. Most evidence suggested that pregnant women did not have different symptoms from the virus than nonpregnant individuals but if they developed severe disease, the clinical course was heightened and worsened [21]. Pregnant women symptomatic with COVID with severe disease were at increased risks for intensive care unit (ICU) admission, need for mechanical ventilation and ventilatory support, and death compared with nonpregnant women of the same age [21].

UNDERSTANDING THE SEVERE ACUTE RESPIRATORY SYNDROME CORONAVIRUS 2

Understanding how to best attack and mitigate this virus requires an understanding of the molecular makeup of this novel coronavirus. Further, an understanding of how the virus binds and invades host cells is imperative to finding neutralizing targets.

Viral makeup

Coronaviruses, in general, are spherical, enveloped viruses containing a helical symmetry nucleocapsid and a single-stranded RNA genome [22,23]. SARS-CoV-2 shares approximately 80% genome sequence identity with SARS-CoV [23]. Similar to other coronaviruses, the SARS-CoV-2 RNA genome contains 6 functional open reading frames. These ORFs are arranged in order from 5' to 3': replicase (ORF1a/ORF1b), spike (S), envelope (E), membrane (M), and nucleocapsid (N) [23]. Another 7 ORFs are scattered throughout the viral genome and likely code for accessory proteins. Although many of these genes are similar to counterparts in other coronaviruses [23], the S-gene, coding for the spike protein, diverges and has a very different sequence [24]. As with attempts at therapeutics to neutralize previous coronaviruses, the spike protein of SARS-CoV-2 has become the target for preventative and therapeutic options [25]. The S protein of SARS-CoV-2 is a class I fusion protein that protects its fusion domain. This protein keeps the binding domain hidden and inactive until the virus finds a host cell with an appropriate receptor, and targets that cell for infection [25]. The fusion protein is then enzymatically cleaved, revealing a hook-shaped structure that is necessary for viral binding and incorporation into the membrane of the target cell [26,27]. It is suspected that nucleotide polymorphisms and mutations within the spike protein alter viral transmissibility and virus–host cell interactions [26]. The speed and efficiency of these mutations is remarkable.

SARS-CoV-2 can rapidly mutate and alter its conformation in order to adapt to its current environment [28]. Mutations in the SARS-CoV-2 genome have allowed for changes in disease severity, viral transmission, and host immunity evasion. As such, containment attempts of SARS-CoV-2 have involved worldwide population vaccination coverage and physical mitigation methods (social distancing, hand washing, mask wearing) to control the spread of the virus. History will be able to determine the extent to which these methods were able to control viral transmission.

COVID-19 receptor

In humans, SARS-CoV-2 enters cells using the same receptor as SARS-CoV, a receptor known as angiotensin-converting enzyme 2 (ACE2). ACE2 is a type I membrane glycoprotein responsible for the conversion of angiotensin II into angiotensin 1. This receptor is highly expressed in the lungs, nose, heart, intestine, and kidneys of humans [29]. The SARS-CoV-2 S-protein receptor binding domain (RBD), a 211 amino acid sequence, has been the target for neutralizing antibodies, both host and manufactured. By neutralizing the SARS-CoV-2 RBD, it is felt that one could effectively block the virus and prevent worsening of symptoms and progression of disease. Although similar to that of SARS-CoV, the RBD of SARS-CoV-2 functionally facilitates a much stronger interaction and tighter bond between itself and the host cell [29].

SEVERE ACUTE RESPIRATORY SYNDROME CORONAVIRUS 2 PATHOGENESIS

There is a wide range of SARS-CoV-2 clinical pathologic conditions in humans, spanning from asymptomatic infection to mild symptoms to severe respiratory failure and death. Asymptomatic infections have been well-documented [30,31]. One review performed before the introduction of COVID-19 vaccination estimated that 33% of people with SARS-CoV-2 infection never develop symptoms [31]. Asymptomatic infections were a confounder early in the pandemic because it had been believed that only symptomatic individuals had viral loads high enough to transmit infection. This theory proved false, and as the pandemic thrived, asymptomatic spread of disease was a major contributor to community positivity rates [31].

The original COVID-19 and several subsequent variants would bind to airway epithelial cells via the ACE2 receptor in the upper respiratory tract. Replicating and releasing from the upper airway cells, SARS-CoV-2 migrated into the lower airways. Here, SARS-CoV-2 would enter lung alveolar epithelial cells [32]. The rapid replication of SARS-CoV-2 in the alveoli triggers a strong immune response that precipitates a cytokine storm syndrome, which ultimately leads to acute respiratory distress syndrome and respiratory failure, a principal cause of death in COVID-19 patients [32]. Although far from universal, older patients (aged >60 years) and those with serious preexisting diseases (particularly obesity, pulmonary complications, and diabetes) have demonstrated a greater risk of progressing to severe COVID-19 disease and death.

All ages and genders are susceptible to SARS-CoV-2 infection. The median age of COVID-19 infection is around 50 years, and clinical manifestations can differ dramatically with age. To date, 78% of hospitalizations and approximately 75% of all deaths related to COVID have occurred in the older than 65 years demographic [33]. Older men with comorbidities tend to develop severe disease, whereas most young people and children have only mild symptoms (nonpneumonia or mild pneumonia), if they have any symptoms at all. When infected with COVID-19, the most common symptoms are fever, fatigue, and dry cough, with sputum production, headache, hemoptysis, diarrhea, anorexia, sore throat, chest pain, chills. Nausea and vomiting are somewhat less common symptoms [34]. In the age of delta and omicron, a sore throat and persistent cough have been commonly described [35]. Self-reported olfactory and taste disorders were also reported by patients in Italy, and subsequently described worldwide [36]. Viral incubation period was about 3 to 5 days because most people showed signs of viral infection on day 6 to 10 after exposure. Symptoms of dyspnea and pneumonia developed within a median time of 8 days from illness onset [37].

The degree of SARS-CoV-2 contagiousness may be due to certain virologic features of SARS-CoV-2. Human-to-human transmission can occur through respiratory droplets containing SARS-CoV-2 particles and can spread by speech, coughing, or sneezing [38]. The recipient mucous membranes of the eyes, nose, or mouth are viral portals. Additionally, transmission can occur by direct contact with contaminated surfaces because the virus is able to survive outside of the host for at least several hours [38–40]. Typically, respiratory viruses have the highest transmission rate from human to human while the infected person has viral symptoms. It is thought that the virus is at its peak during this time. COVID-19 is also thought to be most transmissible during the symptomatic period as well [41]. However, the possibility of viral transmission from an asymptomatic individual [42] exists as there is clear evidence of asymptomatic or presymptomatic spread of SARS-CoV-2 demonstrated by colonization and replication in a human throat during the initial infection [43,44]. In fact, it is possible that unknown and asymptomatic infections might account for approximately 80% of transmitted cases because of this high viral transmissibility during the asymptomatic period [42]. Asymptomatic period infectiousness, aerosolized particles, and viral survivability outside of the host likely contribute greatly to the rapid global spread of the virus. Public health mitigation interventions to reduce transmission have proven successful in China and several other countries, such as South Korea.

Severe acute respiratory syndrome coronavirus 2 diagnosis

The COVID-19 pandemic has highlighted the imperative nature of prompt and accurate viral diagnosis. Currently, polymerase chain reaction (PCR) genomic amplification methods represent the gold standard [45–48]. PCR testing, although accurate, is very expensive due to the complexity of the process and the required technical elements. Requirements for testing include PCR reaction reagents, expensive analysis machines, and experienced laboratory technicians [45]. Early in the pandemic, important supplies including nasopharyngeal swabs used for sample collection were in short supply greatly limiting the ability to test symptomatic people adequately and efficiently. An inability to adequately test patients in the first days of the pandemic likely contributed to the rapid transmission of the virus as people could not be isolated and contact tracing was not possible. Further complicating the testing deficiencies in the United States, PCR reaction reagents were lacking, and supply did not meet demand. Eventually, as the supply of collection equipment and of PCR reagents production was increased, efficient testing was generally made widely available. Mass testing centers were set up throughout the country so that people could quickly be screened for COVID-19 if they had contact with a known COVID-19 patient or if they had symptoms of COVID-19.

PCR testing in developing countries has been particularly challenging. Economic disparities in developing and underdeveloped countries prevent effective mass PCR testing programs. As such, other methods are required to screen symptomatic people. Rapid antigen and antibody tests and immunoenzymatic serologic tests became inexpensive to produce and easy to use. Rapid testing has become the most widely used technique for monitoring the spread of SARS-CoV-2 infection. These low-cost point-of-care tests enabled for effective viral surveillance systems. Yet, in other countries where COVID-19 tests (either Rapid or PCR tests) were in short supply, other systems needed to be developed to screen patients. In the absence of diagnostic testing, it became necessary to consider the patient's symptoms, contact history, and also the patient's medical history. The integration of all of these elements provides a solid foundation for adequately diagnosing COVID-19 infection and effectively managing and containing the COVID-19 pandemic [49].

Accurate and early COVID-19 diagnosis is crucial for controlling its spread. Testing 36 to 72 hours following a known exposure is recommended, especially if one is symptomatic and is at high risk for becoming symptomatic. False-negative results can also arise when nasopharyngeal or oral swabs are improperly used by collection technicians, therefore multiple detection methods should be available to confirm a COVID-19 diagnosis. One such alternative method was chest computed tomography (CT). COVID-19 patients demonstrated typical CT features including bilateral multilobar ground-glass opacities with a peripheral or posterior distribution. Thus, it has been suggested that CT scanning combined with repeated swab tests should be used for individuals with high clinical suspicion of COVID-19 but are testing negative for the virus [50].

With an understanding of SARS-CoV-2 from a molecular and pathogenic standpoint, and diagnostics and mitigation methods in place, the next frontier to conquer was therapeutics. Patients hospitalized were being treated symptomatically, although no therapeutics had been developed to combat the virus. The collaboration of private and public sectors was brought together in an effort known as WARP SPEED. The goal of WARP SPEED was to have these sectors work together to rapidly develop and trial therapeutics.

OPERATION WARP SPEED

In response to the COVID-19 pandemic, the US government quickly activated Operation Warp Speed (OWS). OWS created a partnership between the Department of Health and Human Services and the Department of Defense (DOD) with the goal of accelerating the development of a COVID-19 vaccine [51]. This partnership decided the best strategy would be to use different private companies to use different vaccine platforms to generate expeditious delivery of safe and effective vaccines. These companies also took steps, such as starting large-scale manufacturing during clinical trials and combining clinical trial phases or running them concurrently. Clinical trials gathered data on safety and efficacy, with more participants in each successive phase (eg, phase 3 has more participants than phase 2) [51,52]. Common to each of these companies was the compressed timelines. To meet OWS timelines, some vaccine companies relied on data from other vaccines using the same platforms, where available, or conducted certain animal studies at the same time as clinical trials. However, as is done in a nonpandemic environment, all vaccine companies gathered initial safety and antibody response data with a small number of participants before proceeding into large-scale human studies (eg, phase 3 clinical trials) [51,52]. There was no compromise of safety and effectiveness in the development of these vaccines.

Anti-COVID-19 therapeutics

When COVID-19 first came to the United States, we were ill prepared to treat the disease. Since then, convalescent plasma, monoclonal antibodies, intravenous antivirals, and oral antivirals have become commonplace for early intervention. The only late intervention therapy that has proven useful once a person is mechanically ventilated is steroid use.

CHLOROQUINE AND HYDROXYCHLOROQUINE

Although not a WARP SPEED initiative, anecdotal evidence from around the world suggested a potential use for the drugs, chloroquine and hydroxychloroquine. These antimalarial and immune altering medicines were thought to elicit a therapeutic benefit by the inhibition of cellular entry by the virus [53]. These medicines are known to inhibit the glycosylation of cellular receptors and prevent, at least partially, virus–host receptor binding. Further, they can increase the endosomal pH to inhibit membrane fusion [54]. It is currently accepted that these medicines provide no clinical benefit to effectively treat patients with COVID-19 [54,55]. Even though some studies showed they can inhibit SARS-CoV-2 infection in vitro, clinically this has not proven to occur. Further, 2 clinical studies demonstrated no association with death rates in patients receiving chloroquine or hydroxychloroquine compared with those not receiving the drug [54]. On 15 June 2020, owing to the side effects observed in clinical trials, the US Food and Drug Administration (FDA) revoked the emergency use authorization (EUA) for chloroquine and hydroxychloroquine as a treatment of COVID-19 [56].

PASSIVE IMMUNITY AND CONVALESCENT PLASMA

Without effective treatments available to combat COVID-19, a group of scientists and physicians looked to a historical therapy that had been used to treat previous viral disease including measles and Ebola. This therapy relied on having donors who had recovered from COVID-19 and were likely to have levels of neutralizing antibodies in their plasma. Collecting this plasma and transfusing it into a sick person would potentially provide therapeutic benefit to the sick patient [57].

Under the guidance of the Mayo Clinic Expanded Access Program, convalescent plasma could be collected and administered to hospitalized patients. The program was expanded to nearly 2900 hospitals in every state and several countries, and more than 70,000 patients were transfused 1 or 2 units of plasma. Although never designed to be a randomized clinical trial, the Mayo EAP became the largest trial testing the safety of convalescent plasma transfusions [58]. Several randomized controlled trials, including the large RECOVERY trial in the United Kingdom [59], failed to establish survival benefit to transfused patients versus controls. Others have pointed to trial deficiencies to explain the lack of effect. First, convalescent plasma was usually administered to patients when they had already developed severe disease while hospitalized. Second, plasma antibody titers were not adequately measured. More recently, high-titer convalescent plasma was used to treat outpatients with COVID-19 in a randomized controlled trial [60]. Using convalescent plasma in this manner reduced hospitalizations by 50%. As convalescent plasma will be readily available and inexpensive to collect in any area where a COVID-19 spike is occurring, the WHO should reevaluate its position and allow convalescent plasma to be used in countries where monoclonal antibodies are not in plentiful supply.

PASSIVE IMMUNITY AND MONOCLONAL ANTIBODIES

Arising from the work done with convalescent plasma, and with knowledge from past experiences with viruses including Ebola, monoclonal antibodies were developed as therapeutic options for the treatment and potential prophylaxis for COVID-19 [61]. Similar to convalescent plasma, monoclonal antibodies are a form of passive immunity where laboratory generated antibodies are targeted to specific epitopes on the virus. In the case of SARS-CoV-2, multiple antibodies were created to bind the viral spike protein to prevent viral binding and invasion of the host cell. In contrast with convalescent plasma, which consists of many antibodies contained in plasma, monoclonal antibodies are directed toward specific targets and selected specifically for their ability to neutralize the virus [24,62].

Bamlanivimab (Eli Lily) was the first monoclonal antibody given a EUA by the FDA in November 2020. This single monoclonal antibody was approved to treat mild COVID-19 disease in outpatients who were at risk of developing severe disease and being hospitalized. Specifically, Bamlanivimab (Bam) is a neutralizing human IgG1κ monoclonal antibody [63]. In a clinical trial known as the BLAZE-1 trial in patients with mild-to-moderate COVID-19, this monoclonal antibody showed an effect of on reducing viral loads in treated patients versus untreated control patients. More important than the viral load reduction, however, was that the treated patients showed less emergency room visits and reduced hospitalizations compared with untreated control patients [64]. In the highest risk of developing severe disease group of patients (body mass index >35 or aged >65 years), there was a sharp contrast between the treated and untreated with treated patients showing pronounced reductions in emergency room visits and hospitalizations [64].

Unfortunately, because of the rapid rate in which SARS-CoV-2 can mutate its spike protein, this monoclonal antibody became less effective as variants began to circulate. The large number of COVID-19 variants developed resistance to bamlanivimab neutralization. This led the FDA and CDC to revoke the EUA for this monoclonal antibody because it was no longer useful in the treatment against COVID-19 variants beta and gamma [65]. Bamlanivimab did demonstrate effectiveness against the Delta variant when combined with a second monoclonal (Etesevimab) and its use was briefly resumed but stopped again because it had little efficacy versus the Omicron variant [63].

A second authorized monoclonal therapeutic consisted of the 2 monoclonal antibodies casirivimab and imdevimab and was developed by Regeneron. Similar to the Lily monoclonal, this novel monoclonal antibody cocktail had directed activity versus the SARS-CoV-2 spike protein and was distributed under the name REGEN-COV. This cocktail was trialed as both an infusion and a subcutaneous injection [66]. In November, 2020, the FDA issued an EUA for REGN-COV to be used in at risk patients with COVID-19 who currently had mild-to-moderate symptoms. In clinical trials, more than 4000 outpatients with mild-to-moderate COVID-19 and at least one risk factor for severe disease were randomized to receive either REGEN-COV or placebo [67]. The REGEN-COV treatment groups showed sharp reductions in COVID-19–related hospitalization or all-cause death, and a more rapid resolution of COVID-19 symptoms compared with placebo. The EUA was then amended to include its use as a postexposure prophylactic treatment because treated individuals demonstrated a profound decrease in developing symptomatic COVID-19 compared with untreated controls in clinical trial. In a postexposure prophylaxis arm of the clinical trial, 1505 participants who lived in a household with a patient infected with COVID-19 but were asymptomatic and had a negative SARS-CoV-2 test. The treatment group demonstrated an 81% risk reduction in the development of PCR-confirmed COVID-19 infection through 29 days [68]. This would be particularly important for nursing home patients, and others who live in close quarters with a person infected with COVID-19, as well as for COVID-19 negative immunocompromised people with a strong exposure to COVID.

Similar to the Lily monoclonal antibody, REGEN-COV proved less effective against increasing COVID-19 variants, and the EUA was eventually withdrawn for this treatment. Other monoclonal antibodies have been granted

EUA by the FDA for use against various COVID-19 variants. One such monoclonal, sotrovimab was created from an antibody identified in 2003 in a survivor of SARS [69]. This monoclonal, developed by Glaxo Smith Kline, showed initial effectiveness against Delta and Omicron variants in the COMET-ICE clinical trial. This trial, similar to others, demonstrated effectiveness in outpatients with COVID-19 experiencing mild-to-moderate symptoms but who were at risk of developing severe disease. Ultimately, the SARS-CoV-2 variants evaded this monoclonal, and the EUA was withdrawn. Finally, Astra Zeneca has developed a 2 monoclonal antibody cocktail called Evusheld that is being trialed as a prophylaxis drug for immune compromised patients who are either resistant to a COVID-19 vaccine, or unable to mount a robust antibody response to the vaccine. It is thought that this passive immunity can provide up to 6 months of protection against developing symptomatic COVID-19 [70].

DEXAMETHASONE

Treatments for patients with severe disease from COVID-19 requiring high flow oxygen or mechanical ventilation have been a challenge. Neither convalescent plasma nor monoclonal antibodies demonstrated any survival benefit to patients with this late-stage COVID-19. Further, neither treatment demonstrated a reduction in days on the ventilator or days hospitalized once the virus had caused severe disease. With treatments limited, physicians looked to dexamethasone, a corticosteroid that suppresses the immune response. It was felt that by suppressing the cytokine storm, dexamethasone could provide benefit [71]. A large clinical trial known as the RECOVERY trial in the United Kingdom demonstrated that when patients with severe COVID-19 were treated with dexamethasone (6 mg once daily for up to 10 days), they saw a reduction in 28-day mortality. No benefit was observed in patients not requiring oxygen. This trial changed clinical practice, which had dictated that corticosteroids were contraindicated and rewrote the clinical treatment guidelines so that COVID-19 patients requiring supplemental oxygen could be administered dexamethasone [72].

Antivirals

Until recently, remdesivir had been the only antiviral medicine approved by the FDA to be used in COVID-19 patients. Two large randomized clinical trials have been performed using remdesivir, a study carried out by the VA and the ACTT-1 trial. The ACTT-1 trial found that IV remdesivir provided no survival benefit but patients who recovered from COVID-19 were able to be discharged earlier from the hospital [73]. The VA study also showed no survival benefit but demonstrated that patients stayed in the hospital longer than untreated patients. It has been speculated that the VA study did not follow the same protocol as the ACTT-1 trial, specifically that patients stayed in the hospital for the full length of their remdesivir course [74]. In ACTT-1, patients were discharged from the trial when they met the trial endpoint, no further infusions were administered. This detail may have not been properly communicated and could explain the longer hospital stays observed in the VA trial.

An oral antiviral medicine known as Paxlovid has just come to market. This oral pill is administered to a person with very early COVID-19 twice per day for 5 days. Paxlovid has many medication interactions with other medicines, so its use is limited to people with no contraindications [74]. The clinical trial investigating Paxlovid in outpatients with risk factors for developing severe disease, demonstrated a marked reduction in hospitalizations (70%) compared with untreated control patients, and no deaths. More recently, several patients have found themselves with rebound COVID-19 infections following their 5-day course of Paxlovid. This is a phenomenon that requires further study [75,76].

ACTIVE IMMUNITY AND VACCINES

As soon as COVID-19 was declared a public health emergency and classified as a pandemic, an intense worldwide effort was undertaken to develop safe and effective COVID-19 vaccines. Vaccines generated were from several different "classes"; however, their general principle was all the same–to force the human immune system to generate anti-COVID antibodies in the absence of active infection. The antibodies, then, would serve to survey and protect a person should they contract the virus. The development of the vaccines had to be expeditious, and the clinical trials had to be incredibly efficient in order to deliver these too naive populations within a finite timeline.

MESSENGER RNA VACCINES

Scientists have developed a new type of vaccine that uses a genetic molecule called messenger RNA (mRNA) that codes for a portion of the virus rather than a part of an actual bacteria or virus. These novel vaccines had been developed for other viruses but had never been manufactured on a large scale. Their premise is to use mRNA, a genetic molecule necessary for protein production. In essence, these vaccines are delivering a genetic blueprint to human cells to make a protein designated by the mRNA and then the body develops antibodies against the produced protein. Once cells finish making a protein, the mRNA quickly breaks down by cellular enzymes. mRNA from vaccines does not enter a cell's nucleus and does not alter native DNA.

PFIZER VACCINE

This mRNA vaccine was the first COVID-19 vaccine to receive EUA. Similar to other mRNA vaccines, it has an mRNA message to build the spike protein. This mRNA is enclosed within a lipid envelope. A US clinical trial involving 43,548 participants, funded by BioNTech and Pfizer, demonstrated that this vaccine (2 doses, 3 weeks apart) was very effective in preventing symptomatic COVID-19. In fact, 95% of individuals administered the vaccine did not contract COVID-19 [77]. A clinical trial was also performed in Israel with 1.2 million people and the efficacy of the vaccine was confirmed [78]. Side effects were minimal, usually consisting of fatigue, arm soreness, headache, and/or fever. A rare but significant side effect following vaccination can include myocarditis (inflammation of the heart muscle) and pericarditis (inflammation of the tissue surrounding the heart) [79]. These side effects are more likely following the second dose of the vaccine and occur more commonly in teenage boys. As immunity begins to wane somewhere around 5 to 6 months after dose 2, it is recommended that a third shot be administered as a booster dose. This has shown in studies to restore immunity back to the high efficacy level seen after the second shot. Especially in people with compromised immune systems, a fourth shot is recommended as a second booster as well.

More recently, the Pfizer mRNA vaccine has been approved for children aged 5 to 11 years. The side effect profile is like that in adults, although the incidence of myocarditis seems much lower. Overall efficacy is similar to what is seen in adults, despite the dose being approximately one-third the dose that the adult receives. Again, waning immunity after 5 to 6 months has prompted to recommendation to issue a booster shot at that time [80].

MODERNA MESSENGER RNA VACCINE

The second COVID-19 vaccine to be granted EUA by the FDA and CDC also used an mRNA platform and came from Moderna. Although it has a very similar makeup to the Pfizer vaccine, they differ in the amount of mRNA (30 mcg Pfizer vs 100 mcg Moderna) and the lipid envelope is manufactured using slightly different lipids. In a US clinical phase 2/3 trial involving more than 30,000 individuals, only 11 developed symptomatic COVID-19 following 2 doses 1 month apart [81]. The vaccine had a 94% efficacy rate and was 100% effective against severe illness, hospitalization, and death from COVID-19 [81]. The trial population included more than 7000 people aged older than 65 years, and another 5000 who were aged 65 years or younger but had comorbidities that placed them in a group most at risk of developing severe COVID-19. Paramount to the success of these clinical trials to be completed in the contracted timeline was the need to ensure that all ages, genders, and diversity of communities were appropriately represented and reflected the US population. Although the Moderna was thought to have longer lasting immunity compared with the Pfizer vaccine, antibody levels did begin to wane after approximately 6 months and a booster was recommended.

The Moderna vaccine clinical trial for children, aged 11 to 17 years had been completed in the United States but no EUA was initially authorized because of concerns of myocarditis and pericarditis, in especially teenage boys. Data has now been collected worldwide and Moderna was deemed safe and effective in a unanimous vote by the FDA advisory committee on June 14, 2020. Overall, the incidence of myocarditis in this age group is very rare but a warning has been attached to the vaccine label listing this as a potential adverse effect, especially after the second shot [79].

JOHNSON AND JOHNSON ADENOVIRAL VACCINE

The J&J/Janssen COVID-19 vaccine contains a piece of a modified SARS-CoV-2 viral DNA coding for the COVID-19 spike protein. The vector adenovirus, which typically causes the common cold, has been modified so that it cannot reproduce itself and thus is nonpathogenic. This adenovirus vector serves as a shuttle to move the spike protein DNA into cells where the cells then use their own machinery to synthesize the spikes [82]. The body then generates antibodies to these spike proteins to produce both acute and lasting immune responses to deter symptomatic COVID-19. The Johnson and Johnson vaccine had a lower efficacy rate for preventing symptomatic COVID-19 when compared with the mRNA vaccines (74%–78%) but this was billed as a one shot vaccine [82]. Real life data from this vaccine uncovered a rare but significant side effect where people developed blood clots with diminished platelet counts, and the FDA has now limited its use in favor of the mRNA vaccines. Further waning immunity after 5 to 6 months suggested the need for a booster to restore immunity levels, and the FDA and CDC issued a statement that receiving an mRNA booster would be recommended.

SUMMARY

Although there is plenty of room for criticism around the response by the United States to the COVID-19 pandemic, much was accomplished in a relatively short period of time. Beginning with the genomic sequence published by the Chinese before COVID-19 invading every country on earth, the United States had already begun to understand and characterize the pathogen. In relatively quick fashion, the response included an understanding of the virus itself, the development of testing to be able to provide early and efficient viral diagnoses, the development of effective treatments to help prevent people from dying from severe COVID-19, the development of treatments to help prevent disease progression and hospitalizations, the development of treatments to act as prophylaxis agents in close contacts, and finally the development of safe and effective vaccines to provide the world population immunity to protect them from severe disease, hospitalization, and death from COVID-19. The study continues, however, as evolving COVID-19 variants continue to find ways to evade immunity. Potential areas for future research include the development of newer vaccines with variant mRNA "blueprints" to better fight off infection and newer treatments, both antiviral medications and monoclonal antibodies to continue to treat people sick from COVID-19. Highlighted in this plan and in the future directions is the need to continue to be able to perform large and efficient clinical trials accurately representing the population of the United States, so that we can build the best treatments, build the best preventatives, and develop the best vaccines to keep all people, young and old, safe, and virus-free.

Disclosure

The author has nothing to disclose.

References

[1] Holmes EC, Goldstein SA, Rasmussen AL, et al. The origins of SARS-CoV-2: A critical review. Cell 2021;184(19):4848–56.

[2] Available at: https://www.cdc.gov/coronavirus/2019-ncov/index.html.
[3] Sharun K, Dhama K, Pawde AM, et al. SARS-CoV-2 in animals: potential for unknown reservoir hosts and public health implications. Vet Q 2021;41(1):181–201.
[4] Dhama K, Khan S, Tiwari R, et al. Coronavirus Disease 2019-COVID-19. Clin Microbiol Rev 2020;33(4):e00028-20.
[5] Sharma A, Ahmad Farouk I, Lal SK. COVID-19: A Review on the Novel Coronavirus Disease Evolution, Transmission, Detection, Control and Prevention. Viruses 2021;13(2):202.
[6] Drosten C, Günther S, Preiser W, et al. Identification of a novel coronavirus in patients with severe acute respiratory syndrome. Engl J Med 2003;348:1967–76.
[7] Lau LT, Fung YWW, Wong FPF, et al. A real-time PCR for SARS-coronavirus incorporating target gene pre-amplification. Biochem Biophys Res Commun 2003;312:1290–6.
[8] Zaki AM, Van Boheemen S, Bestebroer TM, et al. Isolation of a novel coronavirus from a man with pneumonia in Saudi Arabia. N Engl J Med 2012;367:1814–20.
[9] Song HD, Tu CC, Zhang GW, et al. Cross-host evolution of severe acute respiratory syndrome coronavirus in palm civet and human. Proc Natl Acad Sci U S A 2005;102:2430–5.
[10] Azhar EI, El-Kafrawy SA, Farraj SA, et al. Evidence for Camel-to-Human Transmission of MERS Coronavirus. N Engl J Med 2014;370:2499–505.
[11] Liu K, Pan X, Li L, et al. Binding and molecular basis of the bat coronavirus RaTG13 virus to ACE2 in humans and other species. Cell 2021;184(13):3438–51.e10.
[12] Allam Z. The First 50 days of COVID-19: A Detailed Chronological Timeline and Extensive Review of Literature Documenting the Pandemic. Surveying the Covid-19 Pandemic and its Implications. 2020:1–7. https://doi.org/10.1016/B978-0-12-824313-8.00001-2.
[13] Mercatelli D, Giorgi FM. Geographic and Genomic Distribution of SARS-CoV-2 Mutations. Front Microbiol 2020;11:1800.
[14] Rahman S, Montero MTV, Rowe K, et al. Epidemiology, pathogenesis, clinical presentations, diagnosis and treatment of COVID-19: a review of current evidence. Expert Rev Clin Pharmacol 2021;14(5):601–21.
[15] Bambra C, Riordan R, Ford J, et al. The COVID-19 pandemic and health inequalities. J Epidemiol Community Health 2020;74(11):964–8.
[16] Zhang JY, Shang T, Ahn D, et al. How to Best Protect People With Diabetes From the Impact of SARS-CoV-2: Report of the International COVID-19 and Diabetes Summit. J Diabetes Sci Technol 2021;15(2):478–514.
[17] The Lancet. The plight of essential workers during the COVID-19 pandemic. Lancet 2020;395(10237):1587.
[18] Nicola M, Alsafi Z, Sohrabi C, et al. The socio-economic implications of the coronavirus pandemic (COVID-19): A review. Int J Surg 2020;78:185–93.
[19] Devakumar D, Shannon G, Bhopal SS, et al. Racism and discrimination in COVID-19 responses. Lancet 2020;395(10231):1194.
[20] Dykgraaf SH, Matenge S, Desborough J, et al. Protecting Nursing Homes and Long-Term Care Facilities From COVID-19: A Rapid Review of International Evidence. J Am Med Dir Assoc 2021;22(10):1969–88.
[21] Di Mascio D, Buca D, Berghella V, et al. Counseling in maternal-fetal medicine: SARS-CoV-2 infection in pregnancy. Ultrasound Obstet Gynecol 2021;57(5):687–97.
[22] Pal M, Berhanu G, Desalegn C, et al. Severe Acute Respiratory Syndrome Coronavirus-2 (SARS-CoV-2): An Update. Cureus 2020;12(3):e7423.
[23] Das A, Ahmed R, Akhtar S, et al. An overview of basic molecular biology of SARS-CoV-2 and current COVID-19 prevention strategies. Gene Rep 2021;23:101122.
[24] Du L, He Y, Zhou Y, et al. The spike protein of SARS-CoV–a target for vaccine and therapeutic development. Nat Rev Microbiol 2009;7(3):226–36.
[25] Zhu C, He G, Yin Q, et al. Molecular biology of the SARs-CoV-2 spike protein: A review of current knowledge. J Med Virol 2021;93(10):5729–41.
[26] Li L, Petrovsky N. Molecular mechanisms for enhanced DNA vaccine immunogenicity. Expert Rev Vaccin 2016;15:313–29.

[27] Peacock TP, Goldhill DH, Zhou J, et al. The furin cleavage site in the SARS-CoV-2 spike protein is required for transmission in ferrets. Nat Microbiol 2021;6(7):899–909.
[28] Guruprasad L. Human SARS CoV-2 spike protein mutations. Proteins 2021;89(5):569–76.
[29] Yan R, Zhang Y, Li Y, et al. Structural basis for the recognition of SARS-CoV-2 by full-length human ACE2. Science 2020;360:1444–8.
[30] Oran DP, Topol EJ. Prevalence of Asymptomatic SARS-CoV-2 Infection : A Narrative Review. Ann Intern Med 2020;173(5):362–7.
[31] Oran DP, Topol EJ. The Proportion of SARS-CoV-2 Infections That Are Asymptomatic : A Systematic Review. Ann Intern Med 2021;174(5):655–62.
[32] Du L, Bouzidi MS, Gala A, et al. Human Galectin-9 Potently Enhances SARS-CoV-2 Replication and Inflammation in Airway Epithelial Cells. bioRxiv [Preprint] 2022; https://doi.org/10.1101/2022.03.18.484956 2022.03.18.484956.
[33] Available at: https://www.cdc.gov/coronavirus/2019-ncov/covid-data/investigations-discovery/hospitalization-death-by-age.html.
[34] Alimohamadi Y, Sepandi M, Taghdir M, et al. Determine the most common clinical symptoms in COVID-19 patients: a systematic review and meta-analysis. J Prev Med Hyg 2020;61(3):E304–12.
[35] Available at: https://www.deseret.com/coronavirus/2022/3/11/22972900/new-covid-variant-delta-omicron-symptoms-coronavirus.
[36] Giacomelli A, Pezzati L, Conti F, et al. Self-reported olfactory and taste disorders in SARS-CoV-2 patients: a cross-sectional study [published online ahead of print, 2020 Mar 26]. Clin Infect Dis 2020;71:889–90.
[37] Elias C, Sekri A, Leblanc P, et al. The incubation period of COVID-19: A meta-analysis. Int J Infect Dis 2021;104:708–10.
[38] Doremalen N, Bushmaker T, Morris D, et al. Aerosol and surface stability of HCoV-19 (SARS-CoV-2) compared to SARS-CoV-1. Engl J Med 2020;382:1564–7.
[39] Fan J, Liu X, Pan W, et al. Epidemiology of coronavirus disease in gansu province, China, 2020. Emerg Infect Dis 2020;26:1257–65.
[40] Xiang Ong SW, Tan YK, Chia PW, et al. Air, surface environmental, and personal protective equipment contamination by severe acute respiratory syndrome coronavirus 2 (SARS-CoV-2) from a symptomatic patient. JAMA 2020;323:1610–2.
[41] Zhou F, Yu T, Du R, et al. Clinical course and risk factors for mortality of adult inpatients with COVID-19 in Wuhan, China: a retrospective cohort study. Lancet 2020;395:1054–62.
[42] Bai Y, Yao L, Wei T, et al. Presumed asymptomatic carrier transmission of COVID-19. J Am Med Assoc 2020;323:1406–7.
[43] Arons MM, Hatfield KM, Reddy SC, et al. Presymptomatic SARS-CoV-2 infections and transmission in a skilled nursing facility. N Engl J Med 2020;382:2081–90.
[44] Pan Y, Zhang D, Yang P, et al. Viral load of SARS-CoV-2 in clinical samples. Lancet Infect Dis 2020;20:411–2.
[45] Murad D, Chandrasekaran S, Pillai A, et al. SARS-CoV-2 Infection Detection by PCR and Serologic Testing in Clinical Practice. J Clin Microbiol 2021;59(7):e0043121.
[46] Safiabadi Tali SH, LeBlanc JJ, Sadiq Z, et al. Tools and Techniques for Severe Acute Respiratory Syndrome Coronavirus 2 (SARS-CoV-2)/COVID-19 Detection. Clin Microbiol Rev 2021;34(3):e00228-20.
[47] Available at: https://www.washingtonpost.com/investigations/2020/04/18/timeline-coronavirus-testing/.
[48] Adeel M, Farooq T, Shakoor N, et al. COVID-19 and Nanoscience in the Developing World: Rapid Detection and Remediation in Wastewater. Nanomaterials (Basel) 2021;11(4):991.
[49] Kabir MA, Ahmed R, Iqbal SMA, et al. Diagnosis for COVID-19: current status and future prospects. Expert Rev Mol Diagn 2021;21(3):269–88.
[50] Jalaber C, Lapotre T, Morcet-Delattre T, et al. Chest CT in COVID-19 pneumonia: A review of current knowledge. Diagn Interv Imaging 2020;101(7–8):431–7.

[51] Lancet Commission on COVID-19 Vaccines and Therapeutics Task Force Members. Operation Warp Speed: implications for global vaccine security. Lancet Glob Health 2021;9(7): e1017–21.
[52] McDougle L. Ensuring Safety of Operation Warp Speed Vaccines for COVID-19. J Natl Med Assoc 2020;112(5):446–7.
[53] Hernandez AV, Roman YM, Pasupuleti V, et al. Hydroxychloroquine or Chloroquine for Treatment or Prophylaxis of COVID-19: A Living Systematic Review. Ann Intern Med 2020;173(4):287–96.
[54] Singh B, Ryan H, Kredo T, et al. Chloroquine or hydroxychloroquine for prevention and treatment of COVID-19. Cochrane Database Syst Rev 2021;(2):CD013587. Accessed June 14, 2022.
[55] Gupta A, Malviya A. Chloroquine and hydroxychloroquine for COVID-19: time to close the chapter. Postgrad Med J 2021;97:676–7.
[56] Available at: https://www.fda.gov/drugs/drug-safety-and-availability/fda-cautions-against-use-hydroxychloroquine-or-chloroquine-covid-19-outside-hospital-setting-or.
[57] Brown BL, McCullough J. Treatment for emerging viruses: Convalescent plasma and COVID-19. Transfus Apher Sci 2020;59(3):102790.
[58] Joyner MJ, Bruno KA, Klassen SA, et al. Safety Update: COVID-19 Convalescent Plasma in 20,000 Hospitalized Patients. Mayo Clin Proc 2020;95(9):1888–97.
[59] RECOVERY Collaborative Group. Convalescent plasma in patients admitted to hospital with COVID-19 (RECOVERY): a randomised controlled, open-label, platform trial. Lancet 2021;397(10289):2049–59.
[60] Sullivan DJ, Gebo KA, Shoham S, et al. Randomized Controlled Trial of Early Outpatient COVID-19 Treatment with High-Titer Convalescent Plasma. medRxiv 2021;2021:12.10.21267485.
[61] Nelson PN, Reynolds GM, Waldron EE, et al. Monoclonal antibodies. Mol Pathol 2000;53(3):111–7.
[62] Hussain A, Hasan A, Nejadi Babadaei MM, et al. Targeting SARS-CoV2 Spike Protein Receptor Binding Domain by Therapeutic Antibodies. Biomed Pharmacother 2020;130: 110559.
[63] Nathan R, Shawa I, De La Torre I, et al. A Narrative Review of the Clinical Practicalities of Bamlanivimab and Etesevimab Antibody Therapies for SARS-CoV-2. Infect Dis Ther 2021;10(4):1933–47.
[64] Gottlieb RL, Nirula A, Chen P, et al. Effect of Bamlanivimab as Monotherapy or in Combination With Etesevimab on Viral Load in Patients With Mild to Moderate COVID-19: A Randomized Clinical Trial. JAMA 2021;325(7):632–44.
[65] Hemmer CJ, Löbermann M, Reisinger EC. COVID-19: Epidemiologie und Mutationen : Ein Update [COVID-19: epidemiology and mutations : An update]. Radiologe 2021;61(10): 880–7, German.
[66] Kreuzberger N, Hirsch C, Chai KL, et al. SARS-CoV-2-neutralising monoclonal antibodies for treatment of COVID-19. Cochrane Database Syst Rev 2021;9(9):CD013825.
[67] Weinreich DM, Sivapalasingam S, Norton T, et al. Trial Investigators. REGEN-COV Antibody Combination and Outcomes in Outpatients with Covid-19. N Engl J Med 2021;385(23):e81.
[68] O'Brien MP, Forleo-Neto E, Musser BJ, et al. Covid-19 Phase 3 Prevention Trial Team. Subcutaneous REGEN-COV Antibody Combination to Prevent Covid-19. N Engl J Med 2021;385(13):1184–95.
[69] Gupta A, Gonzalez-Rojas Y, Juarez E, et al. COMET-ICE Investigators. Effect of Sotrovimab on Hospitalization or Death Among High-risk Patients With Mild to Moderate COVID-19: A Randomized Clinical Trial. JAMA 2022;327(13):1236–46.
[70] Levin MJ, Ustianowski A, De Wit S, et al, PROVENT Study Group. Intramuscular AZD7442 (Tixagevimab-Cilgavimab) for Prevention of Covid-19. N Engl J Med 2022;386(23): 2188–200.

[71] Maláska J, Stašek J, Duška F, et al, REMED Study Group. Effect of dexamethasone in patients with ARDS and COVID-19 - prospective, multi-centre, open-label, parallel-group, randomised controlled trial (REMED trial): A structured summary of a study protocol for a randomised controlled trial. Trials 2021;22(1):172.
[72] RECOVERY Collaborative Group, Horby P, Lim WS, Emberson JR, et al. Dexamethasone in Hospitalized Patients with Covid-19. N Engl J Med 2021;384(8):693–704.
[73] Beigel JH, Tomashek KM, Dodd LE, et al, ACTT-1 Study Group Members. Remdesivir for the Treatment of Covid-19 - Final Report. N Engl J Med 2020;383(19):1813–26.
[74] Ohl ME, Miller DR, Lund BC, et al. Association of Remdesivir Treatment With Survival and Length of Hospital Stay Among US Veterans Hospitalized With COVID-19. JAMA Netw Open 2021;4(7):e2114741.
[75] Drożdżal S, Rosik J, Lechowicz K, et al. An update on drugs with therapeutic potential for SARS-CoV-2 (COVID-19) treatment. Drug Resist Updat 2021;59:100794.
[76] Singh AK, Singh A, Singh R, et al. An updated practical guideline on use of molnupiravir and comparison with agents having emergency use authorization for treatment of COVID-19. Diabetes Metab Syndr 2022;16(2):102396.
[77] Polack FP, Thomas SJ, Kitchin N, et al. C4591001 Clinical Trial Group. Safety and Efficacy of the BNT162b2 mRNA Covid-19 Vaccine. N Engl J Med 2020;383(27):2603–15.
[78] Bar-On YM, Goldberg Y, Mandel M, et al. Protection of BNT162b2 Vaccine Booster against Covid-19 in Israel. N Engl J Med 2021;385(15):1393–400.
[79] Singh B, Kaur P, Cedeno L, et al. COVID-19 mRNA Vaccine and Myocarditis. Eur J Case Rep Intern Med 2021;8(7):002681.
[80] Woodworth KR, Moulia D, Collins JP, et al. The Advisory Committee on Immunization Practices' Interim Recommendation for Use of Pfizer-BioNTech COVID-19 Vaccine in Children Aged 5-11 Years - United States, November 2021. MMWR Morb Mortal Wkly Rep 2021;70(45):1579–83.
[81] Baden LR, El Sahly HM, Essink B, et al, COVE Study Group. Efficacy and Safety of the mRNA-1273 SARS-CoV-2 Vaccine. N Engl J Med 2021;384(5):403–16.
[82] Sadoff J, Le Gars M, Shukarev G, et al. Interim Results of a Phase 1-2a Trial of Ad26.-COV2.S Covid-19 Vaccine. N Engl J Med 2021;384(19):1824–35.

Advances in Anesthesia 40 (2022) 63–69

ADVANCES IN ANESTHESIA

Building Anesthesia Capacity in the Developing World

Kaylyn Sachse, MD

Department of Anesthesiology, Vanderbilt University Medical Center, 1301 Medical Center Drive, 4648 The Vanderbilt Clinic, Nashville, TN 37232-5614, USA

Keywords

• Global anesthesia • Global health equity • Anesthesia capacity building

Key points

- Access to safe anesthesia is often limited in low- and middle-income countries (LMICs), where basic operating room necessities such as pulse oximeters and oxygen may not be available.
- Short-term medical missions are traditionally well funded by high-income countries (HICs), but they may have unintended negative consequences on the communities they seek to help.
- Education initiatives that form partnerships between HICs and LMICs have had success improving anesthesia safety and access to care.
- Ideal aid initiatives in the developing world should focus on education and building sustainable local capacity.

BACKGROUND

The Lancet Commission on Global Surgery defines surgery as both an integral and indispensable part of health care [1]. However, it is estimated that more than 70% of the world's population (approximately 5 billion people) do not have access to safe and affordable surgical and anesthetic care, with most of those affected living in low- and middle-income countries (LMICs) [2]. Although the poorest countries make up one-third of the world's population, only 6% of the 313 million procedures performed every year are undertaken in these countries. In places like the United States, there are almost 21 physician anesthesiologists per 100,000 people, whereas most of sub-Saharan Africa has fewer than 1 physician anesthesiologist provider per 100,000 people [3]. The problem of limited access to anesthesia and surgical providers is further

No financial or commercial disclosures.

E-mail address: kaylyn.sachse@vumc.org

https://doi.org/10.1016/j.aan.2022.07.009
0737-6146/22/

compounded by insufficient infrastructure and supplies. In a 2016 review of anesthesia care capacity in 22 LMICs, only half of the hospitals surveyed reported reliable electricity, and 61% had reliable oxygen supplies. In total, only 56% of hospitals that reported anesthesia capacity were able to perform general anesthesia [4]. Although it is often difficult to precisely measure anesthesia-related mortality in LMICs, it is estimated that it may be more than 100 times higher than in high-income countries (HICs) [5,6]. The impact of these statistics is staggering and seems almost impossible to overcome. So, what can we, as anesthesiologists, do in HICs to help bridge the chasm of inequity in global health?

SHORT-TERM MEDICAL MISSIONS

Traditionally, most of the funding and resources from HICs for global health have been focused on short-term medical missions (STMMs). Before the COVID pandemic, the estimated cost of sending US providers on STMM trips was approximately $3.7 billion annually [7]. Despite the large amount of funding dedicated to these projects, there are few data to support their quality or the overall impact on the communities they seek to help [8]. In fact, there is growing concern that there may be unintended negative consequences, especially when STMMs are performed without engaging with local health care providers [9,10]. Who will provide follow-up or multidisciplinary care for patients once the teams return home to HICs? Who will treat potential complications? How does the presence of these teams affect the local health care infrastructure? What happens when a global pandemic puts a complete stop to STMMs? These are just a few of the reasons we must reevaluate this antiquated model for global health and explore more sustainable ways to provide aid.

Historical models for global health have often failed to make their intended impact because they have been developed in HICs without the guidance of those living and working in LMICs [11]. To be successful and sustainable, these efforts must be a true partnership that starts with those who have dedicated their lives to providing care for their neighbors in LMICs. Needs assessments must be led by LMIC providers who have a deep, context-sensitive understanding of the problems faced in their region. What is needed or has been successful in urban America will not necessarily translate to the needs in rural sub-Saharan Africa. With all projects, steps must be taken to ensure the interventions are building the capacity of the local health care systems and not inadvertently weakening them. Instead of focusing on how many cases can be completed during an STMM, the goal should be to help improve the sustainability of safe surgery in LMICs.

EDUCATION INITIATIVES

One the most important means of building local capacity is increasing the specialty trained workforce through education. With such limited numbers of anesthesiologists in LMICs, practitioners bear heavy clinical burdens and are often not able to devote much time to the education of trainees. This is where LMIC-HIC partnerships can flourish, and they have taken a variety of shapes over the years. These partnerships have formed between the governments of LMICs and HICs, between academic institutions in HICs and LMICs, and even between societal organizations and nonprofit organizations and LMIC providers.

In a 2008 collaboration of more than 100 international experts, including surgeons, anesthesiologists, nurses, engineers, and public health personnel, the World Health Organization (WHO) released consensus guidelines for safe surgery [12]. From these recommendations, the Safe Surgery Saves Lives Program was formed, which implemented a quick and widely applicable surgical safety checklist with the goal of reducing major surgical complications worldwide. Implementation of this preoperative, intraoperative, and postoperative safety checklist instills a culture of thorough communication and teamwork and requires minimal funding or infrastructure. The initial 8 hospitals that participated in the Safe Surgery Saves Lives Program were from a diverse range of geographic and socioeconomic backgrounds, 4 in LMICs and 4 in HICs. Investigators engaged with local teams to introduce the checklist to all operating room teams using in-person lectures, teleconferences, instructional videos, and hands-on guidance. After implementation of the checklist, statistically significant decreases were seen in overall complications, in-hospital deaths, surgical site infections, and unplanned reoperations [13]. All sites showed varying rates of decrease in overall postoperative complications and mortality, with an average of a 36% decrease in complications and a 46% decrease in mortality. The decrease in major complications remained significant even after adjusting for location (HIC vs LMIC) and case mix. The benefits of the surgical safety checklist also can be applied to the pediatric population in LMICs. In prospectively collected data on 7-day perioperative mortality in Kenya, lower pediatric mortality was associated with compliance with the surgical safety checklist. More than 10 years after the initial release of the WHO surgical safety checklist, it has seen wide adoption in HICs and growing use in LMICs. In the African Surgical Outcomes Study (ASOS), which included 25 countries in Africa, the surgical checklist was used in a little more than half of cases [14]. Continued education as well as thoughtful implementation of the surgical safety checklist in LMICs has the potential for substantial improvements in complication and mortality rates [15].

The only monitoring equipment mentioned in the WHO surgical safety checklist is a pulse oximeter. Although the presence of a pulse oximeter is often taken for granted in HIC operating rooms, 1 study found that only 51% of hospitals in the surveyed LMICs had a functioning pulse oximeter [4]. In 2011, the global nonprofit Lifebox was formed, with the goal of making reliable and affordable pulse oximeters widely available. Their teams developed and manufactured a durable pulse oximeter specifically targeted for use in LMICs. Since the nonprofit began, they have successfully distributed more than 28,000 Lifebox pulse oximeters to low resource settings [16]. In addition to delivering critical equipment, Lifebox also comes with training on how to use the pulse oximeter and encourages use of the surgical safety checklist. The Lifebox organization has also expanded to include an initiative aimed at surgical site infections called Clean Cut. According to ASOS data, the most common postoperative complication was infection, occurring in approximately 10% of all patients undergoing surgery in Africa [14]. The Clean Cut program was piloted at a tertiary hospital in Ethiopia where the teams used process mapping to identify barriers to compliance and develop context-specific solutions [17]. The program, which includes team building and a surgical safety checklist, was implemented with local providers over a period of 6 months using very few resources. After implementation, compliance with infection prevention standards had significantly improved, and the risk of postoperative complications decreased by 35% [18]. Alongside the Ethiopian Federal Ministry of Health, the Clean Cut program has expanded to 11 hospitals in Ethiopia, with plans for further expansion in Africa, Central America, and Asia [19].

OBSTETRIC ANESTHESIA

According to WHO estimates, 295,000 women died of causes related to childbirth in 2017 and the vast majority of those deaths occurred in LMICs. Women in low-income countries are at 130 times higher risk of pregnancy-related deaths compared with women in HICs [20]. Unfortunately, a large percentage of these deaths are believed to be preventable. Although the leading causes of global maternal mortality are related to hemorrhage, hypertensive disorders, and infection, one recent meta-analysis estimated that anesthesia was responsible for 3.5% of all direct maternal deaths and 13.8% of deaths following cesarean delivery [21]. Investigators found that maternal mortality was 3 times higher when general anesthesia was performed for cesarean delivery instead of neuraxial anesthesia. More than half (54%) of the anesthesia deaths in which a cause was reported were attributed to airway complications. Additional risk factors for anesthesia-related mortality included anesthesia being administered by nonphysician providers with no formal training. Education initiatives have the potential to reduce maternal mortality risk. The World Federation of Societies of Anaesthesiolgists and the Association of Anaesthetists together developed Safer Anesthesia from Education-Obstetrics (SAFE-OB), a 3-day continuing education course for both physician and nonphysician providers focusing on the most common clinical scenarios that result in maternal deaths in LMICs. Initial studies in Ethiopia, Madagascar, and the Republic of Congo have shown lasting changes in practice and improvements in knowledge and skills even a year after the SAFE-OB course [22,23]. Nonprofit organizations such as Kybele have sponsored long-term educational partnerships in the Republic of Armenia that have resulted in significant increases in the use of neuraxial anesthesia for cesarean delivery and the development of national practice guidelines [24].

REGIONAL ANESTHESIA

Studies looking at perioperative mortality in LMICs have found lower mortality rates associated with neuraxial and regional anesthesia compared with general anesthesia. When Médecins Sans Frontières (MSF or Doctors Without Borders) looked at more than 75,000 anesthetics performed by trained staff in LMICs between 2008 and 2014, there was a 1.69% mortality rate with general anesthesia with intubation, compared with 0.04% and 0.06% with neuraxial and regional anesthesia, respectively [25]. Regional anesthesia techniques have several advantages in LMIC environments, including avoiding general anesthesia and the need for airway manipulation and anesthesia machines, as well as providing improved analgesia and muscle relaxation in settings where medications are limited. Despite these potential benefits and decreased mortality rates, regional anesthesia is underused in LMICs because of a lack of trained providers and equipment [26]. In a survey of anesthesia providers in Nigeria, 92.9% of the 147 providers queried reported regularly using spinal anesthesia, compared with 2.9% using peripheral nerve blocks regularly [27]. Several recent partnerships have been established to help address this need for increased regional anesthesia education. In 2016, Rwandan and Canadian anesthesiologists together established a locally run and sustainable regional anesthesia service at the University Teaching Hospital of Kigali [26]. Anesthesiologists at the Hospital for Special Surgery in New York developed and implemented a 3-week, in-person regional anesthesia training program (GRACE: Global Regional Anesthesia Curricular Engagement) for physician anesthesiologists at Komfo Anokye Teaching Hospital (KATH) in Kumasi, Ghana. The physicians at KATH reported high satisfaction with GRACE, and there was statistically significant improvement in knowledge-based testing. In the 3 months after completion of GRACE, the number of peripheral nerve blocks performed at KATH increased to 118 from 48 in the 3 months before the training [28]. Similar success has been seen after implementation of a 4-week regional anesthesia curriculum in Ethiopia [29]. After the start of the COVID pandemic, travel to perform these in-person, hands-on workshops became difficult to impossible. Researchers at Toronto Western Hospital expanded and developed a telesimulation course that linked instructor and trainee stimulators remotely over the Internet. With minimal equipment in each location (ultrasound, computer, web cams, video converters, nerve block phantom model, and Skype), a remote, hands-on femoral nerve block workshop was successfully taught to orthopedic and emergency medicine residents at Black Lion Hospital in Ethiopia [30].

SUMMARY

There are large disparities in the anesthesia care available to those in LMICs compared with those in HICs. In addition to a lack of trained anesthesia providers, LMICs often lack common operating room necessities such as oxygen, airway supplies, and pulse oximeters. Efforts from HICs to extend aid to LMICs should focus on building local capacity through education. Many successful partnerships have formed between academic institutions, professional societies, and nonprofits in HICs and local providers in LMICs. Those looking to get involved can contact some of these existing organizations or look to their example when creating new partnerships. Importantly, these partnerships must strive to be sustainable and not hinder the development of local systems.

CLINICS CARE POINTS

- Large disparities exist between the anesthesia and surgical care available in HICs and LMICs.- While HICs have historically spent most of their aid funding for LMICs on short-term medical missions, these trips may have unintended negative consequences and are likely not the most efficient use of resources.- Education partnerships between HICs and LMICs should strive for sustainability and build local capacity in LMICs.

References

[1] Meara JG, Hagander L, Leather AJM. Surgery and global health: a Lancet Commission. Lancet 2014;383(9911):12–3.
[2] Meara JG, Leather AJM, Hagander L, et al. Global Surgery 2030: evidence and solutions for achieving health, welfare, and economic development. Lancet 2015;386(9993): 569–624.
[3] Workforce Map - WFSA. Available at: https://wfsahq.org/resources/workforce-map/. Accessed April 19, 2022.
[4] Hadler RA, Chawla S, Stewart BT, et al. Anesthesia care capacity at health facilities in 22 low- and middle-income countries. World J Surg 2016;40(5):1025–33.
[5] Newton MW, Hurt SE, McEvoy MD, et al. Pediatric perioperative mortality in Kenya a prospective cohort study from 24 hospitals. Anesthesiology 2020;452–60; https://doi.org/10.1097/ALN.0000000000003070.
[6] Uribe-Leitz T, Jaramillo J, Maurer L, et al. Variability in mortality following caesarean delivery, appendectomy, and groin hernia repair in low-income and middle-income countries: a systematic review and analysis of published data. The Lancet 2016;4:e165–74. Available at: www.thelancet.com/lancetgh.
[7] Caldron PH, Impens A, Pavlova M, et al. Economic assessment of US physician participation in short-term medical missions. Globalization and Health 2016;12(1); https://doi.org/10.1186/s12992-016-0183-7.
[8] Martiniuk AL, Manouchehrian M, Negin JA, et al. Brain gains: a literature review of medical missions to low and middle-income countries. BMC Health Serv Res 2012;12. Available at: http://www.biomedcentral.com/1472-6963/12/134.
[9] Hendriks TCC, Botman M, Rahmee CNS, et al. Impact of short-term reconstructive surgical missions: a systematic review. BMJ Glob Health 2019;4(2); https://doi.org/10.1136/bmjgh-2018-001176.
[10] Caldron PH, Impens A, Pavlova M, et al. A systematic review of social, economic and diplomatic aspects of short-term medical missions. BMC Health Serv Res 2015;15(1); https://doi.org/10.1186/s12913-015-0980-3.
[11] Nthumba PM, Newton MW, Gathuya Z. Global surgery in the 21st century: the voice from Africa - We need a new model. Paediatr Anaesth 2021;31(5):510–2.
[12] World Health Organization. WHO guidelines for safe surgery 2009. Safe surgery saves lives. Geneva, Switzerland: World Health Organization; 2009. Available at. https://www.who.int/publications/i/item/9789241598552. Accessed April 20,2022.
[13] Haynes AB, Weiser TG, Berry WR, et al. A surgical safety checklist to reduce morbidity and mortality in a global population. New Engl J Med 2009;360(5):491–9.

[14] Biccard BM, Madiba TE, Kluyts HL, et al. Perioperative patient outcomes in the African Surgical Outcomes Study: a 7-day prospective observational cohort study. Lancet 2018;391(10130):1589–98.
[15] Weiser TG, Haynes AB. Ten years of the surgical safety checklist. Br J Surg 2018;105(8): 927–9.
[16] Pulse oximetry - Lifebox. Available at: https://www.lifebox.org/what-we-do/pulse-oximetry/. Accessed April 19, 2022.
[17] Forrester JA, Koritsanszky LA, Amenu D, et al. Developing process maps as a tool for a surgical infection prevention quality improvement initiative in resource-constrained settings. J Am Coll Surg 2018;226(6):1103–16.e3.
[18] Forrester JA, Starr N, Negussie T, et al. Clean Cut (adaptive, multimodal surgical infection prevention programme) for low-resource settings: a prospective quality improvement study. 10.1002/bjs.11997
[19] Clean Cut – Lifebox. Available at: https://www.lifebox.org/clean-cut/. Accessed April 19, 2022.
[20] The Global Health Observatory - Maternal and reproductive health. Available at: https://www.who.int/data/gho/data/themes/maternal-and-reproductive-health. Accessed April 19, 2022.
[21] Sobhy S, Zamora J, Khan KS, et al. Multidisciplinary Evidence Synthesis Hub (MEsh) (prof anaesthesia-related maternal mortality in low-income and middle-income countries: a systematic review and meta-analysis), 4, 2016. Available at: www.thelancet.com/lancetgh.
[22] Moore JN, Morriss WW, Asfaw G, et al. The impact of the Safer Anaesthesia from Education (SAFE) obstetric anaesthesia training course in Ethiopia: a mixed methods longitudinal cohort study. Anaesth Intensive Care 2020;48(4):297–305.
[23] White MC, Rakotoarisoa T, Cox NH, et al. A mixed-method design evaluation of the SAFE obstetric anaesthesia course at 4 and 12-18 months after training in the Republic of Congo and Madagascar. Anesth Analgesia 2019;129(6):1707–14.
[24] Yuill G, Amroyan A, Millar S, et al. Establishing obstetric anesthesiology practice guidelines in the Republic of Armenia: a global health collaboration. Anesthesiology 2017;127(2): 220–6.
[25] Ariyo P, Trelles M, Helmand R, et al. Providing anesthesia care in resource-limited settings: a 6-year analysis of anesthesia services provided at Médecins Sans Frontières facilities. Anesthesiology 2016;124(3):561–9.
[26] Ho M, Livingston P, Bould MD, et al. Barriers and facilitators to implementing a regional anesthesia service in a low-income country: a qualitative study. Pan Afr Med J 2019;32; https://doi.org/10.11604/pamj.2019.32.152.17246.
[27] Rukewe A, Fatiregun A. The use of regional anesthesia by anesthesiologists in Nigeria. Anesth Analg 2010;110(1):243–4.
[28] Brouillette MA, Aidoo AJ, Hondras MA, et al. Regional anesthesia training model for resource-limited settings: a prospective single-center observational study with pre-post evaluations. Reg Anesth Pain Med 2020;45(7):528–35.
[29] Moll V, Schmidt PC, Amos C, et al. Building regional anesthesia capacity in limited-resource settings: a pilot study evaluating a 4-week curriculum. Pain Manag 2021;11(1):29–37.
[30] Liu M, Salmon M, Zaidi R, et al. Ultrasound-guided regional anesthesia: feasibility and effectiveness of teaching via telesimulation in Ethiopia. Reg Anesth Pain Med 2021;46(8): 722–6.

Advances in Anesthesia 40 (2022) 71–92

ADVANCES IN ANESTHESIA

Updates in the Management of Perioperative Vasoplegic Syndrome

Kaitlyn A. Brennan, DO, MPH[a], Monica Bhutiani, MD, MEd[b], Meredith A. Kingeter, MD[c], Matthew D. McEvoy, MD[d,*]

[a]Department of Anesthesiology, Vanderbilt University Medical Center, 1211 21st Avenue South, MAB 422, Nashville, TN 37212, USA; [b]Department of Anesthesiology, Vanderbilt University Medical Center, 1211 21st Avenue South, VUH 4107, Nashville, TN 37212, USA; [c]Anesthesia Residency, Vanderbilt University Medical Center, 1215 21st Avenue South, Suite 5160 MCE NT, Nashville, TN 37212, USA; [d]VUMC Enhanced Recovery Programs, Department of Anesthesiology, Vanderbilt University Medical Center, 1301 Medical Center Drive, TVC 4648, Nashville, TN 37232, USA

Keywords

• Vasoplegia syndrome • Hypotension • Shock • ACE inhibitor • Vasopressin • Methylene blue • Hydroxycobalamin

Key points

- Vasoplegia is a common cause of refractory hypotension in the perioperative period, especially in cardiac surgery, liver transplant, and sepsisVasoplegia is driven by both central, cellular, and intracellular pathways, and treatment should be geared toward the purported causeTreatment ranges from routine vasopressor support to more specific targeted agents, such as methylene blue and angiotensin II

BACKGROUND

Vasoplegic syndrome (VS) is a constellation of signs characterized by hypotension (typically mean arterial pressure [MAP] <50 mm Hg without vasopressor support), low systemic vascular resistance (SVR), normal-to-high-cardiac output, and a reduced response to vasoactive medications [1]. Although most closely associated with cardiac surgery and cardiopulmonary bypass (CPB)

*Corresponding author. Vanderbilt University Medical Center, Department of Anesthesiology, 1211 21st Avenue South, Nashville, TN 37212. *E-mail address:* matthew.d.mcevoy@vumc.org

https://doi.org/10.1016/j.aan.2022.07.010

[2], VS is frequently seen in patients during liver transplantation, notably following reperfusion of the donor graft [1,3]. Additionally, there have been reports of perioperative VS in the setting of sepsis, recent use of angiotensin blocking medications, anaphylaxis, and a variety of other clinical settings that will be discussed below. There have been several reported treatments of VS, including high-dose vasopressors, inotropes, corticosteroids, methylene blue (MB), angiotensin II, and high-dose vitamin B12 or C, all with varying results [1,4,5].

Although understanding the complex central, cellular, and intracellular pathways that maintain vascular tone can shed light on factors that drive dysregulation leading to VS, an in-depth review of all of these mechanisms lies outside the scope of this review. Instead, we will focus on 3 etiologic categories in order to provide a mental construct for evaluating the likely cause of VS in a given patient and the implications for treatment. To that end, we have grouped causes of VS into 3 broad categories: pharmacologic, ischemia/reperfusion (I/R), and immunomodulation.

CAUSES

Normally, SVR is determined largely by levels of intracellular calcium (Ca^{2+}). Increased cytosolic Ca^{2+} leads to vascular smooth muscle contraction and increased SVR, whereas decreased cytosolic levels result in vascular smooth muscle relaxation and a decrease in SVR. Vascular tone, therefore, depends on the balance between the influx and removal of Ca^{2+} from the cytosolic space, which is regulated by central (sympathetic nervous system, vasoactive hormones), cellular (G-protein coupled receptors [GPCRs]), and intracellular mechanisms (secondary messenger pathways) (eg, nitric oxide [NO], prostacyclin, endothelin). There have been several recent in-depth reviews of these physiologic pathways that we commend to the reader [6,7]. Here, we will summarize the pathways pertinent to our discussion of causes and treatment modalities of VS. See Fig. 1 for a visual representation of these pathways.

Neuromodulation and immunomodulation play key roles in maintaining central vascular tone during stress and shock states. Cytokines such as tumor necrosis factor alpha (TNF-α), interleukin-1, and interleukin-6 stimulate the sympathetic nervous system, adrenal medulla, and hypothalamic pituitary axis to increase the levels of norepinephrine, epinephrine, cortisol, vasopressin, and angiotensin II in the systemic circulation. However, sustained activation of these pathways can lead to dysautonomia, adrenoreceptor downregulation or desensitization, and a proinflammatory state, ultimately resulting in hyporesponsiveness of vasopressor agents and possible VS [8,9].

GPCRs are the ultimate targets of centrally produced vasopressors and predominately regulate vascular tone at a cellular level [10]. Agonist activation of these proteins initially increases cytosolic calcium. However, sustained activation of these receptors result in GPCR phosphorylation by GPCR kinases leading to desensitization and ultimately downregulation. Clinically, this resembles vasopressor hyporesponsiveness [11].

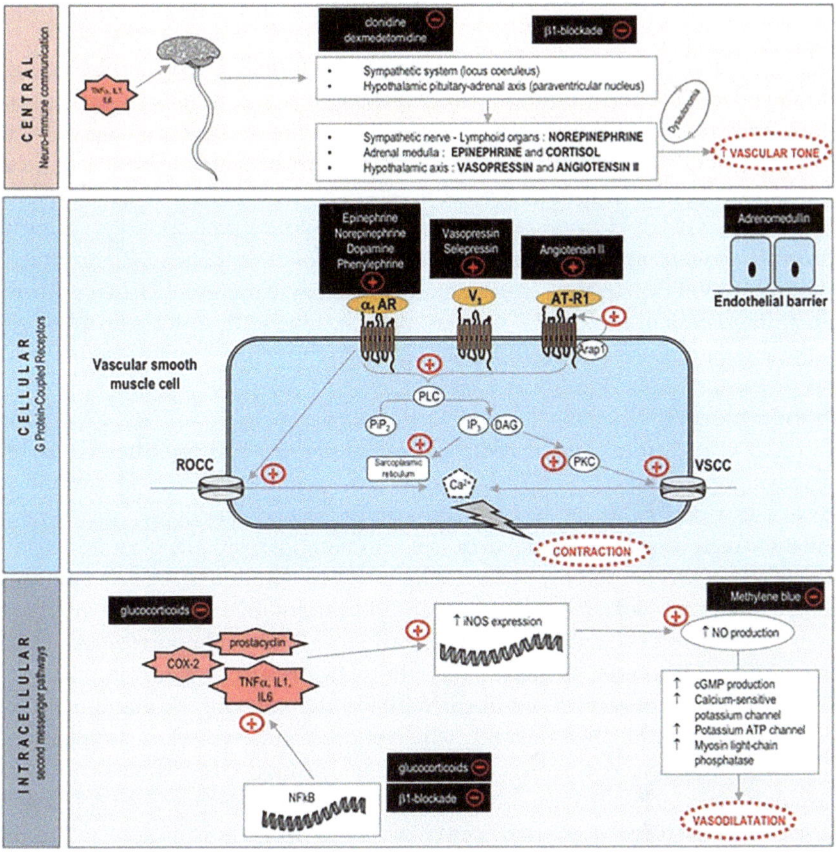

Fig. 1. The principal mechanisms involved in the regulation of vascular tone during vasoplegia as well as treatment options at the central, cellular, and intracellular levels. Central level: Inflammatory triggers such as TNFα (interleukin (IL)-1 and IL-6 activate the neuro-immune system. This activation leads to norepinephrine, epinephrine, cortisol, vasopressin, and indirectly angiotensin II production in order to counteract vasoplegia. Overactivation of this system may be treated at this integrative level with α2 agonists and selective β1 blockers. Cellular level: G-protein-coupled receptors are predominantly involved in vascular smooth muscle cell contraction: α1 adrenoceptors (α 1 AR), vasopressin 1 receptors (V1R), and angiotensin type 1 receptors (AT-R1). These receptors activate phospholipase C (PLC) with generation of inositol 1,4,5 trisphosphate (IP3) and diacylglycerol (DAG) from phosphatidyl inositol 4,5 bisphosphate (PiP 2). DAG stimulates protein kinase C (PKC), which in turn activates voltage-sensitive calcium channels, whereas IP3 activates sarcoplasmic reticulum calcium channels. α1ARs increase intracellular calcium by receptor-operated calcium channels (ROCC) stimulation. Available treatments at this level are epinephrine, norepinephrine, dopamine, phenylephrine, selepressin, vasopressin (V1), and angiotensin II. Adrenomedullin primarily acts on endothelial cells. Intracellular level: Translocation of nuclear factor-κB (NF-κB) into the nucleus induces proinflammatory cytokine production. These cytokines enhance iNOS expression and overproduction of NO. This molecule activates cyclic guanosine monophosphate production as a mediator of vasodilation. Available treatments at this level are glucocorticoids (at different steps), β1 blockade, and methylene blue. Vascular sensitive calcium channel (VSCC). (*From* Levy B, Fritz C, Tahon E, Jacquot A, Auchet T, Kimmoun A. Vasoplegia treatments: the past, the present, and the future. Crit Care. 2018 Feb 27;22(1):52.)

Intracellular mechanisms of vascular tone are largely controlled by endothelial secretions, the most important of which is NO. Calcium-independent nitric oxide synthase (NOS) generates NO, which induces cyclic guanosine monophosphate (cGMP)-mediated vasodilation [12]. Inflammatory mediators similar to bradykinin and thrombin increase levels of endothelial NOS, causing a mild increase in cGMP. However, inflammatory cytokines and lipopolysaccharides can also activate an inducible NOS (iNOS), which increases NO production roughly 1000-fold, leading to major vascular dysfunction [13,14]. Although other intracellular molecules such as prostacyclin and endothelin play roles in the regulation of vascular tone, no current treatments target those pathways.

Pharmacologic

Refractory and unexplained hypotension under general anesthesia has been increasingly attributed to VS. Although most commonly seen in cardiac surgery, it can occur during any general anesthetic and has higher incidences in patients treated with antagonists of the renin-angiotensin-aldosterone pathway (RAAS), such as angiotensin converting enzyme inhibitors (ACE-I) and angiotensin receptor blockers (ARBs) [1,6,15]. Normally, blood pressure homeostasis is maintained by 3 interactive systems: the RAAS, the adrenergic system (sympathetic nervous system), and the vasopressin system [6,7,16]. The RAAS pathway generates angiotensin II via the cleaving of angiotensinogen by renin to generate angiotensin I, which subsequently converts to angiotensin II via the angiotensin converting enzyme [17]. Angiotensin II acts to increase vascular resistance and sympathetic activity while also promoting both aldosterone secretion from the adrenal cortex and antidiuretic hormone secretion from the posterior pituitary. The resultant effect is intravascular volume expansion and arteriolar vasoconstriction [18]. Blockade of this pathway via ACE-Is or ARBs therefore results in decreased SVR, often resulting in increased cardiac output and increased vascular capacitance.

Most anesthetic drugs decrease sympathetic output resulting in an increased reliance on the RAAS and vasopressin systems for blood pressure control under general anesthesia [19].

Furthermore, if patients are treated with RAAS antagonists (ACE-I or ARB) blood pressure regulation predominantly relies on the vasopressin system placing them at an increased risk for developing refractory hypotension under general anesthesia [6,19]. In the cardiac surgery population, the incidence of VS increases from 8% to 10% to 46% for patients on RAAS antagonists, and RAAS antagonists are an independent risk factor for postoperative VS when used concomitantly with heparin and calcium channel blockers [4,20]. Although cases of VS are well documented following reperfusion of the donor liver during transplantation, no studies to date explore the relationship of this phenomenon with ACE-Is and ARBs.

Currently, the decision to hold RAAS inhibitors perioperatively to prevent VS is controversial. These drugs vary greatly in their duration of action and possess some pharmacologic differences. Therefore, although some studies suggest cessation of RAAS blockers the day before surgery may attenuate VS, that course of action may not effectively attenuate the effect of drugs with a longer duration of action [21,22]. Finally, there is currently a paucity of prospective research examining the possible harm associated with discontinuation of these drugs in the perioperative period.

Ischemia-Reperfusion

VS can result after absolute or relative ischemia and subsequent reperfusion because the ischemic injury disrupts the normal physiologic response to hypotension through vasoactive hormonal regulators. We will discuss reperfusion VS with respect to the 3 clinical settings in which this is commonly reported: cardiac surgery with CPB, hepatic reperfusion during liver transplantation, and return of spontaneous circulation (ROSC) after cardiac arrest.

VS frequently occurs during and after cardiac surgery with reported incidences as high as 46%, depending on definition and risk factors [23]. In this population, it is associated with an increase in both morbidity and mortality and thus warrants discussion of causes and risk factors [24,25]. The pathophysiology of VS after heart surgery is complex and multifactorial.

Historically, VS in the cardiac operating room was thought to be due to the exposure of blood to an extracorporeal circuit, initiating the inflammatory cascade with increased inflammatory mediators and production of vasoactive molecules such as NO, endothelins, platelet-activating factors, thromboxane A2, prostaglandins, and other cytokines [26]. In patients with VS, exposure to these molecules pathologically alters endothelial vasomotor response, leading to the loss of vasomotor tone and subsequent hypotension [27]. This theory is refuted at least in part as VS is also seen in off-pump coronary artery bypass surgeries; thus the presence CPB and subsequent inflammatory provocation does not completely account for the VS frequently seen in cardiac surgery [28]. Instead, neurohormonal modulation also plays a contributory role. Vasopressin secretion is increased on CPB resulting in a relative depletion of vasopressin stores. This leads to reduced plasma vasopressin levels in patients who develop VS [29].

Additionally, peripheral alpha-1 receptors are downregulated in severe chronic illness, such as ongoing myocardial injury; subsequent surgical stress in this setting can lead to norepinephrine depletion and receptor resistance [9]. As noted, decreased agonism at alpha-1, vasopressin-1, and angiotensin II receptors results in decreased cytoplasmic calcium and reduced vascular tone [7].

Despite varying definitions and mechanisms of VS leading to heterogeneity in studies examining the topic, overarching patient-specific and surgery-specific factors have been identified to predict the likelihood of VS during and after CPB. Several studies have described patient-specific characteristics associated with the development of VS after cardiac surgery; these include reduced left ventricular ejection fraction less than 35% and/or ventricular assist device [30], elevated creatinine or presence of renal failure [2,30,31], and overall higher euroSCORE [24]. Certain medications used preoperatively also contribute to the risk for VS, including intravenous heparin [20], ACE-I [4,20,24], amiodarone [32], and beta-blockers [24]. There are also operation-specific factors that place patients at increased risk of VS, including the type of procedure and procedural components. An isolated coronary artery bypass grafting and aortic graft/repair surgeries are associated with lower rates of VS, whereas valve surgeries, redo cardiac surgeries, and cases intended to treat heart failure (Left vetricular assist device [LVAD] implantation, heart transplantation) are associated with higher rates of VS [2,24,29,32]. Furthermore, longer time on CPB, longer aortic cross-clamp time, and administration of blood products increase the risk for VS [24,30,31], whereas lower core temperatures on CPB were protective against VS, possibly due to blunting of the inflammatory cascade [24].

The diagnosis of VS in cardiac surgery is particularly challenging given the broad differential diagnosis for post-CPB hypotension in this population, including cardiac tamponade, right and/or left ventricular dysfunction, hemorrhagic shock, aortic dissection, or even site-dependent blood pressure monitoring errors (direct aortic measurement vs femoral vs radial). However, when these diagnoses have been ruled out, findings of low SVR with normal-to-high cardiac output should prompt the recognition and rapid treatment of VS.

Liver Transplant

Patients requiring liver transplantation for end-stage liver disease are often decompensated with sequelae of cirrhosis and portal hypertension, such as hepatic encephalopathy, esophageal varices, ascites, and hepatorenal syndrome. Before transplantation, these patients typically have a hyperdynamic cardiovascular system with supranormal cardiac output, low SVR, and low vascular reactivity resulting in systemic hypotension [33,34]. During liver transplantation, patients may experience additional hemodynamic perturbations including postreperfusion syndrome (PRS) after portal vein unclamping and generalized VS. These can compound an already decreased SVR, further worsening refractory hypotension and concerns for end-organ hypoperfusion.

PRS is superficially similar to VS and is commonly defined as a $\geq$ 30% decrease in MAP below the patient's baseline, occurring within the first 5 to 10 minutes after graft reperfusion, and lasting $\geq$ 1 minute [35,36]. Although VS and PRS similarly present as significant hypotension, they are differentiated by filling pressures, pulmonary artery pressures, and cardiac output. In VS, central filling pressures (right atrial pressure [RAP], left atrial pressure [LAP]) are low as a result of pure, dysregulated vasodilation; cardiac output is normal/high without any cardiac dysfunction (low PCWP), and there is no increase in PVR or PAP [4,37,38]. In PRS, an element of cardiac stunning and dysfunction occurs secondary to the cold, ischemic, acidotic perfusate that donor live sends into circulation, along with blood return from the relatively ischemic mesentery and lower body secondary to portal vein and inferior vena cava clamping. Although cardiac output may still be normal or high compared with the average patient, it is a decrease from baseline for the recipient, with decreased lusitropy, impaired diastolic function, and elevated filling pressures.

Furthermore, a component of newly elevated PVR/PAP caused by the acidotic perfusate can precipitate right heart dysfunction and decreased cardiac output [35,38–42].

Liver transplant recipients may develop PRS, VS, or both during their perioperative course. Fortunately, the mainstay of treatment of both VS and PRS is fluids and vasopressors. However, in a patient with a fresh hepatic anastomosis, guarding against decreased flow in the hepatic artery during treatment is vital. Low-flow in the hepatic artery, due to either lower cardiac output or subsequent splanchnic vasoconstriction due to pressors, is associated with lower graft survival and higher arterial complications, such as thrombosis [43–45]. Therefore, after the initial stabilization of perfusion pressures, using goal-directed volume resuscitation and weaning of vasoactive medications with a focus of promoting hepatic blood flow helps minimize adverse graft outcomes.

Return of Spontaneous Circulation After Cardiac Arrest

Metabolic derangements and multiorgan dysfunction occur frequently after ROSC from cardiac arrest because of myocardial depression and systemic inflammatory response [46,47]. In 2008, a consensus statement on Post-Cardiac Arrest Syndrome defined the syndrome as a constellation of pathophysiologic processes stemming from the ischemia-reperfusion insult of cardiac arrest and ROSC [48]. In addition to cardiac and neurologic injury, the ischemia and subsequent reperfusion initiates an inflammatory cascade that leads to thrombosis, adrenal suppression, impaired tissue oxygenation, and increased risk of infection [48]. Furthermore, the endothelial damage, impaired vasoregulation, intravascular volume depletion, and subsequent hypotension that frequently follows ROSC are pertinent to the current discussion of VS [48–50].

The definition of "postcardiac arrest shock" (PCAS) is not universally agreed on in the literature. Pragmatically, it is defined as hypotension with systolic blood pressure (SBP) of 90 mm Hg or lesser or MAP of 65 mm Hg or lesser, necessitating continuous vasoactive medications [51–53]. Mechanistically, the pathophysiology of PCAS is similar to septic shock [53]. The ischemia-reperfusion injury leads to cytokine release and NOS expression that triggers relaxation of vascular smooth muscle [54,55]. In combination with metabolic acidosis, loss of alpha-1 receptor responsiveness and sympathetic tone, and temperature derangements, this can result in VS [9,56]. As many as 70% of patients meet this definition of PCAS after ROSC [51–53,57], and PCAS is linked to increased morbidity and mortality, which publications report to be as high as 75% [46,47,58,59]. Some predictors of PCAS include male patients, longer arrest time before ROSC, out-of-hospital arrest (vs in-hospital), hypotension on admission, presence of diabetes mellitus, and higher sequential organ failure assessment (SOFA) score [51,58,60,61].

Immunomodulation

Sepsis and septic shock are major causes of morbidity and mortality in intensive care unit (ICU) patients [62].

Patients that develop septic shock have a 40% higher mortality rate than those who do not develop hypotension associated with their sepsis [63]. The development of sepsis dysregulates the normal vasoconstrictive response to hypotension, at times making the response to traditional vasopressors ineffective [12]. Sepsis is associated with the development of a proinflammatory state driven primarily by nuclear factor kappa B [64], leading to an increase in iNOS and cyclooxygenase-2 [65]. iNOS in turn increases NO production, which induces vascular smooth muscle relaxation via cGMP [66]. Despite this dysregulation in proinflammatory and anti-inflammatory markers, attempts at decreasing the inflammatory response to sepsis have not shown to improve mortality substantially, with only a 3.5% decrease in mortality noted after the administration of anti-TNFα antibodies [67].

Interestingly, patients with sepsis and septic shock develop a downregulation of nearly all catecholamine receptors, including vasopressin receptors, angiotensin receptors, and adrenergic receptors [68–70]. In addition to the downregulation in vasopressin receptors, sepsis also induces a decrease in circulating levels of vasopressin [71]. Combined with the vascular smooth muscle relaxation from proinflammatory cytokines, this receptor downregulation and decreased vasopressin availability can lead to VS. Norepinephrine remains the mainstay of vasopressor therapy for sepsis-associated VS [72]. Vasopressin is a reasonable second vasopressor to add if norepinephrine is inadequate to maintain MAP greater than 65 mm Hg, but does not show superiority over norepinephrine when used an s a solo agent [73]. Similarly, epinephrine shows no benefit as a solo agent but may have benefit in the septic patient with sepsis-associated heart failure [74].

Dopamine, once considered the mainstay of therapy in septic shock, has been showed to increase mortality when used as a first-line agent [75].

Anaphylaxis

Anaphylaxis in the perioperative period is primarily immunoglobin E (IgE) mediated, although nonimmunomodulated anaphylactoid reactions may occur. The initial diagnosis is often presumptive and usually is based on the proximity to induction of anesthesia (the most common time for anaphylaxis to occur) and the clinical symptoms, with severe reactions more likely to occur within minutes of induction [76]. The mechanism behind the development of anaphylaxis helps to explain why VS may play a substantial role in the development of this clinical syndrome. On subsequent exposure to a previously sensitized substrate, 2 IgE molecules are cross-linked by the allergen, signaling a cascade of proinflammatory mediators, including histamine and tryptase. Histamine specifically is known to increase NO production. Other molecules known to increase NO, such as platelet activating factor and TNFα are also released during an anaphylactic response [77]. As discussed previously, NO increases the activation of guanylyl cyclase, which increases cGMP and causes smooth muscle relaxation [78].

Mainstays of treatment include the removal of the offending substance (if possible) along with fluid and vasopressor administration to counteract the increased vascular capacitance and decreased SVR. Epinephrine is often required for the treatment of severe reactions [79]. Given the increase in NO production, MB has been posited to specifically treat the VS associated with anaphylaxis and may be helpful, although current data is extrapolated only from case reports [77,79]. Animal studies have suggested that an epinephrine-MB treatment combination may be more effective than epinephrine alone [80].

Other

Several other entities, such as pancreatitis, burns, and adrenal insufficiency either mimic VS or may have a component of VS underlying the hemodynamic derangements associated with the clinical process. Patients with pancreatitis have both proinflammatory and anti-inflammatory responses to disease [81]. Given the hypotension that can occur with severe pancreatitis, it was postulated that increasing NO may play a role in the development of VS related to acute pancreatitis. Currently, there are no human studies to support this. Additionally, patients with severe acute pancreatitis and vasopressor-resistant hypotension may respond to corticosteroids, suggesting induced adrenal insufficiency as the cause of hypotension versus VS [82]. Burn patients often have a profound proinflammatory response precipitating increased NO production. The increased production of NO occurs relatively early in burn injury, and production is seemingly proportional to total body surface area [83,84]. Although fluid administration corrects the profound hypotension that can occur in many of these patients, a subset remain hypotensive despite adequate volume resuscitation and administration of vasopressors. VS associated with burns is becoming a more widely described phenomenon with treatment modalities extrapolated mostly from the cardiac surgery population. Multiple case reports have described MB as an effective pharmacologic treatment, although large-scale studies have not been completed [85,86]. It is worth noting that adrenal insufficiency may mimic the vasopressor-resistant hypotension present in VS. Steroids may play a role in the treatment of VS outside of the correction of adrenal insufficiency, which is discussed below.

TREATMENT

When VS is encountered in any of the clinical settings referenced above, rapid diagnosis and action is needed to counteract the profound hypotension and resultant hypoperfusion. A review of the current treatment options, including several novel options, with practical advice for using these agents is presented below. See Table 1 for an overview applying these agents in the clinical setting.

Table 1
Causes of vasolplegia syndrome, etiologies, and potential treatments

Problem	Cellular Location and Cause of VS		Treatment
ACEI/ARB use	Cellular	Antagonism of RAAS pathway	Norepinephrine Vasopressin
Postreperfusion			
Postbypass	Cellular	Downregulation of catecholamine receptors	Adrenergic agents
	Intracellular	Increased NO production	Methylene blue
	Cellular, intracellular	Downregulation of catecholamine receptors, increased NO production	Angiotensin II
Liver transplant	Cellular	Cardiac stunning	Adrenergic agents
Post-ROSC	Cellular	Impaired vasoregulation	Adrenergic agents
	Intracellular	Increased NO production	Methylene blue
Sepsis	Cellular	Downregulation of catecholamine receptors	Norepinephrine and other adrenergic agents
	Intracellular	Increased NO production	Methylene blue
	Cellular, intracellular	Downregulation of catecholamine receptors, increased NO production	Angiotensin II
Anaphylaxis	Cellular, intracellular	IgE linkage leading to increased NO production	Epinephrine Methylene blue
Other			
Pancreatitis	Central	Acute adrenal insufficiency mimicking VS	Corticosteroid replacement
Burn	Intracellular	Increased NO production	Methylene blue

Vasopressors

Adrenergic agents

Catecholamines, endogenous adrenergic substances, are synthesized in the hypothalamus and adrenal glands and act on alpha 1, vasopressin 1, and angiotensin II receptors throughout the body to produce vasoconstriction [7]. In the setting of vascular tone dysregulation, medications are available to act on these receptors to increase SVR and MAP, namely phenylephrine, dopamine, norepinephrine, epinephrine, vasopressin, terlipressin, and angiotensin II. The cornerstone of catecholamine therapy is norepinephrine, and it should be considered a first-line agent for the treatment of hypotension [87]. Norepinephrine primarily acts on the alpha 1 receptor resulting in potent vasoconstriction and secondarily acts on beta 1 receptors with an increase in cardiac output, typically without a compensatory increase in heart rate or myocardial oxygen demand.

Norepinephrine is preferred over phenylephrine for its additional beta agonism. Although there is no difference in gut perfusion and mixed data on cardiopulmonary performance, there is an association between phenylephrine and mortality in patients presenting in septic shock when compared with norepinephrine [88–91]. Norepinephrine is strongly preferred over dopamine, as dopamine is more arrhythmogenic and associated with higher numbers of adverse events, in-hospital mortalities, ICU length of stay, and mortality [75,92]. Epinephrine can be used independently when cardiac dysfunction presents with VS [87,93]. However, with pure VS and normal cardiac output, epinephrine offers no difference in outcomes compared with norepinephrine [7,94]. It can, however, be added as a third agent to norepinephrine and vasopressin if MAP goals are still not met [87]. Additionally, the increase in serum lactate levels associated with epinephrine use makes lactate a less reliable marker of adequate resuscitation [95].

Vasopressin and terlipressin

Vasopressin is a catecholamine sparing agent that acts on vasopressin receptors and results in vasoconstriction, through vasopressin-1. There are several large, randomized control trials looking at the difference between vasopressin and norepinephrine in the setting of both septic shock and cardiac surgery. The VASST trial found no difference between vasopressin and norepinephrine with respect to 28-day mortality, 90-day mortality, or serious adverse events in patients presenting in septic shock [73]. In less severe shock, there were trends in favor of the vasopressin group for both 28-day and 90-day mortality compared with the norepinephrine only group. The VANISH trial was designed to look at kidney failure in septic patients randomized to vasopressin and steroids, vasopressin and placebo, norepinephrine and steroids, or norepinephrine and placebo, and found no difference between the groups [96]. Finally, the VANCS trial looked at a composite outcome of mortality and severe complications in norepinephrine only versus vasopressin only in vasoplegic shock after cardiac surgery [97]. There was a statistically significant decrease in the composite outcome as well as the incidence of postoperative atrial fibrillation in the vasopressin-only group, suggesting that cardiac surgery patients may benefit from vasopressin as first-line therapy for postoperative VS. The VANCS II group then looked at sepsis in patients with cancer and found no 28-day mortality benefit for vasopressin-only therapy [98]. The Surviving Sepsis guidelines still advocate for first-line norepinephrine treatment. If the MAP is still inadequate (ie, $<$65 mm Hg), the guidelines suggest adding vasopressin [87].

Terlipressin is a synthetic vasopressin analog. With a higher vasopressin-1 receptor affinity, it is more selective for vasoconstriction and has theoretically less electrolyte and coagulation side effects than vasopressin [99]. However, it is not approved by the US Food and Drug Administration, and although it has been historically used in hepatorenal syndrome, its use for the treatment of vasoplegia is lacking trials and data [100].

Angiotensin II

Angiotensin II is a synthetic analog of the naturally occurring hormone angiotensin. This hormone has wide-ranging effects, including exocrine, paracrine, autocrine, and intracrine activity. Its existence has been postulated since 1898 but due at least in part to its rapid breakdown, initial studies failed to identify the compound. It was eventually isolated in the 1930s [101]. Although its potential as a vasopressor was described in animal studies during the 1960s, initial descriptions of angiotensin II used clinically in humans as a vasopressor are seen in several case studies published in the 1990s concerning its use as a successful treatment of ACE-I overdose [102–104]. It has since been recognized as a potent method to increase arterial blood pressure via peripheral stimulation of type 1 angiotensin receptors and resulting vasoconstriction [105].

Angiotensin II was approved for use in the United States in 2018 after the ATHOS 3 trial, a large phase 3 study. The primary outcome of this study was MAP greater than 75 mm Hg or increased greater than 10 mm Hg from baseline within 3 hours of angiotensin II initiation. In addition, the authors found a decreased in the SOFA score [69]. The study was not powered to detect a mortality benefit. Although 80.7% of the patients in the ATHOS 3 cohort were diagnosed with sepsis, a post hoc analysis did show similar benefit in cardiac surgery-associated VS [69,106]. The initial clinical use of angiotensin II after ATHOS 3 was described mostly via case reports [107]. In 2021, a large multicenter postmarketing study showed 67% of patients had a positive hemodynamic response to angiotensin II infusion, including increase in MAP and decrease in other vasopressor requirements. They also noted a decrease in 30-day mortality in patients that responded favorably to angiotensin II (0.50, 95% CI, 0.35–0.7) [107].

Deleterious side effects of angiotensin II are derived almost exclusively from data gleaned from the ATHOS 3 trial. There may be an increased risk of thrombotic events, potentially secondary to direct release of plasminogen activator 1 [69,108]. There is potential for transaminitis, although the clinical significance of this is unknown [107]. There are reports of arrythmias, with 10% of patients in the previously mentioned postmarketing use study developing an arrythmia while receiving angiotensin II, although the rate of arrhythmogenicity was no different in treatment versus control groups in ATHOS 3 [69,107].

The angiotensin II dosing strategy described in ATHOS 3 has been subsequently adopted by many institutions. The drug is given at 20 ng/kg/min. If the MAP is less than 60 mm Hg after 5 minutes, the dosage is increased to 80 ng/kg/min. If the MAP is between 60 and 74, the dosage is increased by 10 ng/kg/min every 15 minutes to achieve the desired MAP. If the MAP is greater than 85, the dosage is decreased by 10 ng/kg/min every 15 minutes to achieve the desired MAP. This dosing strategy is contingent on the patient being within the first 3 hours of drug initiation. The maximum dose described in ATHOS 3 during the first 3 hours of drug administration was 200 ng/kg/min. After 3 hours, the maximal dose is decreased to 40 ng/kg/min. Titration is similar, patients with a MAP less than 59 are moved to the 40 ng/kg/min dose after 5 minutes. For patients with a MAP greater than 60 mm Hg, the drug is titrated by 10 ng/kg/min every 15 minutes to achieve the desired MAP. The minimum dose is 2.5 ng/kg/min, although there are some hyperresponders that require even slower down titration. Those patients may require 1.25 ng/kg/min dosing before angiotensin II is discontinued [69].

A major deterrent for angiotensin II use has been cost, which varies slightly by institution. A cost-effectiveness analysis published in 2020 showed that angiotensin II saved 0.8 lives at day 28 compared with standard therapy, and the cost per life saved was estimated a US$108,884 [109].

Methylene blue

MB was first used to treat symptomatic, severe methemoglobinemia.

However, it has since gained traction as a rescue treatment of hypotension refractory to vasopressors and fluid administration and has been proposed for prophylactic use in patients at high risk for VS syndrome [37,110]. MB acts mostly on the NO/cGMP second messenger pathway that results in vasodilation. MB scavenges NO, inhibits NO synthase, and inhibits guanylate cyclase, the enzyme that synthesizes cGMP and causes calcium reuptake and smooth muscle relaxation [111,112]. Most commonly, side effects of MB are benign and include discoloration of urine and interruption of pulse oximeter readings. As a monoamine oxidase inhibitor (MAOI), concomitant use with antidepressants (SSRIs or MAOis) carries a risk of serotonin syndrome. Because MB results in vasoconstriction via decreased NO production, caution should be taken in patients with pulmonary hypertension, right ventricular dysfunction, or coronary artery disease due to risk of increased PVR and coronary vasospasm. MB can also precipitate hemolytic anemia in patients with G6PD deficiency [113].

There are no large randomized controlled trials (RCTs) investigating the effects of MB on morbidity and mortality. Much of the current literature is retrospective and consists of case reports, cohort studies, and small meta-analyses. There are a few RCTs investigating the effects of MB on hemodynamic improvement (increased MAP and decreased vasoactive medications) in cardiac, liver, and critical care settings, with some reporting improved clinical outcomes [85,86,111,114–118]. However, the current evidence is not definitive.

Hydroxocobalamin (vitamin B12)

Intravenous hydroxocobalamin is a well-recognized treatment of acute cyanide toxicity in Europe and has been approved recently in the United States for the same indication [119]. The understood mechanism of hydroxocobalamin therapy in this setting involves direct binding to cyanide to form cyanocobalamin, which deactivates the effect of cyanide and allows for subsequent renal excretion of the cyanocobalamin compound [119]. The mechanism behind the hemodynamic effects of hydroxocobalamin is less clear. There is a consistent increase in blood pressure, primarily diastolic blood pressure, associated with hydroxocobalamin use in humans and animals that seems to be related to its effectiveness as a scavenger of NO [120]. There may be some additional effects related to hydroxocobalamin binding to hydrogen sulfide, thus inhibiting the binding of adenosine triphosphate-sensitive potassium channels, leading to hypotension [120]. Further downstream modulation of cytokine pathways has also been implicated, which may explain the prolonged effects of hydroxocobalamin in experimental models of septic shock [121].

The primary adverse effect of hydroxocobalamin administration is increased blood pressure, which, in the case of VS, is beneficial. Other named adverse reactions to hydroxocobalamin include transient chromaturia, erythema, rash, nausea, headaches, and injection site reactions [119]. To date, there are 3 reports illustrating the hemodynamic benefits of hydroxocobalamin, with and without trialing MB, in the setting of liver transplantation [122]. The previously published case reports demonstrated the use of hydroxocobalamin in liver transplantation with lower doses of hydroxocobalamin (125-mg and 250-mg bolus doses), followed by hydroxocobalamin infusions (250–500 mg/h) for VS. Boettcher and colleagues [5] reported lower doses of hydroxocobalamin but a more limited duration of response, thus requiring the initiation of a hydroxocobalamin infusion.

Vitamin C

Vitamin C is a water-soluble vitamin involved in many basic cellular processes and an integral cofactor in important antioxidant functions. Humans lack the ability to synthesize vitamin C, and thus are entirely dependent on dietary sources [123]. It came to be known as ascorbic acid as its original discovered use, in the 1920s, was as the treatment of scurvy, hence the Latin translation of against-scurvy, or "a-scorbitus" [124]. Its functions include scavenging both reactive oxygen and nitrogen species. In addition, it can help to preserve endothelial integrity via modulation of cGMP levels, and it has been shown to be integral to maintenance of endogenous norepinephrine levels [123,125]. Oxidative stress in increased in VS, making vitamin C an attractive potential treatment.

Oxidative stress is also implicated in septic shock, and the original studies concerning high-dose vitamin C as a treatment of hypotension were performed in patients with sepsis. Original retrospective data suggested that high-dose vitamin C administration (defined as 1.5 G IV every 6 hours for 4 days or until ICU discharge), along with thiamine and hydrocortisone, resulted in both a significantly decreased vasopressor requirement, and a significantly decreased mortality rate [126]. Subsequent RCTs, including the VITAMINS trial and the VICTAS trial failed to replicate this treatment benefit, with both studies showing no difference in vasopressor or ventilator-free days [127,128]. There is at least one additional ongoing RCT to further examine any link between vitamin C administration and organ dysfunction [129].

Studies of vitamin C supplementation are limited to a small case series describing high-dose vitamin C treatment in 3 postcardiac surgery patients with refractory VS. The authors used a dosing strategy of 1500 mg IV 3 times a day. They reported a reduction in norepinephrine requirements, with 2 of 3 patients liberated entirely from norepinephrine within 24 hours of vitamin C administration. Toxicity associated with vitamin C administration is rare, although several side effects have been described, most at very high doses. These include kidney stone formation, specifically oxalate stone formation in patients prone to renal stones.

This is related to the small amount of metabolism to oxalate and has been shown to be both mostly related to a long-term use and is more common in those with preexisting renal dysfunction [130,131]. In addition, osmotic diarrhea and resulting abdominal pain has been described with very high oral intake [132]. Hemolysis in specific patient populations, including those with G6PD deficiency and those with paroxysmal nocturnal hemoglobinuria [132,133].

Steroids

Steroids have the potential to improve responsiveness to vasopressors in shock, and their ability to modulate the production of iNOS has been described [134]. The data surrounding steroid use in septic shock, which may have a VS component, is mixed [135,136]. These large studies did not specifically separate patients into those with and without VS, and it is unknown whether steroid therapy directly improves hemodynamics or outcomes in patients with VS.

FUTURE RESEARCH

There is much research to be done on this topic and much that is currently ongoing.

Currently, there are 3 large prospective RCTs underway that will help inform perioperative use of ACE-I or ARB medications and thus perioperative avoidance of hypotension. These are the GUARDIAN trial (NCT04884802), POISE-3 trial (NCT03505723), and a trial from Soochow University in China [137,138]. These trials are focusing on major noncardiac surgery. Additional research is still needed to better determine effective treatments for postbypass VS as well as postreperfusion VS in liver transplant and when achieving ROSC.

However, the latter 2 may prove difficult due to lower numbers of cases overall and the unpredictable nature of in-hospital cardiac arrest, where post-ROSC treatments could be tested. For all causes of VS, specifically evaluating MB and high-dose vitamin B12 with combinations of adrenergic agents and/or vasopressin would be informative.

SUMMARY

In conclusion, VS occurs fairly frequently in cardiac surgery, liver transplant, major noncardiac surgery, and in post-ROSC situations. It is paramount for the anesthesiologist to understand the pathophysiology of these causes and the different treatment strategies available for rescuing a patient from life-threatening hypotension.

CLINICS CARE POINTS

- Vasoplegia is defined by hypotension, low SVR, normal or high cardiac output, and reduced response to vasoactive medications.
- INitric oxide production drives much of the symptomatology seen in vasoplegic syndrome.
- Traditional vasopressors, especially norepinephrine, are appropriate first line agents.More specific medications, such as methylene blue and angiotensin II, are appropriate second line agents for persistent vasoplegia.

Disclosure

The authors have nothing to disclose.

References

[1] Liu H, Yu L, Yang L, et al. Vasoplegic syndrome: An update on perioperative considerations. J Clin Anesth 2017;40:63–71.
[2] Tsiouris A, Wilson L, Haddadin AS, et al. Risk assessment and outcomes of vasoplegia after cardiac surgery. Gen Thorac Cardiovasc Surg 2017;65:557–65.
[3] Koelzow H, Gedney JA, Baumann J, et al. The effect of methylene blue on the hemodynamic changes during ischemia reperfusion injury in orthotopic liver transplantation. Anesth Analg 2002;94:824–9, table of contents.
[4] Shanmugam G. Vasoplegic syndrome–the role of methylene blue. Eur J Cardiothorac Surg 2005;28:705–10.
[5] Boettcher BT, Woehlck HJ, Reck SE, et al. Treatment of Vasoplegic Syndrome With Intravenous Hydroxocobalamin During Liver Transplantation. J Cardiothorac Vasc Anesth 2017;31:1381–4.
[6] Lambden S, Creagh-Brown BC, Hunt J, et al. Definitions and pathophysiology of vasoplegic shock. Crit Care 2018;22:174.
[7] Levy B, Fritz C, Tahon E, et al. Vasoplegia treatments: the past, the present, and the future. Crit Care 2018;22:52.
[8] Kimmoun A, Ducrocq N, Levy B. Mechanisms of vascular hyporesponsiveness in septic shock. Curr Vasc Pharmacol 2013;11:139–49.
[9] Hwang TL, Lau YT, Huang SF, et al. Changes of alpha 1-adrenergic receptors in human liver during intraabdominal sepsis. Hepatology 1994;20:638–42.
[10] Althoff TF, Offermanns S. G-protein-mediated signaling in vascular smooth muscle cells implications for vascular disease. J Mol Med (Berl) 2015;93:973–81.
[11] Schmidt C, Höcherl K, Kurt B, et al. Blockade of multiple but not single cytokines abrogates downregulation of angiotensin II type-I receptors and anticipates septic shock. Cytokine 2010;49:30–8.
[12] Landry DW, Oliver JA. The pathogenesis of vasodilatory shock. N Engl J Med 2001;345:588–95.
[13] Lange M, Enkhbaatar P, Nakano Y, et al. Role of nitric oxide in shock: the large animal perspective. Front Biosci (Landmark Ed 2009;14:1979–89.

[14] Saha BK, Burns SL. The Story of Nitric Oxide, Sepsis and Methylene Blue: A Comprehensive Pathophysiologic Review. Am J Med Sci 2020;360:329–37.
[15] Carrel T, Englberger L, Mohacsi P, et al. Low systemic vascular resistance after cardiopulmonary bypass: incidence, etiology, and clinical importance. J Card Surg 2000;15: 347–53.
[16] Omar S, Zedan A, Nugent K. Cardiac vasoplegia syndrome: pathophysiology, risk factors and treatment. Am J Med Sci 2015;349:80–8.
[17] Arendse LB, Danser AHJ, Poglitsch M, et al. Novel Therapeutic Approaches Targeting the Renin-Angiotensin System and Associated Peptides in Hypertension and Heart Failure. Pharmacol Rev 2019;71:539–70.
[18] Papazisi O, Palmen M, Danser AHJ. The Use of Angiotensin II for the Treatment of Post-cardiopulmonary Bypass Vasoplegia. Cardiovasc Drugs Ther 2022;36:739–48.
[19] Lange M, Van Aken H, Westphal M, et al. Role of vasopressinergic V1 receptor agonists in the treatment of perioperative catecholamine-refractory arterial hypotension. Best Pract Res Clin Anaesthesiol 2008;22:369–81.
[20] Mekontso-Dessap A, Houel R, Soustelle C, et al. Risk factors for post-cardiopulmonary bypass vasoplegia in patients with preserved left ventricular function. Ann Thorac Surg 2001;71:1428–32.
[21] Roshanov PS, Rochwerg B, Patel A, et al. Withholding versus Continuing Angiotensin-converting Enzyme Inhibitors or Angiotensin II Receptor Blockers before Noncardiac Surgery: An Analysis of the Vascular events In noncardiac Surgery patIents cOhort evaluatioN Prospective Cohort. Anesthesiology 2017;126:16–27.
[22] Smith I, Jackson I. Beta-blockers, calcium channel blockers, angiotensin converting enzyme inhibitors and angiotensin receptor blockers: should they be stopped or not before ambulatory anaesthesia? Curr Opin Anaesthesiol 2010;23:687–90.
[23] Asleh R, Alnsasra H, Daly RC, et al. Predictors and Clinical Outcomes of Vasoplegia in Patients Bridged to Heart Transplantation With Continuous- Flow Left Ventricular Assist Devices. J Am Heart Assoc 2019;8:e013108.
[24] Levin MA, Lin HM, Castillo JG, et al. Early on- cardiopulmonary bypass hypotension and other factors associated with vasoplegic syndrome. Circulation 2009;120:1664–71.
[25] Gomes WJ, Carvalho AC, Palma JH, et al. Vasoplegic syndrome after open heart surgery. J Cardiovasc Surg (Torino) 1998;39:619–23.
[26] Wan S, LeClerc JL, Vincent JL. Inflammatory response to cardiopulmonary bypass: mechanisms involved and possible therapeutic strategies. Chest 1997;112:676–92.
[27] Abou-Arab O, Martineau L, Bar S, et al. Postoperative Vasoplegic Syndrome Is Associated With Impaired Endothelial Vasomotor Response in Cardiac Surgery: A Prospective, Observational Study. J Cardiothorac Vasc Anesth 2018;32:2218–24.
[28] Sun X, Zhang L, Hill PC, et al. Is incidence of postoperative vasoplegic syndrome different between off-pump and on-pump coronary artery bypass grafting surgery? Eur J Cardiothorac Surg 2008;34:820–5.
[29] Colson PH, Bernard C, Struck J, et al. Post cardiac surgery vasoplegia is associated with high preoperative copeptin plasma concentration. Crit Care 2011;15:R255.
[30] Sun X, Boyce SW, Herr DL, et al. Is vasoplegic syndrome more prevalent with open-heart procedures compared with isolated on-pump CABG surgery? Cardiovasc Revasc Med 2011;12:203–9.
[31] Dayan V, Cal R, Giangrossi F. Risk factors for vasoplegia after cardiac surgery: a meta-analysis. Interact Cardiovasc Thorac Surg 2019;28:838–44.
[32] Mehaffey JH, Johnston LE, Hawkins RB, et al. Methylene Blue for Vasoplegic Syndrome After Cardiac Operation: Early Administration Improves Survival. Ann Thorac Surg 2017;104:36–41.
[33] Moller S, Hobolth L, Winkler C, et al. Determinants of the hyperdynamic circulation and central hypovolaemia in cirrhosis. Gut 2011;60:1254–9.

[34] Moller S, Bendtsen F. The pathophysiology of arterial vasodilatation and hyperdynamic circulation in cirrhosis. Liver Int 2018;38:570–80.
[35] Aggarwal S, Kang Y, Freeman JA, et al. Postreperfusion syndrome: cardiovascular collapse following hepatic reperfusion during liver transplantation. Transpl Proc 1987;19:54–5.
[36] van Rijn R, Schurink IJ, de Vries Y, et al. Hypothermic Machine Perfusion in Liver Transplantation - A Randomized Trial. N Engl J Med 2021;384:1391–401.
[37] Ozal E, Kuralay E, Yildirim V, et al. Preoperative methylene blue administration in patients at high risk for vasoplegic syndrome during cardiac surgery. Ann Thorac Surg 2005;79: 1615–9.
[38] de Armas LC, Castillo YA. Is it possible to distinguish between vasoplegic syndrome and postreperfusion syndrome during liver graft reperfusion? Anesth Analg 2010;110: 969–70 [author reply 970-1].
[39] Siniscalchi A, Aurini L, Spedicato S, et al. Hyperdynamic circulation in cirrhosis: predictive factors and outcome following liver transplantation. Minerva Anestesiol 2013;79:15–23.
[40] Ripoll C, Catalina MV, Yotti R, et al. Cardiac dysfunction during liver transplantation: incidence and preoperative predictors. Transplantation 2008;85:1766–72.
[41] Hilmi I, Horton CN, Planinsic RM, et al. The impact of postreperfusion syndrome on short-term patient and liver allograft outcome in patients undergoing orthotopic liver transplantation. Liver Transpl 2008;14:504–8.
[42] Paugam-Burtz C, Kavafyan J, Merckx P, et al. Postreperfusion syndrome during liver transplantation for cirrhosis: outcome and predictors. Liver Transpl 2009;15:522–9.
[43] Abbasoglu O, Levy MF, Testa G, et al. Does intraoperative hepatic artery flow predict arterial complications after liver transplantation? Transplantation 1998;66:598–601.
[44] Marin-Gomez LM, Bernal-Bellido C, Alamo-Martinez JM, et al. Intraoperative hepatic artery blood flow predicts early hepatic artery thrombosis after liver transplantation. Transpl Proc 2012;44:2078–81.
[45] Kim P, Klintmalm G. Importance of hepatic flows in liver transplantation. J Hepatol Gastroint Dis 2016;2:2–3.
[46] Kilgannon JH, Roberts BW, Reihl LR, et al. Early arterial hypotension is common in the post-cardiac arrest syndrome and associated with increased in-hospital mortality. Resuscitation 2008;79:410–6.
[47] Trzeciak S, Jones AE, Kilgannon JH, et al. Significance of arterial hypotension after resuscitation from cardiac arrest. Crit Care Med 2009;37:2895–903 [quiz: 2904].
[48] Nolan JP, Neumar RW, Adrie C, et al. Post-cardiac arrest syndrome: epidemiology, pathophysiology, treatment, and prognostication. A Scientific Statement from the International Liaison Committee on Resuscitation; the American Heart Association Emergency Cardiovascular Care Committee; the Council on Cardiovascular Surgery and Anesthesia; the Council on Cardiopulmonary, Perioperative, and Critical Care; the Council on Clinical Cardiology; the Council on Stroke. Resuscitation 2008;79:350–79.
[49] Fink K, Schwarz M, Feldbrügge L, et al. Severe endothelial injury and subsequent repair in patients after successful cardiopulmonary resuscitation. Crit Care 2010;14:R104.
[50] Bro-Jeppesen J, Johansson PI, Kjaergaard J, et al. Level of systemic inflammation and endothelial injury is associated with cardiovascular dysfunction and vasopressor support in post-cardiac arrest patients. Resuscitation 2017;121:179–86.
[51] Lemiale V, Dumas F, Mongardon N, et al. Intensive care unit mortality after cardiac arrest: the relative contribution of shock and brain injury in a large cohort. Intensive Care Med 2013;39:1972–80.
[52] Dumas F, Bougouin W, Geri G, et al. Emergency Percutaneous Coronary Intervention in Post-Cardiac Arrest Patients Without ST-Segment Elevation Pattern: Insights From the PROCAT II Registry. JACC Cardiovasc Interv 2016;9:1011–8.
[53] Jozwiak M, Bougouin W, Geri G, et al. Post-resuscitation shock: recent advances in pathophysiology and treatment. Ann Intensive Care 2020;10:170.

[54] Adrie C, Adib-Conquy M, Laurent I, et al. Successful cardiopulmonary resuscitation after cardiac arrest as a "sepsis-like" syndrome. Circulation 2002;106:562–8.
[55] Adrie C, Laurent I, Monchi M, et al. Postresuscitation disease after cardiac arrest: a sepsis-like syndrome? Curr Opin Crit Care 2004;10:208–12.
[56] Peberdy MA, Callaway CW, Neumar RW, et al. Part 9: post- cardiac arrest care: 2010 American Heart Association Guidelines for Cardiopulmonary Resuscitation and Emergency Cardiovascular Care. Circulation 2010;122:S768–86.
[57] Argaud L, Cour M, Dubien PY, et al. Effect of Cyclosporine in Nonshockable Out-of-Hospital Cardiac Arrest: The CYRUS Randomized Clinical Trial. JAMA Cardiol 2016;1: 557–65.
[58] Hästbacka J, Kirkegaard H, Søreide E, et al. Severe or critical hypotension during post cardiac arrest care is associated with factors available on admission - a post hoc analysis of the TTH48 trial. J Crit Care 2021;61:186–90.
[59] Issa MS, Grossestreuer AV, Patel H, et al. Lactate and hypotension as predictors of mortality after in-hospital cardiac arrest. Resuscitation 2021;158:208–14.
[60] Roberts BW, Kilgannon JH, Chansky ME, et al. Multiple organ dysfunction after return of spontaneous circulation in postcardiac arrest syndrome. Crit Care Med 2013;41: 1492–501.
[61] Matsuda J, Kato S, Yano H, et al. The Sequential Organ Failure Assessment (SOFA) score predicts mortality and neurological outcome in patients with post-cardiac arrest syndrome. J Cardiol 2020;76:295–302.
[62] Martin GS, Mannino DM, Eaton S, et al. The epidemiology of sepsis in the United States from 1979 through 2000. N Engl J Med 2003;348:1546–54.
[63] Singer M, Deutschman CS, Seymour CW, et al. The Third International Consensus Definitions for Sepsis and Septic Shock (Sepsis-3). Jama 2016;315:801–10.
[64] Altavilla D, Squadrito G, Minutoli L, et al. Inhibition of nuclear factor-kappaB activation by IRFI 042, protects against endotoxin-induced shock. Cardiovasc Res 2002;54:684–93.
[65] Abraham E. Nuclear factor-kappaB and its role in sepsis-associated organ failure. J Infect Dis 2003;187(Suppl 2):S364–9.
[66] Donati A, Conti G, Loggi S, et al. Does methylene blue administration to septic shock patients affect vascular permeability and blood volume? Crit Care Med 2002;30:2271–7.
[67] Marshall JC. Such stuff as dreams are made on: mediator-directed therapy in sepsis. Nat Rev Drug Discov 2003;2:391–405.
[68] Bucher M, Hobbhahn J, Taeger K, et al. Cytokine-mediated downregulation of vasopressin V(1A) receptors during acute endotoxemia in rats. Am J Physiol Regul Integr Comp Physiol 2002;282:R979–84.
[69] Khanna A, English SW, Wang XS, et al. Deane AM: Angiotensin II for the Treatment of Vasodilatory Shock. N Engl J Med 2017;377:419–30.
[70] Forse RA, Saint-Vil D, Gagner M, et al. Intra-abdominal sepsis and adrenergic receptor response. J Trauma 1992;32:564–9.
[71] Landry DW, Levin HR, Gallant EM, et al. Vasopressin deficiency contributes to the vasodilation of septic shock. Circulation 1997;95:1122–5.
[72] Rhodes A, Evans LE, Alhazzani W, et al. Surviving Sepsis Campaign: International Guidelines for Management of Sepsis and Septic Shock: 2016. Intensive Care Med 2017;43: 304–77.
[73] Russell JA, Walley KR, Singer J, et al. Vasopressin versus norepinephrine infusion in patients with septic shock. N Engl J Med 2008;358:877–87.
[74] Avni T, Lador A, Lev S, et al. Vasopressors for the Treatment of Septic Shock: Systematic Review and Meta-Analysis. PLoS One 2015;10:e0129305.
[75] De Backer D, Biston P, Devriendt J, et al. Comparison of dopamine and norepinephrine in the treatment of shock. N Engl J Med 2010;362:779–89.
[76] Dewachter P, Mouton-Faivre C, Emala CW. Anaphylaxis and anesthesia: controversies and new insights. Anesthesiology 2009;111:1141–50.

[77] Evora PR, Simon MR. Role of nitric oxide production in anaphylaxis and its relevance for the treatment of anaphylactic hypotension with methylene blue. Ann Allergy Asthma Immunol 2007;99:306–13.
[78] Kawada T, Ishibashi T, Sasage H, et al. Modification by LY 83583 and methylene blue of relaxation induced by nitric oxide, glyceryl trinitrate, sodium nitroprusside and atriopeptin in aortae of the rat, guinea-pig and rabbit. Gen Pharmacol 1994;25:1361–71.
[79] Mertes PM, Tajima K, Regnier-Kimmoun MA, et al. Perioperative anaphylaxis. Med Clin North Am 2010;94:761–89, xi.
[80] Zheng F, Barthel G, Collange O, et al. Methylene blue and epinephrine: a synergetic association for anaphylactic shock treatment. Crit Care Med 2013;41:195–204.
[81] Hynninen M, Valtonen M, Markkanen H, et al. Intramucosal pH and endotoxin and cytokine release in severe acute pancreatitis. Shock 2000;13:79–82.
[82] Eklund A, Leppäniemi A, Kemppainen E, et al. Vasodilatory shock in severe acute pancreatitis without sepsis: is there any place for hydrocortisone treatment? Acta Anaesthesiol Scand 2005;49:379–84.
[83] Gamelli RL, George M, Sharp-Pucci M, et al. Radisavljevic Z: Burn-induced nitric oxide release in humans. J Trauma 1995;39:869–77 [discussion: 877–8].
[84] Carter EA, Derojas-Walker T, Tamir S, et al. Nitric oxide production is intensely and persistently increased in tissue by thermal injury. Biochem J 1994;304(Pt 1):201–4.
[85] Church JT, Posluszny JA, Hemmila M, et al. Methylene blue for burn-induced vasoplegia: case report and review of literature. J Burn Care Res 2015;36:e107–11.
[86] Jaskille AD, Jeng JC, Jordan MH. Methylene blue in the treatment of vasoplegia following severe burns. J Burn Care Res 2008;29:408–10.
[87] Evans L, Rhodes A, Alhazzani W, et al. Surviving sepsis campaign: international guidelines for management of sepsis and septic shock 2021. Intensive Care Med 2021;47: 1181–247.
[88] Ducrocq N, Kimmoun A, Furmaniuk A, et al. Comparison of equipressor doses of norepinephrine, epinephrine, and phenylephrine on septic myocardial dysfunction. Anesthesiology 2012;116:1083–91.
[89] Krejci V, Hiltebrand LB, Sigurdsson GH. Effects of epinephrine, norepinephrine, and phenylephrine on microcirculatory blood flow in the gastrointestinal tract in sepsis. Crit Care Med 2006;34:1456–63.
[90] Morelli A, Ertmer C, Rehberg S, et al. Phenylephrine versus norepinephrine for initial hemodynamic support of patients with septic shock: a randomized, controlled trial. Crit Care 2008;12:R143.
[91] Vail E, Gershengorn HB, Hua M, et al. Association Between US Norepinephrine Shortage and Mortality Among Patients With Septic Shock. Jama 2017;317:1433–42.
[92] Suzuki R, Uchino S, Sasabuchi Y, et al. Dopamine use and its consequences in the intensive care unit: a cohort study utilizing the Japanese Intensive care PAtient Database. Crit Care 2022;26:90.
[93] Annane D, Vignon P, Renault A, et al. Norepinephrine plus dobutamine versus epinephrine alone for management of septic shock: a randomised trial. Lancet 2007;370:676–84.
[94] Myburgh JA, Higgins A, Jovanovska A, et al. A comparison of epinephrine and norepinephrine in critically ill patients. Intensive Care Med 2008;34:2226–34.
[95] Levy B, Bollaert PE, Charpentier C, et al. Comparison of norepinephrine and dobutamine to epinephrine for hemodynamics, lactate metabolism, and gastric tonometric variables in septic shock: a prospective, randomized study. Intensive Care Med 1997;23:282–7.
[96] Gordon AC, Mason AJ, Thirunavukkarasu N, et al. Effect of Early Vasopressin vs Norepinephrine on Kidney Failure in Patients With Septic Shock: The VANISH Randomized Clinical Trial. JAMA 2016;316:509–18.
[97] Hajjar LA, Vincent JL, Barbosa Gomes Galas FR, et al. Vasopressin versus Norepinephrine in Patients with Vasoplegic Shock after Cardiac Surgery: The VANCS Randomized Controlled Trial. Anesthesiology 2017;126:85–93.

[98] Hajjar LA, Zambolim C, Belletti A, et al. Vasopressin Versus Norepinephrine for the Management of Septic Shock in Cancer Patients: The VANCS II Randomized Clinical Trial. Crit Care Med 2019;47:1743–50.
[99] Kam PC, Williams S, Yoong FF. Vasopressin and terlipressin: pharmacology and its clinical relevance. Anaesthesia 2004;59:993–1001.
[100] Ortoleva J, Shapeton A, Vanneman M, et al. Vasoplegia During Cardiopulmonary Bypass: Current Literature and Rescue Therapy Options. J Cardiothorac Vasc Anesth 2020;34: 2766–75.
[101] Basso N, Terragno NA. History about the discovery of the renin-angiotensin system. Hypertension 2001;38:1246–9.
[102] Jackson T, Corke C, Agar J. Enalapril overdose treated with angiotensin infusion. Lancet 1993;341:703.
[103] Trilli LE, Johnson KA. Lisinopril overdose and management with intravenous angiotensin II. Ann Pharmacother 1994;28:1165–8.
[104] Derrick JR, Anderson JR, Roland BJ. Adjunctive use of a biologic pressor agent, angiotensin, in management of shock. Circulation 1962;25:263–7.
[105] Hall A, Busse LW, Ostermann M. Angiotensin in Critical Care. Crit Care 2018;22:69.
[106] Klijian A, Khanna AK, Reddy VS, et al. Treatment With Angiotensin II Is Associated With Rapid Blood Pressure Response and Vasopressor Sparing in Patients With Vasoplegia After Cardiac Surgery: A Post-Hoc Analysis of Angiotensin II for the Treatment of High-Output Shock (ATHOS-3) Study. J Cardiothorac Vasc Anesth 2021;35:51–8.
[107] Wieruszewski PM, Wittwer ED, Kashani KB, et al. Angiotensin II Infusion for Shock: A Multicenter Study of Postmarketing Use. Chest 2021;159:596–605.
[108] Bauer SR, Sacha GL, Lam SW. Safe Use of Vasopressin and Angiotensin II for Patients with Circulatory Shock. Pharmacotherapy 2018;38:851–61.
[109] Busse LW, Nicholson G, Nordyke RJ, et al. Angiotensin II for the treatment of distributive shock in the intensive care unit: A US cost-effectiveness analysis. Int J Technol Assess Health Care 2020;36:145–51.
[110] Maslow AD, Stearns G, Butala P, et al. The hemodynamic effects of methylene blue when administered at the onset of cardiopulmonary bypass. Anesth Analg 2006;103:2–8, table of contents.
[111] Hosseinian L, Weiner M, Levin MA, et al. Methylene Blue: Magic Bullet for Vasoplegia? Anesth Analg 2016;122:194–201.
[112] Shaefi S, Mittel A, Klick J, et al. Vasoplegia After Cardiovascular Procedures-Pathophysiology and Targeted Therapy. J Cardiothorac Vasc Anesth 2018;32:1013–22.
[113] Clifton J 2nd, Leikin JB. Methylene blue. Am J Ther 2003;10:289–91.
[114] Pasin L, Umbrello M, Greco T, et al. Methylene blue as a vasopressor: a meta-analysis of randomised trials. Crit Care Resusc 2013;15:42–8.
[115] Kofler O, Simbeck M, Tomasi R, et al. Early Use of Methylene Blue in Vasoplegic Syndrome: A 10-Year Propensity Score-Matched Cohort Study. J Clin Med 2022;11.
[116] Petermichl W, Gruber M, Schoeller I, et al. The additional use of methylene blue has a decatecholaminisation effect on cardiac vasoplegic syndrome after cardiac surgery. J Cardiothorac Surg 2021;16:205.
[117] Feih JT, Rinka JRG, Zundel MT. Methylene Blue Monotherapy Compared With Combination Therapy With Hydroxocobalamin for the Treatment of Refractory Vasoplegic Syndrome: ARetrospective Cohort Study. J Cardiothorac Vasc Anesth 2019;33:1301–7.
[118] Mazzeffi M, Hammer B, Chen E, et al. Methylene blue for postcardiopulmonary bypass vasoplegic syndrome: A cohort study. Ann Card Anaesth 2017;20:178–81.
[119] Dey L: Cyanokit® Package Insert. Dey, LP, Napa, CA 2006.
[120] Mustafa AK, Sikka G, Gazi SK, et al. Hydrogen sulfide as endothelium- derived hyperpolarizing factor sulfhydrates potassium channels. Circ Res 2011;109:1259–68.
[121] Sampaio AL, Dalli J, Brancaleone V, et al. Biphasic modulation of NOS expression, protein and nitrite products by hydroxocobalamin underlies its protective effect in endotoxemic

shock: downstream regulation of COX-2, IL-1β, TNF-α, IL-6, and HMGB1 expression. Mediators Inflamm 2013;2013:741804.
[122] Woehlck HJ, Boettcher BT, Lauer KK, et al. Hydroxocobalamin for Vasoplegic Syndrome in Liver Transplantation: Restoration of Blood Pressure Without Vasospasm. A A Case Rep 2016;7:247–50.
[123] Carr AC, Shaw GM, Fowler AA, et al. Ascorbate-dependent vasopressor synthesis: a rationale for vitamin C administration in severe sepsis and septic shock? Crit Care 2015;19:418.
[124] Doseděl M, Jirkovský E, Macáková K, et al. On Behalf Of The O: Vitamin C-Sources, Physiological Role, Kinetics, Deficiency, Use, Toxicity, and Determination. Nutrients 2021;13.
[125] Oudemans-van Straaten HM, Spoelstra-de Man AM, de Waard MC. Vitamin C revisited. Crit Care 2014;18:460.
[126] Marik PE, Khangoora V, Rivera R, et al. Catravas J: Hydrocortisone, Vitamin C, and Thiamine for the Treatment of Severe Sepsis and Septic Shock: A Retrospective Before- After Study. Chest 2017;151:1229–38.
[127] Fujii T, Luethi N, Young PJ, et al. Effect of Vitamin C, Hydrocortisone, and Thiamine vs Hydrocortisone Alone on Time Alive and Free of Vasopressor Support Among Patients With Septic Shock: The VITAMINS Randomized Clinical Trial. Jama 2020;323:423–31.
[128] Sevransky JE, Rothman RE, Hager DN, et al. Effect of Vitamin C, Thiamine, and Hydrocortisone on Ventilator- and Vasopressor-Free Days in Patients With Sepsis: The VICTAS Randomized Clinical Trial. Jama 2021;325:742–50.
[129] Masse MH, Ménard J, Sprague S, et al. Lessening Organ dysfunction with VITamin C (LOVIT): protocol for a randomized controlled trial. Trials 2020;21:42.
[130] Taylor EN, Stampfer MJ, Curhan GC. Dietary factors and the risk of incident kidney stones in men: new insights after 14 years of follow-up. J Am Soc Nephrol 2004;15:3225–32.
[131] Alkhunaizi AM, Chan L. Secondary oxalosis: a cause of delayed recovery of renal function in the setting of acute renal failure. J Am Soc Nephrol 1996;7:2320–6.
[132] Levine M, Rumsey SC, Daruwala R, et al. Criteria and recommendations for vitamin C intake. Jama 1999;281:1415–23.
[133] Iwamoto N, Kawaguchi T, Horikawa K, et al. Haemolysis induced by ascorbic acid in paroxysmal nocturnal haemoglobinuria. Lancet 1994;343:357.
[134] Radomski MW, Palmer RM, Moncada S. Glucocorticoids inhibit the expression of an inducible, but not the constitutive, nitric oxide synthase in vascular endothelial cells. Proc Natl Acad Sci U S A 1990;87:10043–7.
[135] Sprung CL, Annane D, Keh D, et al. Hydrocortisone therapy for patients with septic shock. N Engl J Med 2008;358:111–24.
[136] Annane D, Renault A, Brun-Buisson C, et al. Hydrocortisone plus Fludrocortisone for Adults with Septic Shock. N Engl J Med 2018;378:809–18.
[137] Marcucci M, Painter TW, Conen D, et al. Rationale and design of the PeriOperative ISchemic Evaluation-3 (POISE-3): a randomized controlled trial evaluating tranexamic acid and a strategy to minimize hypotension in noncardiac surgery. Trials 2022;23:101.
[138] Yang YF, Zhu YJ, Long YQ, et al. Withholding vs. Continuing Angiotensin-Converting Enzyme Inhibitors or Angiotensin Receptor Blockers Before Non-cardiac Surgery in Older Patients: Study Protocol for a Multicenter Randomized Controlled Trial. Front Med (Lausanne) 2021;8:654700.

ELSEVIER
MOSBY

Advances in Anesthesia 40 (2022) 93–109

ADVANCES IN ANESTHESIA

Contemporary Perioperative Management of Direct Oral Anticoagulants

Juan G. Ripoll, MD[a], Allan M. Klompas, MB, BCh, BAO[a], Bradford B. Smith, MD[b], Mark M. Smith, MD[a,*]

[a]Department of Anesthesiology and Perioperative Medicine, Mayo Clinic College of Medicine, 200 First Street Southwest, Rochester, MN 55905, USA; [b]Department of Anesthesiology and Perioperative Medicine, Mayo Clinic College of Medicine, 5777 East Mayo Boulevard, Phoenix, AZ 85054, USA

Keywords

• Direct oral anticoagulants • Novel oral anticoagulants • Anticoagulant reversal • Bleeding • Transfusion

Key points

- It is now estimated that more patients in the United States take direct oral anticoagulants (DOACs) than warfarin for approved anticoagulation indications.
- The perioperative management of DOACs has evolved in recent years with regards to discontinuation periods and emergent reversal strategies.
- Reversal agents are available for DOACs; however, a lack of universal availability emphasizes that providers must understand alternative treatment options.

INTRODUCTION

Perioperative coagulopathy and bleeding due to anticoagulant use is directly associated with increased risk for morbidity and mortality. Historically, warfarin has been the most widely used oral anticoagulant worldwide. During the last 2 decades, direct oral anticoagulants (DOACs) have rapidly emerged as an alternative to warfarin in the setting of nonvalvular atrial fibrillation, prevention and treatment of venous thromboembolism and secondary prevention of arterial thrombosis in the setting of coronary and peripheral arterial disease [1]. It is now estimated that more patients in the United States take DOACs than warfarin for the aforementioned indications [1,2]. Studies to date have shown

*Corresponding author. *E-mail address:* Smith.Mark2@mayo.edu

https://doi.org/10.1016/j.aan.2022.06.002

that these drugs are similarly efficacious with perhaps a lower bleeding risk profile than warfarin. In addition, the predictable pharmacologic profile and lack of routine laboratory testing have made such drugs an attractive alternative to warfarin, which means DOACs are here to stay and will likely continue to increase in popularity.

DOACs or sometimes also referred to as novel oral anticoagulants are a group of synthetic anticoagulants that include factor Xa inhibitors (apixaban, rivaroxan, edoxaban, betrixaban) and direct thrombin inhibitors (dabigatran). The pharmacodynamics and pharmacokinetics between these classes of medications are quite different, as is the approach to emergent reversal in the setting of life-threatening bleeding or need for emergent surgery. Although most providers have been long familiar with warfarin reversal strategies that included transfusion of allogenic plasma historically and more recently prothrombin complex concentrates (PCCs), reversal strategies for DOACs are often unfamiliar. The purpose of this review is to provide insight into the currently available DOACs and discuss the management and reversal strategies for patients in the perioperative period.

Direct oral anticoagulants: factor Xa inhibitors

Background

Before the introduction of DOACs, warfarin was the preferred oral anticoagulant for the prevention of clot formation [3]. However, warfarin has multiple limitations because it exhibits a wide pharmacokinetic variability and numerous drug interactions. Moreover, it has a narrow therapeutic window requiring periodic international normalized ratio (INR) monitoring and the adherence to strict dietary restrictions [4–6]. Multiple studies have shown that patients only spend about half of their treatment within the therapeutic INR goal [7]. Due to these limitations, alternative DOACs, such as factor Xa inhibitors (FXaIs), have rapidly gained popularity in the medical field [6]. Contrary to warfarin, FXaIs exhibit a short half-life, rapid onset of action, and predictable pharmacokinetics [5]. In addition, these medications display a wide therapeutic window avoiding the need for routine monitoring of the anticoagulant effect [5]. Due to their superior pharmacodynamic profile, FXaIs are nowadays considered as first-line agents for oral anticoagulation in many clinical conditions [8–11].

Pharmacology

Factor Xa is uniquely positioned at the convergence of both intrinsic and extrinsic coagulation pathways and its activation is pivotal for hemostasis [4–6]. Indeed, one molecule of factor Xa generates approximately 1×10^3 molecules of thrombin [4–6]. Although it exhibits proliferative and proinflammatory activities, the role of factor Xa outside the coagulation cascade is limited [12]. Direct FXaIs are small synthetic molecules with similar chemical structures whose anticoagulant effect is accomplished by binding to the active site pocket of factor Xa in an L-shaped fashion preventing the interaction with prothrombin, thereby blocking the synthesis of thrombin, and interfering with clot formation (Fig. 1) [4,5]. This mechanism of action allows these medications to inhibit both clot-bound and free thrombin, which constitutes a potential advantage over the indirect thrombin inhibitors [12]. Furthermore, they are not neutralized by platelet factor 4, which eliminates the risk of thrombocytopenia [4,5].

The pharmacodynamic and pharmacokinetic profiles of direct FXaIs have several advantages over warfarin. Their rapid onset (time to peak: 1–4 hours) and shorter elimination half-life (5–27 hours) makes them suitable for clinical use due to sustained anticoagulant activity for up to 24 hours and the avoidance of bridging therapies [4–6]. In addition, FXaIs have a lower predisposition to drug–drug interactions, predictable anticoagulation effect and no interactions with food components (do not require restriction on vitamin K-containing products) allowing a fixed-dose administration and limiting the need for periodic monitoring [4–6].

The majority of direct FXaIs undergo hepatic metabolism. The excretion of FXaIs is mainly via the kidneys or biliary system. Because a significant percentage undergoes unchanged renal elimination, periodic monitoring of the kidney function is warranted [4–6]. A summary of the pharmacologic properties of FXaIs is presented in Table 1. Along with the pharmacodynamic benefits, FXaIs have shown favorable clinical results compared with warfarin in large-scale clinical trials [9,11]. As a result, these anticoagulants are approved by

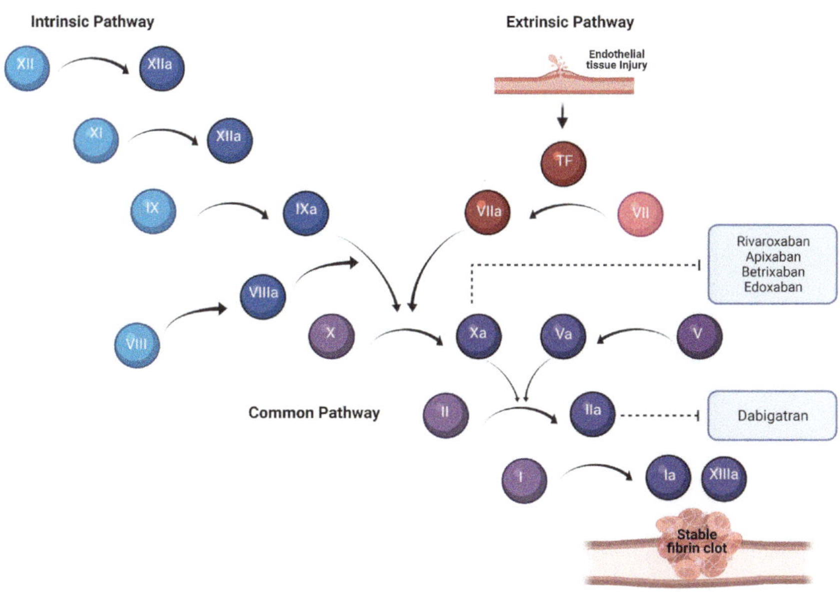

Fig. 1. Direct oral anticoagulants: mechanisms of action. Rivaroxaban, Apixaban, betrixaban, and edoxaban directly inhibit factor Xa. Dabigatran directly inhibits thrombin (factor IIa). TF, tissue factor. Created with BioRender.com.

Table 1
Pharmacologic properties of direct oral anticoagulants

	Dabigatran Pradaxa	Rivaroxaban Xarelto	Apixaban Eliquis	Edoxaban Lixiana and Savaysa	Betrixaban Bevyxxa
Inhibitory target	Factor IIa	Factor Xa	Factor Xa	Factor Xa	Factor Xa
Molecular weight (Da)	627	436	460	548	451
Prodrug	Yes	No	No	No	No
Time to peak (h)	0.5–2	2–4	3–4	1–2	3–4
Bioavailability	3%–7%	80%–100%	50%	62%	34%
Volume of distribution (L)	50–70	50	21	107	32
Half-life (h)	12–17	5–9	12	10–14	19–27
Metabolism	Conjugation	CYP dependent and independent mechanism	CYP dependent mechanism	CYP dependent and independent mechanism	CYP independent mechanism
Active metabolites	Yes, 4 acyl glucuronides	No	No	Yes (<15%)	No
Renal excretion (%)	>80	66	25	35	17.8
Fecal excretion	82%–88%	26.4%	46.7%–56%	62.2%	85%
Dosing	Oral twice daily	Oral once daily	Oral twice daily	Oral once daily	Oral once daily
Dialyzable	Yes	No	No	No	No

Abbreviation: CYP, Cytochrome P450.

The United States Food and Drug Administration (FDA) and suggested by multiple clinical guidelines as preferred therapy for the treatment of stroke and systemic embolism in patients with nonvalvular atrial fibrillation, treatment of acute deep venous thrombosis (DVT) or pulmonary embolism (PE), prevention of venous thromboembolism following knee or hip surgery, and secondary prevention for PE or DVT [8–11]. Furthermore, FXaIs are associated with lower bleeding risks compared with the vitamin K antagonists (eg, warfarin). Large clinical studies have shown an overall lower risk of major bleeding, intracranial hemorrhage, clinically relevant nonmajor bleeding and total bleeding [13].

Measurement of the anticoagulant effect

Antifactor Xa activity. Chromogenic antifactor Xa assays using specific calibrators are the monitoring tests of choice for direct FXaIs. Antifactor Xa activity assays calibrated with drug-specific standards depicts a high degree of linear correlation for edoxaban, apixaban, betrixaban, and rivaroxaban across the on-therapy range [14,15]. Although drug-specific calibration increases accuracy, it is not widely available and is expensive (Table 2) [14,15]. In the absence of a drug-specific calibration curve, using a curve calibrated for either low molecular weight heparin (LMWH) or unfractioned heparin could serve as surrogate for ruling out supratherapeutic anticoagulation levels [14,15].

Prothrombin time. Rivaroxaban and edoxaban prolong the prothrombin time (PT) in a dose-dependent manner mainly due to the interassay variability dependent on the reagents used [14–16]. In fact, PT reagents markedly differ in their sensitivity to rivaroxaban and edoxaban. At best, PT can be used as a qualitative marker because it exhibits insufficient sensitivity to exclude on-therapy levels of both anticoagulants [14–16]. The PT is less sensitive to apixaban than it is for edoxaban and rivaroxaban, and it is not suitable to quantitively or qualitatively assess the effects of the medication [14,15]. This is likely due to greater interassay variability and the fact that apixaban binds to factor Xa more slowly [14,15]. Interestingly, the dilute PT assay (reagent diluted 16 times) for edoxaban has overall improved sensitivity over the conventional PT and displays a similar sensitivity to the antifactor Xa [16].

Activated partial prothrombin time. The activated partial prothrombin time (aPTT) has poor sensitivity for FXaIs and should not be used to assess either quantitively or qualitatively their anticoagulant effect. It has a nonlinear dose-dependent prolongation and a significant interassay variability [14,15].

Other assays. Thromboelastography (TEG) and Rotation thromboelastometry (ROTEM) could detect the presence of on-therapy or supratherapeutic levels of direct FXaIs but lack accuracy and are nonspecific [14].

Periprocedural discontinuation of anticoagulant therapy

Nearly 10% of patients on FXaIs undergo surgical or invasive procedures each year and preoperative elective discontinuation is frequently necessary to

Table 2
Perioperative management of direct oral anticoagulants

Drug	Interval (Days) Between Last Dose and Procedure			Resumption After Procedure		Perioperative Testing	Reversal Agents	
	Low Bleeding Risk		High Bleeding Risk	Low Bleeding Risk	High Bleeding Risk	Specific Tests	Specific (Antidote)	Nonspecific
Dabigatran Pradaxa	CrCl >50 mL/min CrCl 30–50[b] mL/min	2 d 2–3 d	3 d 5 d	24 h (Postoperative day 1)	48–72 h (Postoperative days 2–3)	Chromogenic antifactor IIa assay	Idarucizumab	aPCC PCC Hemodialysis Activated charcoal
Rivaroxaban Xarelto	CrCl >50 or CrCl 30–50 mL/min	2 d	3 d			Chromogenic antifactor Xa assay	Andexanet alfa	PCC aPCC Activated charcoal
Apixaban Eliquis Edoxaban Lixiana and Savaysa Betrixaban Bevyxxa	CrCl >50 mL/min or CrCl <50 mL/min[a]	2 d	3 d					

Abbreviations: aPCC, activated prothrombin complex concentrate; CrCl, creatinine clearance; PCC, prothrombin complex concentrate; rFVIIa, recombinant activated factor VII.
Examples of high bleeding risk procedures: Neurosurgical, urologic, head and neck, orthopedic, and cardiovascular surgeries.
Examples of low bleeding risk procedures: Cholecystectomy, thoracentesis, tooth extractions, pacemaker and defibrillator insertion, abdominal hernia repair.
[a]Edoxaban: avoid use in patients with CrCl <15 mL/min.
[b]Dabigatran: avoid use in patients with CrCl <30 mL/min.

mitigate the bleeding risks [11,17,18]. However, before one can determine whether elective discontinuation of factor Xa-inhibitors is required for a given intervention, it is important to establish the thromboembolic risk of the patient (eg, CHA2DS2VASc score in atrial fibrillation), the periprocedural surgical bleeding risk (high risk–2 day risk of major bleeding 2%–4%; low risk–2 day risk of major bleeding 0%–2%), the clinical effect of bleeding should it occur, and the patient's risk factors that convey an increased bleeding risk (eg, HAS-BLED in atrial fibrillation) [9,17–19]. Furthermore, it is imperative to determine whether the elective interruption of anticoagulation is needed based on clinical judgment considering the unique characteristics of each patient (eg, hepatic and renal function) and the pharmacologic properties of each medication (see Table 1) [9,17,18].

Patients on direct FXaIs who require elective discontinuation will have a shorter perioperative period without anticoagulation when compared with warfarin [9,17,18]. This is mainly due to the rapid resolution of the anticoagulant effect when the medication is discontinued preoperatively coupled with a rapid onset of the peak effect when the medication is resumed postoperatively [17]. Hence, the reliable pharmacologic profiles of FXaIs allow a safe perioperative discontinuation and resumption while maintaining the balance between thromboembolic and bleeding risks [9,17,18].

Clinical evidence is unable to support a uniform guideline and most recommendations guiding periprocedural anticoagulation are solely based on expert consensus [11,15–18,20]. A summary of the current recommendations incorporating the most recent clinical evidence is presented in Table 2.

Bridging therapy. Bridging therapy is not routinely advised in patients on direct FXaIs due to their rapid offset and onset of action [11,15–18,20]. More importantly, discontinuation of FXaIs has not been shown to result in rebound hypercoagulability [11,15–18,20]. Despite the growing evidence about the limited to nonexistent benefits of bridging therapy, its use should be evaluated on a case-by-case basis, particularly in patients with high thromboembolic risk.

Overview of emergent factor Xa inhibitor reversal

Compared with the unpredictability of anticoagulation with vitamin K antagonists, the FXaIs generally work very rapidly after administration with predictable pharmacokinetics allowing many bleeding events to be managed conservatively until the drug effects wear off using supportive measures such as compression, procedural source control, volume resuscitation, and transfusion support [1]. As nicely summarized in the guidelines published by the Anticoagulation Forum, FXaI reversal should only be used for life-threatening bleeding, when conservative measures fail, or when an emergent procedure is required and cannot be performed without reversal due to excessive bleeding risk and there is a high expectation of clinically significant FXaI levels [1]. Before committing to reversal, it may be worthwhile to review the case with pharmacy to determine the predicted kinetics in relation to the timing of the procedure.

In addition to the intended effects of mitigating bleeding, each reversal strategy carries the risk of thromboembolic complications (TEC) both by returning a patient back to their intrinsic "prothrombotic" state as well as direct prothrombotic effects of the reversal itself. Each anticoagulant:reversal pair carries a different risk of TECs that must be weighed against that of continued anticoagulation in each clinical situation.

In general, 4 reversal strategies have been studied: reversal with plasma, PCCs, specific antidotes, or the use of antifibrinolytics (see Table 2). Due to the novelty of this class of medications, these recommendations are rapidly changing; however, consensus seems to have been found. Although no longer first-line recommendations for the reversal of vitamin K antagonists, allogeneic plasma may be used for warfarin reversal when PCCs are unavailable. Importantly, this does *not* extend to FXaI reversal outside of significant hemorrhage requiring a large volume, balanced resuscitation [21,22]. Additionally, the Anticoagulation Forum has suggested that the large volumes of plasma needed to overcome FXa inhibition (if at all) significantly increase the risk of transfusion reactions and volume overload [22]. Despite this consensus, a 2018 survey of North American Anesthesiologists found that plasma was the preferred DOAC reversal strategy by 54% of respondents before emergency surgery and by 68% for major bleeding [21]. Although the reasons for this are likely multifactorial, plasma should not generally be used to reverse FXaI in the setting of emergent surgery or major bleeding unless part of a balanced resuscitation for significant blood loss.

Most of the evidence for reversing FXaIs comes from the off-label use of 4 factor PCCs and more recently, with the factor Xa decoy fragment andexanet alfa in the setting of major bleeding with only limited evidence for preoperative use.

PCCs are highly purified, inactive, heat-treated, nanofiltered, and preservative-free hemostatic blood products made from the cryoprecipitate supernatant of pooled human plasma. Inactive PCCs can be either 3 factor PCCs (factors II, IX, X; Bebulin Baxter Healthcare Corporation, Deerfield, IL) or 4 factor PCCs (factors II, VII, IX, X; Kcentra CSL Behring, King of Prussia, PA) with a resultant overall clotting factor concentration nearly 25 times higher than plasma [23]. In addition to inactive PCCs, there is also an active PCC formulation, antiinhibitor coagulant complex (FEIBA Baxter Healthcare Corporation, Deerfield, IL), which is the sole activated PCC (4 factor) developed for treatment of hemophilia A or B with inhibitors. In addition to activated factor VII, this product contains proenzymes of the prothrombin complex (FII, VII, IX, and X), along with small amounts of the respective activation products. In current clinical practice, inactive 4 factor PCC is the most widely used factor concentrate [24].

Although initially developed for patients with hemophilia B, PCCs gained popularity after the FDA approved the use of the inactive 4 factor PCC Kcentra for warfarin reversal in patients with acute major bleeding and/or need for an urgent surgery or invasive procedure [24,25]. Contemporary off-label uses of these hemostatic agents include the treatment or prophylaxis of bleeding in congenital or acquired deficiency of any vitamin K-dependent coagulation factors, major trauma requiring a massive transfusion, correction of coagulopathy during the perioperative period in patients not on anticoagulation (ie, postcardiopulmonary bypass coagulopathy), and life-threatening hemorrhage in patients on DOACs when antidote therapy is unavailable [25].

In 2018, Levy and colleagues [26] showed that PCCs were able to partially reverse PT and completely reverse endogenous thrombin potential in healthy volunteers anticoagulated with rivaroxaban; however, there was no improvement in bleeding after a hemostatic challenge. Importantly, the same study trialed tranexamic acid monotherapy to aid hemostasis and showed no improvement in PT, thrombin generation, or clinical bleeding, suggesting antifibrinolytics are unhelpful as monotherapy for FXaI reversal [26].

Several prospective cohort studies and retrospective reviews of real-world use have shown the efficacy of PCCs for reversing FXaIs in bleeding patients (usually intracranial and gastrointestinal hemorrhages) with reasonable safety profiles. Effective hemostasis was achieved in 65% to 87.5% of patients with up to 8% experiencing early TECs, with ischemic stroke being the most common [27–29]. A recent retrospective study compared PCCs to activated PCC (aPCC) for FXaI reversal with active hemorrhage [30]. Good or excellent hemostasis was achieved in 87% of aPCC and 89% PCC, with no inpatient TECs, suggesting there may be little benefit to utilizing activated factors for FXaI reversal [30]. Although rarely emphasized, preoperative FXaI reversal with PCC was explicitly evaluated by Santibanez and colleagues [31] as a subset of their retrospective review of 42 total patients requiring FXaI reversal including 36 for bleeding events and 6 for preoperative optimization. Effective hemostasis was achieved in 81% of bleeding patients and 66.7% of preoperative patients while TECs were observed in 5.6% and 16.7%, respectively [31]. A recent meta-analysis on PCC use for the reversal of FXaI related bleeding incorporated 33 studies with 2568 patients with an overall low quality of evidence [32]. Regardless of PCC dose (high vs low), they demonstrated effective hemostasis in about 80% of patients, TECs in 3%, and approximately 15% overall mortality [32].

A huge paradigm shift occurred following the publication of the ANEXXA-4 trial in April 2019. This trial used the factor Xa decoy fragment andexanet alfa to reverse apixaban, rivaroxaban, edoxaban, or LMWH-related acute bleeding in 352 patients within 18 hours of their FXaI dose [33]. In this group, 82% had good or excellent hemostatic efficacy at 12 hours with 10% suffering a TEC within 30 days and a 14% overall mortality at 30 days [33]. Importantly, they showed the in vitro reversal effects were waning within about 4 hours of administration [33]. Together, this foundational study led to andexanet alfa gaining FDA approval for the reversal of rivaroxaban-related and apixaban-related bleeding [1].

Subsequent studies comparing andexanet alfa to PCCs have generally shown comparable results. In a 2020 retrospective review of FXaI reversal for intracranial hemorrhage, excellent or good hemostasis was achieved in 88.9% with andexanet versus 60% in PCCs, whereas TECs were 16.7% versus 9.1%, respectively [34]. Similarly, a 2021 retrospective review of FXaI reversal for hemorrhage found effective hemostasis in 75% with andexanet versus 62.5% with PCCs and TECs rate of 25% and 18.8%, respectively [35]. Following the ANDEXXA-4 trial, Lipari and colleagues [36] retrospectively applied the strict andexanet alfa use criteria to their PCC use for FXaI-related bleeding and demonstrated a clinical success of 90% with a TEC rate of 2.5%. They estimated that had they used andexanet alfa in this patient pool, the per patient costs would increase by US$29,500 [36]. Similarly, other studies have estimated the costs of andexanet alfa use per patient to be greater than US$22,000 compared to around US$5600 with PCCs [34,37]. In a 2021 meta-analysis incorporating 60 studies and 4735 patients receiving DOAC reversal included 936 patients treated with andexanet alfa and 2688 patients treated with PCC. Effective hemostasis was demonstrated in 80.7% in andexanet versus 80.1% with PCCs; however, TECs were found in only 4.3% of PCCs use and 10.7% with andexanet alfa [38].

Although guidelines are rapidly changing as new data emerges, the consistent recommendation to reverse FXaI-related bleeding or before emergent surgery is to use a targeted reversal agent (andexanet alfa) when available, or to consider the off-label use of PCCs when targeted agents are not available [39]. In addition to emergent reversal strategies, activated charcoal should also be considered with recent ingestion to limit additional drug uptake [40].

In addition to the significant difference in cost, perioperative andexanet alfa use may pose real clinical consequences. As a factor Xa decoy molecule, andexanet alfa is an effective inhibitor of heparin and therefore complicates the management of cases where heparin is required for procedural anticoagulation (ie, cardiopulmonary bypass, vascular surgery, and so forth) [39]. In one profound example, a patient that received 2 doses of andexanet alfa for apixaban reversal before emergency cardiac surgery required 80,000 units of heparin to achieve adequate anticoagulation for cardiopulmonary bypass at a cost of nearly US$50,000 [41,42]. If procedural anticoagulation (ie, heparin) is required, we strongly recommend a thorough evaluation and discussion before using andexanet alfa. Often, alternative therapy with PCCs if preoperative reversal is necessary, or delaying andexanet alfa until after periprocedural anticoagulation with heparin has concluded avoids this challenging scenario.

Direct thrombin inhibitors

Background

Direct thrombin inhibitors (DTIs) are a class of medications that directly bind and inactivate thrombin. Oral and intravenous (IV) DTIs are used clinically as anticoagulant alternatives to warfarin or heparin, for venous thromboembolism prophylaxis, during percutaneous coronary intervention (PCI), and in the treatment of heparin-induced thrombocytopenia (HIT) [43,44]. Anesthesia providers should be familiar with DTIs because they may be tasked with caring for patients prescribed these medications or may be required to administer these medications in the perioperative period.

Pharmacology

Thrombin, a critical enzyme in clot formation, is responsible for the conversion of fibrinogen to fibrin, platelet activation, and stimulation of factors V, VIII, and XI [43]. DTIs are unique in their mechanism of action because they bind and inactivate both circulating and clot-bound thrombin (see Fig. 1). Furthermore, DTIs do not rely on cofactors such as antithrombin and do not blind plasma proteins such as PF4, resulting in a predictable anticoagulant response without induction of antiheparin/PF4 antibodies responsible for type II HIT [44].

Dabigatran was first approved by the FDA in 2010 for the prevention and treatment of venous thromboembolism, ischemic heart disease, and stroke prevention in patients with nonvalvular atrial fibrillation [45]. Dabigatran is not approved for patients with mechanical heart valves or during pregnancy. Dosing typically ranges from 75 to 220 mg once or twice daily, based on indication and renal function. Compared with warfarin, dabigatran is thought to have similar if not superior efficacy, with an overall lower severe bleeding risk [46]. As the only oral DTI available clinically, dabigatran is a prodrug converted in the liver that does not bind plasma proteins and has minimal food and drug interactions, resulting in predictable pharmacokinetics (half-life 14–17 hours) without the need for routine laboratory monitoring [47]. Renal elimination is predominant with most of the drug being excreted unchanged in the urine (see Table 1). Given the dependence on renal excretion dose reduction is necessary in patients with renal impairment and administration is not recommended in patients with a creatinine clearance (CrCl) < 30 mL/min [45].

Measurement of the anticoagulant effect

In general, all DTIs prolong the PT/INR, aPTT, and thrombin clot time [48]. The direct thrombin time (dTT) is the most reliable and available test to determine presence or absence of systemic dabigatran. When results of the dTT results are outside of the normal limits in patients taking dabigatran, ongoing anticoagulation effect should be assumed. Although the ecarin clotting time (ECT) can also be beneficial in this regard, most institutions do not offer testing making application in this setting largely impractical. Some institutions offer a dabigatran specific assay (chromogenic antifactor IIa assay); however, this is often a send out test and widespread availability is lacking (see Table 2). Routine monitoring is not recommended in patients taking dabigatran, although renal function and coagulation testing should be evaluated before initiation of therapy. In patients taking dabigatran and presenting for urgent/emergent surgery and/or bleeding patients, coagulation test abnormalities including prolonged PT/INR, aPTT, activated clotting time, and dTT can be helpful to determine drug presence with the latter being most specific. In the perioperative period, TEG may also be clinically useful in the setting of ongoing bleeding because a prolonged R-time would be expected in patients with residual DTI inhibition [49].

Periprocedural discontinuation of dabigatran

In patients taking dabigatran presenting for elective or nonemergent surgery, discontinuation before surgical procedures is dependent on the risk of surgical bleeding as mentioned previously, and patient renal function. Given the known perioperative bleeding risk associated with dabigatran, surgical delay to allow drug clearance is preferred in most elective and nonemergent settings. Patients undergoing surgical procedures with high bleeding risk and normal renal function should receive their last dose of dabigatran 3 days prior, whereas those with high bleeding risk and a CrCl of 30 to 50 mL/min should receive their last dose 5 days prior. Moreover, patients undergoing low bleeding risk procedures with normal or impaired renal function (CrCl 30–50 mL/min) should receive their last dose of dabigatran 2 to 3 days prior (see Table 2) [50]. The American Society of Regional Anesthesia recommends elective discontinuation of dabigatran should occur 3 to 5 days before surgical procedures requiring neuraxial, deep plexus, and deep peripheral nerve blocks and is dependent on renal function as outlined below: Dabigatran should be discontinued for 72 hours in patients with a CrCl of 80 mL or more per minute, discontinued for 96 hours in patients with a CrCl of 50 to 79 mL/min, and discontinued for 120 hours in patients with a CrCl of 30 to 49 mL/min. If neuraxial or peripheral nerve blocks are being considered before these time intervals, dTT or ECT testing should be considered, if clinically available [15]. There is no recommendation regarding an acceptable level of dabigatran inhibition before performing neuraxial or peripheral nerve blocks [51].

Bridging therapy. Bridging therapy is rarely indicated for patients taking dabigatran due to their rapid offset and onset of action [11,15–18,20]. Despite the limited to nonexistent benefits of bridging therapy, its use should be evaluated on a case-by-case basis, particularly in patients with high thromboembolic risk.

Overview of emergent dabigatran reversal

In patients presenting with life-threatening bleeding and/or need for emergent surgery for which delay allowing drug clearance is not practical, dabigatran reversal may be necessary. In 2015, the FDA approved idarucizumab for emergent reversal of dabigatran (see Table 2) [52]. Idarucizumab is a humanized monoclonal antibody fragment that works by binding and neutralizing systemic anticoagulation effects of dabigatran [52]. The dosing for idarucizumab is a 5-gram infusion given in 2 × 2.5 gram doses no more than 15 minutes apart. In the REVERSE-AD study, which led to the FDA approval for idarucizumab, the population consisted of 301 patients presenting with life-threatening bleeding and 202 patients before undergoing urgent/emergent procedures [52]. In a subgroup analysis of the surgical cohort of the REVERSE-AD trial, the results were favorable with regards to normal periprocedural hemostasis in 91% of patients and a 30-day thromboembolic rate of 5%

[53]. This cohort of included patients undergoing the following surgical procedure subtypes; orthopedic (n = 45), abdominal (n = 49), cardiovascular (n = 34), and neurologic (n = 8).

Idarucizumab is currently the only reversal therapy for dabigatran that has been studied in surgical patients. Although the use of idarucizumab would be first-line therapy in the setting of emergent reversal of dabigatran, universal availability at all facilities is lacking. When reversal of dabigatran is required and the antidote idarucizumab is not available, alternative treatment with aPCC or PCC is recommended; however, data supporting efficacy/safety in surgical patients is currently lacking [54,55]. Due to dabigatran's distal inhibition of the coagulation cascade, aPCC may be more efficacious than PCC; however, robust studies in perioperative patients do not exist [56]. Guidance from the Anticoagulation Forum suggests that aPCC at a dose of 50 units/kg be given in these emergent reversal scenarios for which idarucizumab is not available, citing a small study where hemostasis in bleeding patients was reported as good or moderate [1]. Although recombinant-factor VIIa (rFVIIa) and PCCs have been studied in healthy volunteers, animals models and in vitro, there is insufficient data to support the widespread use in surgical setting [1]. Hemodialysis can facilitate the removal of a portion (~50%) of circulating dabigatran; however, the practical use of such therapy in the emergent perioperative setting is unlikely [1]. Activated charcoal should also be considered with recent ingestion to limit additional drug uptake [40]. The use allogenic plasma transfusion to reverse the effects of dabigatran anticoagulation is unlikely to be beneficial outside of massive transfusion scenarios as part of a balanced transfusion ratio to help restore normal blood volume and composition, or in the treatment of factor-mediated coagulopathy that ensues from ongoing bleeding and/or hemodilution.

In summary, patients requiring elective nonurgent surgical procedures who are taking dabigatran should discontinue according to the aforementioned guidance before proceeding to surgery. For patients with life-threatening bleeding and/or need for emergent surgery procedures for which bleeding risk is of concern, active reversal with idarucizumab is recommended. The off-label use aPCC, PCC, and rFVIIa in the setting of dabigatran reversal lacks quality evidence and should only considered when more conservative options are not feasible and/or idarucizumab is unavailable.

SUMMARY

The use of DOACs is rapidly expanding and providers should be familiar with the perioperative management of these anticoagulants. A thorough understanding of the pharmacologic principles, available periprocedural guidelines, drug–drug interactions, effects on laboratory assays and reversal strategies equip clinicians to face the challenges that may arise during elective and nonelective surgical procedures. Further studies are needed to help standardize the perioperative discontinuation and reversal strategies among the different medical societies.

CLINICS CARE POINTS

- DOACs have several advantages over warfarin meaning use and indications will continue to grow.
- Proper perioperative management of DOACs requires an understanding of which patients need therapy discontinuation, how long the discontinuation period should be before surgery, and how to test for residual drug presence and/or emergenty reverse the anticoagulant effects of DOACs when necessary.

Disclosure

Dr Mark Smith was part of investigator initiated clinical trial, which received research support from CSL Behring. ClinicalTrials.gov Identifier: NCT02557672.

References

[1] Cuker A, Burnett A, Triller D, et al. Reversal of direct oral anticoagulants: guidance from the anticoagulation forum. Am J Hematol 2019;94(6):697–709.
[2] Lauffenburger JC, Farley JF, Gehi AK, et al. Factors driving anticoagulant selection in patients with atrial fibrillation in the United States. Am J Cardiol 2015;115(8):1095–101.
[3] Wardrop D, Keeling D. The story of the discovery of heparin and warfarin. Br J Haematol 2008;141(6):757–63.
[4] Becker RC. Factor Xa inhibitors: critical considerations for clinical development and testing. J Thromb Thrombolysis 2021;52(2):397–402.
[5] Schreuder M, Reitsma PH, Bos MHA. Reversal agents for the direct factor xa inhibitors: biochemical mechanisms of current and newly emerging therapies. Semin Thromb Hemost 2020;46(8):986–98.
[6] Yeh CH, Fredenburgh JC, Weitz JI. Oral direct factor Xa inhibitors. Circ Res 2012;111(8): 1069–78.
[7] Baker WL, Cios DA, Sander SD, et al. Meta-analysis to assess the quality of warfarin control in atrial fibrillation patients in the United States. J Manag Care Pharm 2009;15(3):244–52.
[8] Verma A, Ha ACT, Rutka JT, et al. What surgeons should know about non-vitamin K oral anticoagulants: a review. JAMA Surg 2018;153(6):577–85.
[9] January CT, Wann LS, Calkins H, et al. 2019 AHA/ACC/HRS focused update of the 2014 AHA/ACC/HRS guideline for the management of patients with atrial fibrillation: A Report of the American College of Cardiology/American Heart Association Task Force on Clinical Practice Guidelines and the Heart Rhythm Society. Heart Rhythm 2019;16(8):e66–93.
[10] Hindricks G, Potpara T, Dagres N, et al. 2020 ESC Guidelines for the diagnosis and management of atrial fibrillation developed in collaboration with the European Association for Cardio-Thoracic Surgery (EACTS): The Task Force for the diagnosis and management of atrial fibrillation of the European Society of Cardiology (ESC) Developed with the special contribution of the European Heart Rhythm Association (EHRA) of the ESC. Eur Heart J 2021;42(5):373–498.
[11] Stevens SM, Woller SC, Kreuziger LB, et al. Antithrombotic Therapy for VTE Disease: Second Update of the CHEST Guideline and Expert Panel Report. Chest 2021;160(6): e545–608.
[12] Laux V, Perzborn E, Heitmeier S, et al. Direct inhibitors of coagulation proteins - the end of the heparin and low-molecular-weight heparin era for anticoagulant therapy? Thromb Haemost 2009;102(5):892–9.

[13] Chai-Adisaksopha C, Crowther M, Isayama T, et al. The impact of bleeding complications in patients receiving target-specific oral anticoagulants: a systematic review and meta-analysis. Blood 2014;124(15):2450–8.
[14] Samuelson BT, Cuker A. Measurement and reversal of the direct oral anticoagulants. Blood Rev 2017;31(1):77–84.
[15] Horlocker TT, Vandermeuelen E, Kopp SL, et al. Regional anesthesia in the patient receiving antithrombotic or thrombolytic therapy: american society of regional anesthesia and pain medicine evidence-based guidelines (Fourth Edition). Reg Anesth Pain Med 2018;43(3): 263–309.
[16] Narouze S, Benzon HT, Provenzano D, et al. Interventional spine and pain procedures in patients on antiplatelet and anticoagulant medications (second edition): guidelines from the american society of regional anesthesia and pain medicine, the european society of regional anaesthesia and pain therapy, the american academy of pain medicine, the international neuromodulation society, the north american neuromodulation society, and the world institute of pain. Reg Anesth Pain Med 2018;43(3):225–62.
[17] Doherty JU, Gluckman TJ, Hucker WJ, et al. 2017 ACC expert consensus decision pathway for periprocedural management of anticoagulation in patients with nonvalvular atrial fibrillation: a report of the american college of cardiology clinical expert consensus document task force. J Am Coll Cardiol 2017;69(7):871–98.
[18] Tomaselli GF, Mahaffey KW, Cuker A, et al. 2020 ACC expert consensus decision pathway on management of bleeding in patients on oral anticoagulants: a report of the american college of cardiology solution set oversight committee. J Am Coll Cardiol 2020;76(5): 594–622.
[19] Spyropoulos AC, Douketis JD. How I treat anticoagulated patients undergoing an elective procedure or surgery. Blood 2012;120(15):2954–62.
[20] Navas-Blanco JR, Martini A, Fabbro M 2nd. Expert consensus decision pathway of the american college of cardiology on management of bleeding in patients with oral anticoagulants: a review of the 2020 update for perioperative physicians. J Cardiothorac Vasc Anesth 2021;35(8):2471–9.
[21] Levy JH, Connors JM, Steiner ME, et al. Management of oral anticoagulants prior to emergency surgery or with major bleeding: A survey of perioperative practices in North America: communication from the Scientific and Standardization Committees on Perioperative and Critical Care Haemostasis and Thrombosis of the International Society on Thrombosis and Haemostasis. Res Pract Thromb Haemost 2020;4(4):562–8.
[22] Burnett AE, Mahan CE, Vazquez SR, et al. Guidance for the practical management of the direct oral anticoagulants (DOACs) in VTE treatment. J Thromb Thrombolysis 2016;41(1):206–32.
[23] Franchini M, Lippi G. Prothrombin complex concentrates: an update. Blood Transfus 2010;8(3):149–54.
[24] Smith MM, Ashikhmina E, Brinkman NJ, et al. Perioperative use of coagulation factor concentrates in patients undergoing cardiac surgery. J Cardiothorac Vasc Anesth 2017;31(5): 1810–9.
[25] Scharman CD, Shatzel JJ, Kim E, et al. Off-label use of 4-factor prothrombin complex concentrate is common despite little known benefit: a retrospective study. Eur J Haematol 2018;101(3):349–53.
[26] Levy JH, Moore KT, Neal MD, et al. Rivaroxaban reversal with prothrombin complex concentrate or tranexamic acid in healthy volunteers. J Thromb Haemost 2018;16(1): 54–64.
[27] Majeed A, Agren A, Holmstrom M, et al. Management of rivaroxaban- or apixaban-associated major bleeding with prothrombin complex concentrates: a cohort study. Blood 2017;130(15):1706–12.

[28] Marcos-Jubilar M, Garcia Erce JA, Martinez-Calle N, et al. Safety and effectiveness of a prothrombin complex concentrate in approved and off-label indications. Transfus Med 2019;29(4):268–74.
[29] Schulman S, Gross PL, Ritchie B, et al. Prothrombin complex concentrate for major bleeding on factor Xa inhibitors: a prospective cohort study. Thromb Haemost 2018;118(5):842–51.
[30] Castillo R, Chan A, Atallah S, et al. Treatment of adults with intracranial hemorrhage on apixaban or rivaroxaban with prothrombin complex concentrate products. J Thromb Thrombolysis 2021;51(1):151–8.
[31] Santibanez M, Lesch CA, Lin L, et al. Tolerability and effectiveness of 4-factor prothrombin complex concentrate (4F-PCC) for warfarin and non-warfarin reversals. J Crit Care 2018;48:183–90.
[32] Milioglou I, Farmakis I, Neudeker M, et al. Prothrombin complex concentrate in major bleeding associated with DOACs; an updated systematic review and meta-analysis. J Thromb Thrombolysis 2021;52(4):1137–50.
[33] Connolly SJ, Crowther M, Eikelboom JW, et al. Full study report of andexanet alfa for bleeding associated with factor Xa inhibitors. N Engl J Med 2019;380(14):1326–35.
[34] Barra ME, Das AS, Hayes BD, et al. Evaluation of andexanet alfa and four-factor prothrombin complex concentrate (4F-PCC) for reversal of rivaroxaban- and apixaban-associated intracranial hemorrhages. J Thromb Haemost 2020;18(7):1637–47.
[35] Stevens VM, Trujillo TC, Kiser TH, et al. Retrospective Comparison of Andexanet Alfa and 4-Factor Prothrombin Complex for Reversal of Factor Xa-Inhibitor Related Bleeding. Clin Appl Thromb Hemost 2021;27:10760296211039020.
[36] Lipari L, Yang S, Milligan B, et al. Emergent reversal of oral factor Xa inhibitors with four-factor prothrombin complex concentrate. Am J Emerg Med 2020;38(12):2641–5.
[37] Frontera JA, Bhatt P, Lalchan R, et al. Cost comparison of andexanet versus prothrombin complex concentrates for direct factor Xa inhibitor reversal after hemorrhage. J Thromb Thrombolysis 2020;49(1):121–31.
[38] Gomez-Outes A, Alcubilla P, Calvo-Rojas G, et al. Meta-analysis of reversal agents for severe bleeding associated with direct oral anticoagulants. J Am Coll Cardiol 2021;77(24):2987–3001.
[39] Milling TJ, Pollack CV. A review of guidelines on anticoagulation reversal across different clinical scenarios - Is there a general consensus? Am J Emerg Med 2020;38(9):1890–903.
[40] Levy JH, Faraoni D, Spring JL, et al. Managing new oral anticoagulants in the perioperative and intensive care unit setting. Anesthesiology 2013;118(6):1466–74.
[41] Flaherty D, Connors JM, Singh S, et al. Andexanet alfa for urgent reversal of apixaban before aortic surgery requiring cardiopulmonary bypass: a case report. A A Pract 2019;13(7):271–3.
[42] Levy JH, Welsby I. Andexanet alfa use in patients requiring cardiopulmonary bypass: quo vadis? A A Pract 2019;13(12):477.
[43] Di Nisio M, Middeldorp S, Buller HR. Direct thrombin inhibitors. N Engl J Med 2005;353(10):1028–40.
[44] Weitz JI, Eikelboom JW, Samama MM. New antithrombotic drugs: antithrombotic therapy and prevention of thrombosis, 9th ed: American College of chest physicians evidence-based clinical practice guidelines. Chest 2012;141(2 Suppl):e120S–51S.
[45] Lemay A, Kaye AD, Urman RD. Novel anticoagulant agents in the perioperative setting. Anesthesiol Clin 2017;35(2):305–13.
[46] Escobar C, Barrios V, Lip GYH, et al. Effectiveness and safety of dabigatran compared to Vitamin K antagonists in non-asian patients with atrial fibrillation: a systematic review and meta-analysis. Clin Drug Investig 2021;41(11):941–53.
[47] Hauel NH, Nar H, Priepke H, et al. Structure-based design of novel potent nonpeptide thrombin inhibitors. J Med Chem 2002;45(9):1757–66.
[48] Weitz JI, Crowther M. Direct thrombin inhibitors. Thromb Res 2002;106(3):V275–84.

[49] Bliden KP, Chaudhary R, Mohammed N, et al. Determination of non-Vitamin K oral anticoagulant (NOAC) effects using a new-generation thrombelastography TEG 6s system. J Thromb Thrombolysis 2017;43(4):437–45.
[50] Schulman S, Carrier M, Lee AY, et al. Perioperative management of dabigatran: a prospective cohort study. Circulation 2015;132(3):167–73.
[51] Narouze S, Benzon HT, Provenzano DA, et al. Interventional spine and pain procedures in patients on antiplatelet and anticoagulant medications: guidelines from the American Society of Regional Anesthesia and Pain Medicine, the European Society of Regional Anaesthesia and Pain Therapy, the American Academy of Pain Medicine, the International Neuromodulation Society, the North American Neuromodulation Society, and the World Institute of Pain. Reg Anesth Pain Med 2015;40(3):182–212.
[52] Pollack CV Jr, Reilly PA, van Ryn J, et al. Idarucizumab for dabigatran reversal - full cohort analysis. N Engl J Med 2017;377(5):431–41.
[53] Levy JH, van Ryn J, Sellke FW, et al. Dabigatran reversal with idarucizumab in patients requiring urgent surgery: a subanalysis of the RE-VERSE AD Study. Ann Surg 2021;274(3):e204–11.
[54] Diaz MQ, Borobia AM, Nunez MA, et al. Use of prothrombin complex concentrates for urgent reversal of dabigatran in the Emergency Department. Haematologica 2013;98(11): e143–4.
[55] Schulman S, Ritchie B, Goy JK, et al. Activated prothrombin complex concentrate for dabigatran-associated bleeding. Br J Haematol 2014;164(2):308–10.
[56] Ghadimi K, Levy JH, Welsby IJ. Prothrombin complex concentrates for bleeding in the perioperative setting. Anesth Analg 2016;122(5):1287–300.

Advances in Anesthesia 40 (2022) 111–130

ADVANCES IN ANESTHESIA

What Is the Role of Dexmedetomidine in Modern Anesthesia and Critical Care?

Adaora M. Chima, MBBS, MPH[a,b,*], Mohamed A. Mahmoud, MD[a,b], Suryakumar Narayanasamy, MBBS, MD[a,b]

[a]Department of Anesthesiology, Cincinnati Children's Hospital Medical Center, MLC 2001, 3333 Burnet Avenue, Cincinnati, OH 45229, USA; [b]University of Cincinnati, College of Medicine, Cincinnati, OH, USA

Keywords

• Adult • Pediatric • Anesthesia • Procedural sedation • Organ protection • Anti-inflammatory properties • Palliative care sedation • Intensive care unit sedation

Key points

- Currently, there is ample literature on the efficacy and safety of dexmedetomidine for sedation in adults and pediatric patients.
- Dexmedetomidine is one of many drugs that is not FDA (Food and Drug Administration) approved for use in pediatric patients but is used daily in clinical practice.
- Evidence indicates that perioperative administration of dexmedetomidine suppresses surgical stress and inflammation and preserves the immunity of surgical patients.
- Dexmedetomidine has been found to reduce the need for mechanical ventilation in patients who are on noninvasive ventilation and to reduce time to extubation and ICU (Intensive Care Unit) length of stay.

INTRODUCTION

The unique properties of dexmedetomidine (DEX) have sparked new interest in the use of alpha-2 adrenoceptor agonists and have led to a rapid increase in its use in clinical care. In contrast to traditional sedative agents, DEX seems to

*Corresponding author. *E-mail address:* adaora.chima@cchmc.org

https://doi.org/10.1016/j.aan.2022.06.003

provide a neuropharmacological profile that simulates natural sleep pathways. DEX has also been shown to possess anti-inflammatory properties and to provide sympatholysis and anesthetic-sparing effects without relevant respiratory depression. In addition, there is an increasing body of literature showing evidence supporting DEXs organ-protective effects against ischemic and hypoxic injury. DEX is approved only for intravenous (IV) administration but has been administered via intramuscular, buccal, and most recently subcutaneously, in regional blockade. A comprehensive understanding of the predictable side effects, effects of age-related physiologic changes, pharmacokinetic and pharmacodynamic effects of DEX is critical to maximize its safe application in adults and children. This comprehensive review focuses on the growing body of literature around recent advances of clinical applications of DEX in the adult and pediatric population.

DEX is a highly selective, short-acting, alpha-2 adrenoreceptor agonist. DEX has been shown to have a beneficial pharmacologic profile that includes analgesic sparing effects, anxiolysis, sympatholysis, organ-protective effects against ischemic and hypoxic injury, and sedation which parallels natural sleep [1]. In animal studies, DEX has been shown to effectively reduce inflammatory markers and ischemia-reperfusion markers and thus has the potential to mitigate reperfusion sequelae in relevant procedures [2].

The experience and enthusiasm for this novel sedative agent continues to grow. More established treatment regimens describe its use for procedural sedation, as an adjunct to attenuate emergence agitation, as premedication for anxiolysis and as an adjunct to anesthesia (general and regional), palliative care, and for sedation in the intensive care setting. This review focuses on recent literature examining advances in applications of DEX in children and adults.

PERIOPERATIVE APPLICATIONS OF DEXMEDETOMIDINE

A summary of the current adult and pediatric perioperative applications of DEX is provided in Table 1.

PREOPERATIVE APPLICATIONS

DEX is one of many drugs *not* FDA approved for use in pediatric populations, that are commonly used on a daily basis in children.

For pediatric premedication before induction of anesthesia, intranasal administration is preferred. The intranasal route is a well-tolerated, convenient, effective method of administration for many medications and could be an alternative to traditional premedication for the pediatric population. Previous reports have recommended wide ranging intranasal DEX doses from 0.5 to 4 μg/kg [3,4]. The most frequently used doses range from 0.5 to 2 μg/kg and can be administered 30 to 60 minutes before the procedure.

For adult patients, reservations about prescribing sedative premedications due to concerns of delayed recovery from anesthesia have been countered by a Cochrane review that found no evidence to support such concerns in the ambulatory setting [5]. Intranasal DEX at doses of 1 to 1.5 μg/kg [6,7]

Table 1
Current common perioperative applications of dexmedetomidine in children and adults

Applications	Advantage(s)
Pre-Procedure:	
Anxiolysis	Easy and quick arousal from sedation Minimal respiratory depression Attenuates sympathetic hemodynamic response
Intraoperative/Procedural:	
Adjunct to general anesthesia	Reduces Minimum Alveolar Concentration (MAC), inhalational and IV anesthetic requirement Reduces opioid requirement
Adjunct to regional anesthesia	Faster onset of block and longer duration
Airway procedures	
Rigid bronchoscopy	Obtunds airway reflexes while maintaining spontaneous ventilation
MRI sleep studies	Stable hemodynamic and respiratory effects
Drug-induced sleep endoscopy	Maintenance of spontaneous ventilation
Open airway surgeries	Provides sedative properties paralleling natural sleep
Difficult intubation	
Intrathoracic masses with risk of airway compromise	
Bariatric surgery	Potentiates opioid analgesia with minimal additional respiratory depression
Cardiac surgery	Blunts sympathetic response Provides analgesia and sedation postoperatively Expedite extubation
Fetal and obstetric surgery	Sedation for minimally invasive fetal surgeries Ameliorates neuraxial associated itching Neuroprotective may alleviate neurotoxicity from inhalational agents
Neurosurgical procedures	
Brain tumor and epileptic seizure	Preserves epileptiform activity
Awake craniotomy	Allows comfortable and cooperative sedation
Posterior spine fusions	Lowers propofol and inhalational agents requirements Facilitates intraoperative wake-up tests
Vascular surgery	Provides excellent hemodynamics due to its sympatholytic effects
Carotid endarterectomy	
Carotid angioplasty and stenting	
Post–Procedure:	
Patients with obstructive sleep apnea	Reduces opioid requirements Reduces episodes of oxygen desaturation
Postoperative shivering	Reduces incidence with intravenous and neuraxial administration
Postoperative emergence agitation	May reduce the incidence of severe emergence agitation
Sedation in the intensive care	Produces a state of cooperative sedation associated with minimal respiratory depression Facilitates withdrawal from benzodiazepines or opioids
Miscellaneous applications	
Palliative care	May provide a bridge to wean opioid dependence

has been found to be safe and efficacious for premedication in healthy adults. Adults are more likely to have preoperative IV access and can receive IV doses of 0.5 to 2 μg/kg, following careful consideration of age, comorbidities, and hemodynamic effects. A recent prospective randomized controlled trial examined its use as a sedative premedication in 81 adult patients scheduled for elective suspension laryngoscopy and showed that intranasal DEX induced favorable perioperative anxiolysis without prolonging anesthesia recovery [8]. However, when sedating elderly patients, one must consider the effects of age-related physiologic changes to renal and hepatic function, and changes in body composition, which can alter pharmacokinetics. A recent double-blinded, placebo-controlled, single ascending dose study examined the safety and tolerability of intranasal DEX in 48 surgical patients greater than 65 years of age. The investigators concluded that intranasal DEX is not suitable for routine sedation in the elderly due to its high incidence of profound and sustained hypotension irrespective of beta-blocker status [9].

INTRAOPERATIVE APPLICATIONS

In the intraoperative period, DEX is a valuable adjunct due to its sedating, analgesic, sympatholytic, and potentially antiarrhythmic properties. The authors describe the value of intraoperative DEX administration for a variety of surgical specialty scenarios and purposes as follows.

Procedural sedation

Most of 49 systematic reviews/meta-analyses on the pediatric use of DEX report that DEX provides adequate sedation and favorable postoperative recovery [10,11]. In pediatric patients, intranasal DEX administration is a convenient mode of sedation for noninvasive diagnostic procedures such as transthoracic echocardiography or prolonged radiologic imaging such as MRI. Unlike midazolam, intranasal DEX is not painful and is thus easier to administer. Its dosing ranges 2 to 4 μg/kg as a dose of 2 μg/kg can attain a plasma concentration of sedative efficacy within 10 minutes and can reach peak plasma concentration at 47 minutes on average [12], making it suitable for appropriately timed imaging studies. Like other intranasal sedatives, DEX administration by atomizer or drops is equally effective [13]. In these cases, advantages over similarly effective sedatives include non-noxious administration in the absence of IV access, sustained airway patency and respiratory mechanics. Other diagnostic procedures that have been successfully performed under DEX sedation include electroencephalogram (EEG) and auditory brainstem response (ABR). DEX does not hinder EEG interpretation [14] or affect epileptiform activities [15]. Although there are reports of successful DEX sedation for ABRs [16,17], there is little literature on the direct impact of DEX on ABR signals. In the pediatric population, DEX efficacy decreases with increasing age [13]. Thus, it would be prudent to adjust dosing or consider adjuvant medication for additive or synergistic effects.

Table 2
Dexmedetomidine applications and suggested dosing from literature

Preoperative	Route	Dose[a]
Anxiolysis		
Children	Intranasal	2–4 μg/kg
Adults	Intranasal	1–2 μg/kg [116]
	IV	0.5–2 μg/kg [116]
Electroconvulsive therapy		0.5–1 μg/kg [19]
Intraoperative use		
Airway procedures		
Awake fiberoptic	IV	1–2 μg/kg bolus, followed by infusion of 0.3-2 μg/kg/h [23,24]
Abdominal		
Transplant	IV	0.2–0.8 μg/kg/h [44,45]
Bariatric	IV	1 μg/kg followed by 0.5 μg/kg/h [40]
Cardiothoracic	IV	0.5 μg/kg followed by 0.5 μg/kg/h [37]
Dental	Intranasal	1–1.5 μg/kg [56]
		2 μg/kg [57]
	IV	1–2 μg/kg followed by 0.4 μg/kg/h
Neurosurgery (cognitive benefits)	IV	0.3 μg/kg bolus and 0.3 μg/kg/h [32]
Regional adjunct	IV	0.5–1 μg/kg max dose of 150 mcg [62]
	Intrathecal	5–10 μg [117,118]
Postoperative applications		
Emergence agitation	IV	0.3–0.5 μg/kg [74]
Postoperative shivering	IV	0.75–1 μg/kg [81]; 0.3 μg/kg [82,119] (post-spinal anesthesia)

Abbreviation: IV, intravenous.

[a]Doses are suggestions based on available literature and should be adjusted based on age, comorbidities, and infusions should be titrated to effect, adjusting for hemodynamic response. IV boluses should be administered over 10mins to minimize hemodynamic effects.

For procedural sedation in adults, DEX has been used as a primary agent, adjunct to other sedating agents or adjunct to local anesthetic. Its dosing varies widely in the literature (Table 2) and it can be administered as a single bolus, constant infusion or both [18]. Bolus dosing should be administered over 10 to 20 minutes to ameliorate hemodynamic responses (hypotension, bradycardia, less commonly hypertension), and existing comorbidities should inform its use, dose, and titration. In electroconvulsive therapy, premedication with DEX has a dose-dependent effect on the hyperdynamic response to electroconvulsive therapy with variable effects on motor seizure duration. In a study in adults by Limpoon and colleagues, a dose of 1 μg/kg attenuated the sympathetic hemodynamic response but was associated with a slightly shorter motor seizure duration. A dose of 0.5 μg/kg does not have as much of an effect on the hemodynamic response, with minimal effect on motor seizure duration [19]. Similar attenuation was seen in another adult study comparing effects of DEX, esmolol, and lidocaine in electroconvulsive therapy [20]. Thus, DEX may ameliorate cardiac events with electroconvulsive therapy. There have been other studies showing insignificant hemodynamic differences with the use of DEX, but it is unclear what influence sample size or anesthetic regimen had on these findings.

Airway procedures

In adult or pediatric patients with critical airways that require fiberoptic intubation, the goal is to secure the airway while maintaining spontaneous ventilation, minimizing discomfort, and preventing aspiration, obstruction/airway collapse, or injury. Patients are often anxious and require sufficient sedation and analgesia that does not compromise either respiratory mechanics or cognition. Following airway topicalization with local anesthetics, DEX can be used as a sole agent [21] or in conjunction with other sedatives [22] or analgesics to produce optimal conditions for intubation. As a solitary agent, a loading dose of DEX at 1 μg/kg over 10 minutes followed by an IV infusion of 0.3 to 0.7 μg/kg/h (until airway securement) has been found to provide optimal conditions for intubation in adults [23,24]. Its antisialagogue properties make DEX the preferred agent over ketamine in patients with significant airway secretions. This ability to maintain spontaneous ventilation while maintaining upper airway patency makes DEX an attractive choice for drug-induced sleep endoscopy and dynamic airway imaging and planned surgical interventions [25–27].

Neurosurgery

In neurosurgical cases where functional assessments, mapping, or testing stimulation are necessary, an unresponsive patient is undesirable [28]. For example, during deep brain stimulation electrode implantation, intraoperative assessment of accurate electrode placement can be impacted by the type of anesthetic administered. The preferred anesthetic is monitored anesthesia care sedation with agents that are unlikely to abolish the underlying neurologic symptoms. The use of DEX in these surgeries has grown as it provides some analgesia, preserves respiratory drive, and has minimal effect on the multichannel microelectrode recording at recommended doses, while preserving symptoms [29]. At higher doses, there is a risk of abolishing neurologic symptoms and causing bradycardia and hypotension [29,30]. Patients are also easily arousable for interactive neurologic examinations and stimulation tests as DEX provides sedation similar to natural sleep [30,31].

An aging population is associated with an increased incidence of neurovascular disease, necessitating neurovascular interventions such as carotid endarterectomy. Although there is controversy about the effect of a carotid endarterectomy on cognitive function, there is enough concern to consider using anesthesia techniques that mitigate procedure-related cognitive decline. A study examining the cognitive function and cerebral injury/ischemia markers after carotid endarterectomy indicated a neuroprotective effect with the use of intraoperative DEX [32]. At the doses used in this study (0.3 μg/kg bolus and 0.3 μg/kg/h infusion), the relative occurrence of bradycardia and hypotension was statistically insignificant.

Many cranial and spine surgeries require intraoperative neuromonitoring and the use of anesthetic agents that have minimal effects on neurophysiologic responses and evoked potentials. In brainstem and supratentorial cranial surgeries, the inclusion of DEX does not seem to affect somatosensory evoked potentials. However, it significantly decreases transcranial motor evoked potential amplitude [33]. Similar effects on transcranial motor evoked potential were seen in pediatric spine surgeries, although the clinical significance was unclear [34].

Cardiothoracic surgery

DEXs sympatholytic effect suggests its possible utility in preventing intraoperative and postoperative arrhythmias (such as atrial fibrillation) during cardiac surgery cases. However, the Lancet DECADE trial conducted in adult cardiac surgery patients showed that intraoperative and postoperative DEX administration did not reduce the occurrence of atrial fibrillation and was associated with an elevated risk of delirium [35]. An earlier meta-analysis of perioperative use of DEX among cardiac surgery patients had shown that intraoperative DEX was associated with decreased risk of ventricular tachycardia and a higher risk of bradycardia [36].

In pediatric cardiac cases, DEX has been used in the perioperative prophylactic management of junctional ectopic tachycardia [37], an arrhythmia with significant morbidity and mortality. Systematic reviews show that intraoperative DEX can be used for junctional ectopic tachycardia, hemodynamic stability, blunting of the sympathetic stress response and to reduce the duration of mechanical ventilation. Bradycardia and hypotension are potential side effects that have been noted in varying degrees [37,38]. As described above, DEX is also being used in noninvasive sedation when performing transthoracic electrocardiograms in uncooperative children [39].

In thoracic cases necessitating one-lung ventilation, DEX improves oxygenation by preserving hypoxic pulmonary vasoconstriction and decreasing pulmonary shunt [40], which is inhibited by inhalational agents. These effects have been attributed to the attenuation of proinflammatory factors, bronchodilation, and the reduction of minimum alveolar concentration requirements with agents like propofol, which contribute to pulmonary shunting [41].

Abdominal surgery

In a study of surgical gastrointestinal cases, DEX was found to reduce the circulating proinflammatory mediators Interleukin 6 (IL-6), 8, 10, Tumor Necrosis Factor alpha (TNF-alpha), and C-reactive protein [42]. In large quantities, these proinflammatory mediators can trigger severe inflammatory reactions that cause exudation, mechanical obstruction, and cell death, resulting in poor wound healing and increased morbidity. Intraoperative DEX administration reduces the minimum alveolar concentration requirements of volatile agents and opioids, mitigating opioid-related gastrointestinal complications [42] and has been associated with earlier return of bowel function [43]. These effects may be due to DEXs anti-inflammatory effect (Fig. 1) as well as reduced opioid intake.

Several studies have identified the benefits of intraoperative low-dose DEX (0.2–0.8 μg/kg/h) in mitigating inflammation and hepatic ischemic reperfusion

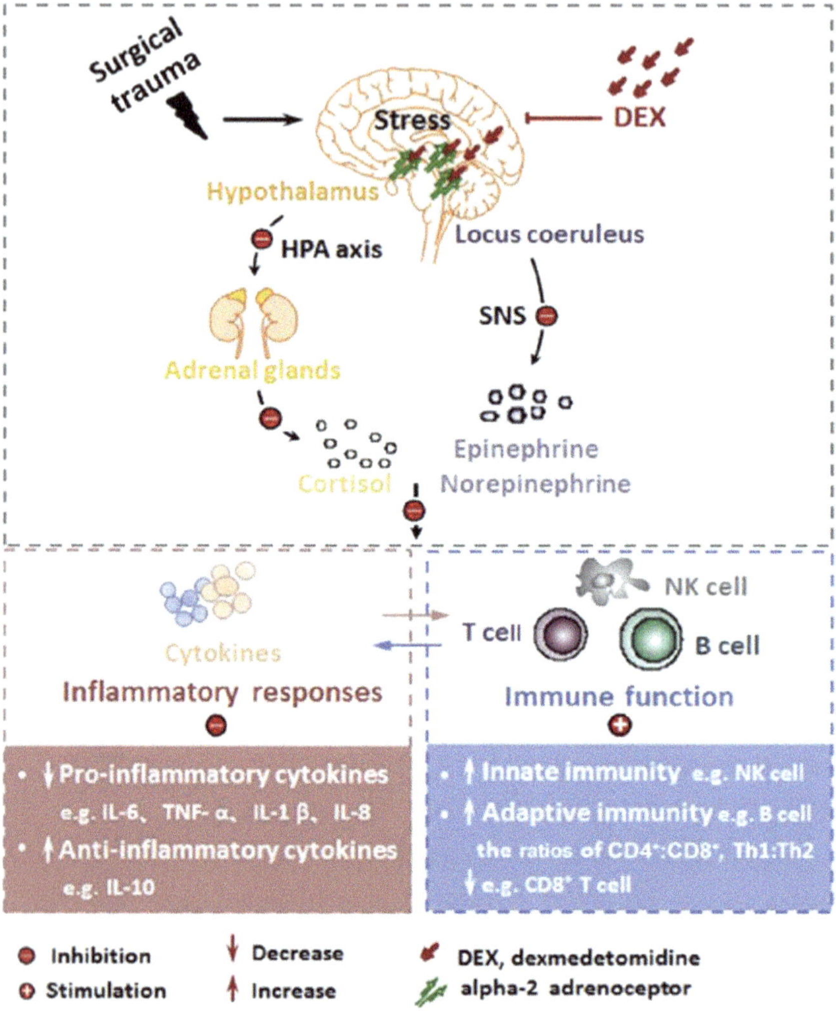

Fig. 1. Schematic that surgical trauma triggers perioperative stress, systemic inflammation, and immune suppression, all of which are negated by dexmedetomidine (DEX). HPA: hypothalamic–pituitary–adrenal; SNS: sympathetic nervous system.From Wang K, Wu M, Xu J, et al. Effects of dexmedetomidine on perioperative stress, inflammation, and immune function: systematic review and meta-analysis. Br J Anaesth. Dec 2019;123(6):777-794. doi:10.1016/j.bja.2019.07.027, with permission.

injury in adult liver transplantation [44] and reducing delayed kidney graft function [45]. Hepatic inflammatory markers and histopathological changes were attenuated in the intervention group as well as extrahepatic sequelae of reperfusion injury. A similar result was found in a retrospective cohort study of pediatric liver transplant recipients of deceased donors, with a reduced frequency of moderate to severe hepatic ischemic reperfusion injury [46].

Fetal surgery

The potentially neuroprotective effect of DEX is a driver for its choice when sedating parturient patients undergoing minimally invasive fetal surgery, with the goal of avoiding neurotoxicity in the fetus. In several animal studies, DEX has been shown to have no neuroapoptotic effect and seems to ameliorate neurotoxic effects from halogenated agent exposure in the developing brain [47,48].

Ambulatory procedures

In gastrointestinal procedures such as diagnostic and interventional endoscopy, DEX infusions have utility in preserving spontaneous ventilation while providing sufficient sedation, anxiolysis, and analgesia compared with benzodiazepines such as midazolam, with no significant difference in cardiopulmonary complications or recovery time. Reported rates range from 0.2 to 0.7 μg/kg/h [49].

A meta-analysis of the use of DEX in adults receiving nonoperating room anesthesia showed similar or higher physician and patient satisfaction compared with various control agents. The investigators reported a lower risk of desaturation below 90% to 92%. Like other studies, a higher incidence of bradycardia and hypotension was noted, and difference in recovery time was not statistically significant [50].

Obesity and bariatric surgery

Among bariatric surgical patients, intraoperative DEX (bolus and or infusion) has been associated with improved oxygenation, higher lung compliance, reduced dead space, and lower plateau pressures [40]. These are all factors that would improve intraoperative ventilation mechanics and reduce the risk of postoperative ventilation requirements.

Multiple studies have shown differing DEX pharmacokinetics and pharmacodynamics between obese and nonobese patients, and as yet, it is unclear what specific weight-based modifications should be made to dosing. Differing study designs and potentially synergistic effects with other administered anesthetic agents make it challenging to compare findings in available publications [51,52]. However, there are consistent reports of reduced clearance in obese patients [53], thus it would be prudent to dose DEX using lean body weight or ideal body weight [54,55] as done with other anesthetic agents that need to be dosed differently in obese patients and titrated to desired effect.

Dental procedures

DEX has been used successfully for premedication and sedation in pediatric dental patients as a solitary agent and an adjunct [56]. In a study comparing a combination of intranasal DEX and oral ketamine with midazolam, the former was found to have a more rapid onset and more efficacy providing anxiolysis and postoperative analgesia [57]. DEX has been shown to ameliorate possible emergence delirium associated with ketamine while ketamine's opposing hemodynamic effect counters DEXs effects of hypotension and bradycardia [58].

Regional anesthesia adjunct

In patients receiving a regional anesthetic as the primary anesthetic for amenable surgeries like orthopedic surgery, DEX can be used as a sedating agent with comparatively lower risk for respiratory compromise [59]. More recently, it has also proven valuable as a local anesthetic adjunct for regional anesthesia. Its addition to a local anesthetic in single shot erector spine blocks not only reduced opioid consumption but also prolonged the duration of the block [60]. A randomized clinical trial (RCT) investigating forearm sensory and motor block effects of ropivacaine and DEX compared with other adjuvants showed similar findings and faster onset of sensory block [61], as did a systematic review of RCTs involving brachial plexus blocks [62]. A meta-analysis of the optimal dose of perineural DEX reported doses ranging 0.5 μg/kg to a max of 150 μg; greater than 60 μg is associated with an increased incidence of bradycardia or hypotension [63].

Vascular surgery

In vascular procedures and surgeries, DEX is of interest because its sympatholytic effects could be protective in patients with cardiac and systemic vascular disease. However, an extensive 2018 Cochrane review did not find strong evidence that DEX or other alpha-adrenergic agents had an impact on perioperative cardiac or all-cause mortality [64,65].

POST-PROCEDURAL APPLICATIONS

Emergence agitation

Emergence agitation is a common postoperative complication after anesthesia in adults and children. Emergence agitation has been shown to increase the risk of injury, unplanned extubation, postoperative bleeding, decrease patient/family satisfaction, and prolong recovery room stay. The reported incidence of emergence agitation ranges from 30% to 50% in preschool-aged children and decreases with increasing age [66–68]. Although the exact mechanism of emergence agitation is poorly understood, possible factors in pediatric patients include rapid emergence following inhalational anesthesia, postoperative pain, type of surgery, patient age, presence of preoperative anxiety, and medications such as anticholinergics, benzodiazepines, and metoclopramide [69]. Risk factors in adult patients include old age, male sex, history of smoking and/or substance abuse, use of inhalational agents for maintenance, presence of a urinary catheter, and postoperative pain [70]. Both non-pharmacological and pharmacologic methods have been used for the prevention and treatment of emergence agitation [71]. In a meta-analysis that included 2549 patients, DEX significantly reduced the risk of emergence agitation, postoperative nausea and vomiting (PONV), and the need for rescue analgesics [72]. DEX was shown to be effective in preventing sevoflurane-related emergence agitation in children [73]. Compared with midazolam and opioids, DEX significantly decreased the incidence of emergence agitation [10]. In pediatric patients undergoing tonsillectomy, 0.3 μg/kg DEX over 10 minutes at the time of induction was shown to prevent almost all emergence agitation [74]. In children, rapid IV bolus of 0.5 μg/kg DEX was shown to reduce the incidence of emergence agitation with a significant decrease in heart rate [75]. In elderly patients, a low-dose DEX infusion at 0.2 μg/kg/h was shown to reduce emergence agitation without any hemodynamic disturbances [76].

Postoperative shivering

DEX has shown to be effective in preventing postoperative shivering when administered via the IV or neuraxial routes [77–79]. However, due to its high cost, its potential side effects, and the availability of less expensive alternatives, DEX may not be first-line agent for prevention of postoperative shivering prevention [77]. When compared with tramadol, DEX was more effective in controlling shivering with a beneficial effect on PONV [80]. Suggested dosing for prophylaxis against postoperative shivering ranges from 0.75 to 1 μg/kg [81]. DEX has also been used for prophylactic management of neuraxial-associated shivering in obstetric patients [82].

Post-anesthesia care unit recovery profile

DEX has a prolonged half-life of 2 to 3 hours which can potentially delay discharge from post-anesthesia care unit (PACU) especially in outpatient settings. In one retrospective cohort study involving outpatient MRI and endoscopic surgeries in pediatric patients with propofol and remifentanil, DEX was found to prolong the PACU stay by 5 to 7 minutes with a potential dose relationship equivalent of 15 minutes delay per microgram per kilogram of DEX administration [83]. Similarly, another study on ambulatory procedures with over 130,000 adult patients showed that DEX was associated with dose-dependent prolonged PACU length of stay mainly due to cardiovascular complications such as hypotension and bradycardia and oversedation [84]. On the other hand, a meta-analysis of 14 studies found that intranasal DEX premedication reduces the incidence of emergence agitation, PONV without increasing the PACU stay time in pediatric patients [85]. More recently, a meta-analysis focused specifically on PACU discharge times involving 33 studies in adult patients found DEX use did not increase in PACU length of stay but reduced emergence agitation, cough, pain, PONV, and shivering in PACU [86]. The benefits of DEX must be carefully weighed against potential cardiovascular changes and over sedation, especially in ambulatory surgical patients. Suggested strategies to mitigate delayed PACU discharge include administering DEX as premedication for pediatric patients or earlier rather than later during the case and using lower doses (0.5 μg/kg or less), especially in elderly patients.

CRITICAL CARE APPLICATIONS

Sedation

DEX is FDA approved for short-term (<24 hours) sedation in the intensive care setting [87]. However, it has also been used for prolonged sedation of mechanically ventilated patients in multiple studies. The PROSDEX trial studied 163 patients (mean age 13 months) who received DEX 0.4 to 0.8 μg/kg/h. DEX was found to improve patient comfort, reduce the usage of other sedative agents, and reduce the risk of withdrawal and delirium [88]. Hemodynamic effects included bradycardia, hypertension at higher doses and hypotension in the lower dose range. Withdrawal symptoms were noted in 5% of patients and were successfully managed by enteral clonidine [89]. A meta-analysis that included 3267 pediatric patients concluded that DEX can be considered relatively safe for prolonged sedation. However, high-quality data are needed on the use of DEX for prolonged sedation including the optimal dosing regimen and weaning protocols [90].

In multiple meta-analyses in adult patients, DEX was found to reduce time to extubation and length of stay in the ICU [91,92]. Similar results were observed in a Cochrane database review that specifically evaluated use of DEX for long-term (>24 hours) sedation [93]. DEX was also found to reduce the need for mechanical ventilation in patients on noninvasive ventilation [94].

DEX withdrawal syndrome after prolonged infusion has been described both in adult and pediatric patients. However, the definition of DEX withdrawal syndrome was not consistent across the studies with reported signs and symptoms of agitation, tachycardia, hypertension, decreased sleep, emesis, loose stools, diaphoresis, positive Confusion Assessment, positive Withdrawal Assessment Tool-1, among others [95]. Enteral or oral clonidine seems to be a promising option for transitioning or weaning from DEX [96]. The addition of clonidine infusion to facilitate DEX weaning did not have an impact on the agitation, duration of weaning, or ICU length of stay in patients with prolonged (>3 days) DEX infusion [97].

Sepsis and septic shock

Patients with septic shock present with decreased vasopressor responsiveness and often receive vasopressor infusions to maintain adequate perfusion. Sedating these patients with DEX can increase the risk of hemodynamic instabilities, such as bradycardia and hypotension. However, due to its central alpha-2 agonist activity, DEX has been shown to increase vasopressor responsiveness. In a recent study involving patients with septic shock requiring vasopressors, DEX was associated with lower vasopressor requirements to maintain target mean arterial pressure [98]. Similarly, in septic shock patients requiring sedation, vasopressor requirements were reduced when DEX was substituted for propofol [99].

Delirium

There are conflicting reports on the effect of DEX on delirium in the ICU. Many studies have shown a reduction in the incidence of delirium among high-risk patients, such as post-cardiac surgery, elderly and traumatic brain injury patients [100–102], and a decrease following low-dose DEX infusions to aid sleep [103]. However, there are conflicting studies that report no effect of DEX on the rate of postop delirium [35,104]. DEX has been described as a second-line therapy in patients with delirium tremens due to alcohol withdrawal [105].

PALLIATIVE CARE APPLICATIONS

Opioids are a mainstay of end of life care, used to increase patient comfort. However, increased opioid doses can have increased side effects without increased analgesic effects and can lead to poor quality of life. In the past decade, the use of DEX to improve quality of life during end of life care has steadily increased [106]. In the palliative care setting, DEX has been shown to reduce opioid requirements while reducing pain scores [107]. DEX has also been used to minimize respiratory distress and improve patient comfort during terminal weaning from mechanical ventilation [108]. Recent reports suggest that in palliative care patients, alternate routes of DEX administration (such as intranasal and continuous subcutaneous infusions) can be considered for procedural sedation for dressing changes and to manage refractory dystonia, baclofen withdrawal, and terminal delirium [109–112].

Cautions/contraindications

Although there are no absolute contraindications to DEX, it is recommended that DEX be avoided in patients with depressed left ventricular function, high-degree atrioventricular block, and volume depletion, in patients receiving digoxin, beta-adrenergic blockers, calcium channel blockers, or other agents which predispose to bradycardia or hypotension.

Caution should also be exercised when administering anticholinergics to treat DEX -associated bradycardia, as IV glycopyrrolate has been shown to elicit immediate, significant hypertension [113]. In dogs, administration of intramuscular atropine with intramuscular DEX reversed heart rate changes and hypotension, but arrhythmias (atrioventricular block, premature ventricular contractions, and bigeminy) were observed [114]. The administration of a prophylactic anticholinergic (atropine or glycopyrrolate) before DEX in pediatric imaging studies did not show any advantage other than a transient clinically insignificant increase in heart rate and systolic blood pressure [115].

SUMMARY

Data regarding the use of DEX in adults and children are promising. As is the case with any novel agent, there is a significant learning curve associated with the use of DEX. An in-depth understanding of the pharmacologic, pharmacokinetic, and pharmacodynamic effects of DEX is critical to maximize its safe use in adults and children. The benign effect of DEX on ventilatory drive is one of its major advantages over other traditional sedative agents. DEX should be strongly considered in patients with respiratory compromise for whom the preservation of spontaneous ventilation and airway tone is preferable and for whom the preservation of patient responsiveness is the goal.

CLINICS CARE POINTS

- Age and comorbidities in adults should be weighed when using DEX. These are very relevant to dosing as well as anticipating potential hemodynamic changes from DEX.
- Although bradycardia and hypotension are known side effects of DEX (especially IV boluses), these effects can be mitigated by appropriate dosing and slow administration over at least 10mins. Hypertension is a less likely side effect that is associated with rapid bolus administration.
- Early intraoperative administration of DEX can minimize emergence delirium without prolonging post op recovery or delaying discharge.
- Intranasal DEX provides a convenient non-noxious, non-invasive mode of administration that can be used in both pediatric and adult patients as premedication and sedation, with or without adjuncts.

Acknowledgments

The authors thank Maria Ashton MS, RPH, MBA for providing writing assistance, editing, and proofreading.

Disclosure

This study was supported by the Department of Anesthesiology at Cincinnati Children's Hospital Medical Center. No financial support was provided other than departmental salary support for the authors.

References

[1] Mahmoud M, Barbi E, Mason KP. Dexmedetomidine: What's New for Pediatrics? A Narrative Review. J Clin Med 2020;9(9); https://doi.org/10.3390/jcm9092724.

[2] Kohli JK, Magoon R, Dey S, et al. Evolving spectrum of dexmedetomidine preconditioning for Ischemia-reperfusion injury amelioration. J Anaesthesiol Clin Pharmacol 2020;36(2): 272–3.

[3] Pasin L, Febres D, Testa V, et al. Dexmedetomidine vs midazolam as preanesthetic medication in children: a meta-analysis of randomized controlled trials. Paediatr Anaesth 2015;25(5):468–76.

[4] Jun JH, Kim KN, Kim JY, et al. The effects of intranasal dexmedetomidine premedication in children: a systematic review and meta-analysis. Can J Anaesth 2017;64(9):947–61, Les effets d'une premedication intranasale de dexmedetomidine chez l'enfant : revue systematique et meta-analyse.

[5] Walker KJ, Smith AF. Premedication for anxiety in adult day surgery. Cochrane Database Syst Rev 2009;(4):CD002192.

[6] Yuen VM, Irwin MG, Hui TW, et al. A double-blind, crossover assessment of the sedative and analgesic effects of intranasal dexmedetomidine. Anesth Analg 2007;105(2): 374–80.

[7] Nooh N, Sheta SA, Abdullah WA, et al. Intranasal atomized dexmedetomidine for sedation during third molar extraction. Int J Oral Maxillofac Surg 2013;42(7):857–62.

[8] Lu C, Zhang LM, Zhang Y, et al. Intranasal Dexmedetomidine as a Sedative Premedication for Patients Undergoing Suspension Laryngoscopy: A Randomized Double-Blind Study. PLoS One 2016;11(5):e0154192.

[9] Barends CRM, Driesens MK, Struys M, et al. Intranasal dexmedetomidine in elderly subjects with or without beta blockade: a randomised double-blind single-ascending-dose cohort study. Br J Anaesth 2020;3; https://doi.org/10.1016/j.bja.2019.12.025.
[10] Rao Y, Zeng R, Jiang X, et al. The Effect of Dexmedetomidine on Emergence Agitation or Delirium in Children After Anesthesia-A Systematic Review and Meta-Analysis of Clinical Studies. Front Pediatr 2020;8:329; https://doi.org/10.3389/fped.2020.00329.
[11] Lian X, Lin Y, Luo T, et al. Comparison of dexmedetomidine with chloral hydrate as sedatives for pediatric patients: A systematic review and meta-analysis. Medicine (Baltimore) 2020;99(31):e21008; https://doi.org/10.1097/MD.0000000000021008.
[12] Miller JW, Balyan R, Dong M, et al. Does intranasal dexmedetomidine provide adequate plasma concentrations for sedation in children: a pharmacokinetic study. Br J Anaesth 2018;120(5):1056–65.
[13] Li BL, Zhang N, Huang JX, et al. A comparison of intranasal dexmedetomidine for sedation in children administered either by atomiser or by drops. Anaesthesia May 2016;71(5): 522–8.
[14] Mason KP, O'Mahony E, Zurakowski D, et al. Effects of dexmedetomidine sedation on the EEG in children. Paediatr Anaesth 2009;19(12):1175–83.
[15] Souter MJ, Rozet I, Ojemann JG, et al. Dexmedetomidine sedation during awake craniotomy for seizure resection: effects on electrocorticography. J Neurosurg Anesthesiol 2007;19(1):38–44.
[16] Godbehere J, Harper S, Loxey T, et al. Auditory brainstem response testing using intranasal dexmedetomidine sedation in children: a pilot study. Int J Audiol 2021;60(7):549–54.
[17] Li BL, Yuen VM, Zhou JL, et al. A randomized controlled trial of oral chloral hydrate vs intranasal dexmedetomidine plus buccal midazolam for auditory brainstem response testing in children. Paediatr Anaesth 2018;28(11):1022–8.
[18] Barends CR, Absalom A, van Minnen B, et al. Dexmedetomidine versus Midazolam in Procedural Sedation. A Systematic Review of Efficacy and Safety. PLoS One 2017;12(1):e0169525.
[19] Subsoontorn P, Lekprasert V, Waleeprakhon P, et al. Premedication with dexmedetomidine for prevention of hyperdynamic response after electroconvulsive therapy: a cross-over, randomized controlled trial. BMC Psychiatry 2021;21(1):408.
[20] Parikh DA, Garg SN, Dalvi NP, et al. Outcome of four pretreatment regimes on hemodynamics during electroconvulsive therapy: A double-blind randomized controlled crossover trial. Ann Card Anaesth 2017;20(1):93–9.
[21] Tang ZH, Chen Q, Wang X, et al. A systematic review and meta-analysis of the safety and efficacy of remifentanil and dexmedetomidine for awake fiberoptic endoscope intubation. Medicine (Baltimore) 2021;100(14):e25324.
[22] Bergese SD, Patrick Bender S, McSweeney TD, et al. A comparative study of dexmedetomidine with midazolam and midazolam alone for sedation during elective awake fiberoptic intubation. J Clin Anesth 2010;22(1):35–40.
[23] Johnston KD, Rai MR. Conscious sedation for awake fibreoptic intubation: a review of the literature. Can J Anaesth 2013;60(6):584–99.
[24] Chu KS, Wang FY, Hsu HT, et al. The effectiveness of dexmedetomidine infusion for sedating oral cancer patients undergoing awake fibreoptic nasal intubation. Eur J Anaesthesiol 2010;27(1):36–40.
[25] Mahmoud M, Gunter J, Donnelly LF, et al. A comparison of dexmedetomidine with propofol for magnetic resonance imaging sleep studies in children. Anesth Analg 2009;109(3): 745–53.
[26] Kandil A, Subramanyam R, Hossain MM, et al. Comparison of the combination of dexmedetomidine and ketamine to propofol or propofol/sevoflurane for drug-induced sleep endoscopy in children. Paediatr Anaesth 2016;26(7):742–51.

[27] Mahmoud M, Jung D, Salisbury S, et al. Effect of increasing depth of dexmedetomidine and propofol anesthesia on upper airway morphology in children and adolescents with obstructive sleep apnea. J Clin Anesth 2013;25(7):529–41.
[28] Tasbihgou SR, Barends CRM, Absalom AR. The role of dexmedetomidine in neurosurgery. Best Pract Res Clin Anaesthesiol 2021;35(2):221–9.
[29] Grant R, Gruenbaum SE, Gerrard J. Anaesthesia for deep brain stimulation: a review. Curr Opin Anaesthesiol 2015;28(5):505–10.
[30] Elias WJ, Durieux ME, Huss D, et al. Dexmedetomidine and arousal affect subthalamic neurons. Mov Disord 2008;23(9):1317–20.
[31] Zhang Z, Ferretti V, Guntan I, et al. Neuronal ensembles sufficient for recovery sleep and the sedative actions of alpha2 adrenergic agonists. Nat Neurosci 2015;18(4):553–61.
[32] Ge YL, Li X, Gao JU, et al. Beneficial effects of intravenous dexmedetomidine on cognitive function and cerebral injury following a carotid endarterectomy. Exp Ther Med 2016;11(3):1128–34.
[33] Pacreu S, Vila E, Molto L, et al. Effect of dexmedetomidine on evoked-potential monitoring in patients undergoing brain stem and supratentorial cranial surgery. Acta Anaesthesiol Scand 2021;65(8):1043–53.
[34] Mahmoud M, Sadhasivam S, Salisbury S, et al. Susceptibility of transcranial electric motor-evoked potentials to varying targeted blood levels of dexmedetomidine during spine surgery. Anesthesiology 2010;112(6):1364–73.
[35] Turan A, Duncan A, Leung S, et al. Dexmedetomidine for reduction of atrial fibrillation and delirium after cardiac surgery (DECADE): a randomised placebo-controlled trial. Lancet 2020;396(10245):177–85.
[36] Geng J, Qian J, Cheng H, et al. The Influence of Perioperative Dexmedetomidine on Patients Undergoing Cardiac Surgery: A Meta-Analysis. PLoS One 2016;11(4):e0152829.
[37] Ghimire LV, Chou FS. Efficacy of prophylactic dexmedetomidine in preventing postoperative junctional ectopic tachycardia in pediatric cardiac surgery patients: A systematic review and meta-analysis. Paediatr Anaesth 2018;28(7):597–606.
[38] Pan W, Wang Y, Lin L, et al. Outcomes of dexmedetomidine treatment in pediatric patients undergoing congenital heart disease surgery: a meta-analysis. Paediatr Anaesth 2016;26(3):239–48.
[39] Sun M, Liu H, Yu Q, et al. A Comparison of Intranasal Dexmedetomidine and Dexmedetomidine-Ketamine Combination Sedation for Transthoracic Echocardiography in Pediatric Patients With Congenital Heart Disease: A Randomized Controlled Trial. J Cardiothorac Vasc Anesth 2020;34(6):1550–5.
[40] Hasanin A, Taha K, Abdelhamid B, et al. Evaluation of the effects of dexmedetomidine infusion on oxygenation and lung mechanics in morbidly obese patients with restrictive lung disease. BMC Anesthesiol 2018;18(1):104.
[41] Xu B, Gao H, Li D, et al. Nebulized dexmedetomidine improves pulmonary shunt and lung mechanics during one-lung ventilation: a randomized clinical controlled trial. PeerJ 2020;8:e9247.
[42] Chen R, Kang Z, Wang Y, et al. The Anti-inflammatory Effect of Dexmedetomidine Administration on Patients Undergoing Intestinal Surgery: A Randomized Study. Drugs R D 2021;21(4):445–53.
[43] Li M, Wang T, Xiao W, et al. Low-Dose Dexmedetomidine Accelerates Gastrointestinal Function Recovery in Patients Undergoing Lumbar Spinal Fusion. Front Pharmacol 2019;10:1509.
[44] Fayed NA, Sayed EI, Saleh SM, et al. Effect of dexmedetomidine on hepatic ischemia-reperfusion injury in the setting of adult living donor liver transplantation. Clin Transpl 2016;30(4):470–82.
[45] Chen J, Perez R, de Mattos AM, et al. Perioperative Dexmedetomidine Improves Outcomes of Kidney Transplant. Clin Transl Sci 2020;13(6):1279–87.

[46] Zhang L, Li N, Cui LL, et al. Intraoperative Low-Dose Dexmedetomidine Administration Associated with Reduced Hepatic Ischemia-Reperfusion Injury in Pediatric Deceased Liver Transplantation: A Retrospective Cohort Study. Ann Transplant 2021;26:e933354; https://doi.org/10.12659/AOT.933354.
[47] Andropoulos DB. Effect of Anesthesia on the Developing Brain: Infant and Fetus. Fetal Diagn Ther 2018;43(1):1–11.
[48] Shan Y, Sun S, Yang F, et al. Dexmedetomidine protects the developing rat brain against the neurotoxicity wrought by sevoflurane: role of autophagy and Drp1-Bax signaling. Drug Des Devel Ther 2018;12:3617–24.
[49] Nishizawa T, Suzuki H, Sagara S, et al. Dexmedetomidine versus midazolam for gastrointestinal endoscopy: a meta-analysis. Dig Endosc 2015;27(1):8–15.
[50] Fonseca FJ, Ferreira L, Rouxinol-Dias AL, et al. Effects of dexmedetomidine in non-operating room anesthesia in adults: a systematic review with meta-analysis. Braz J Anesthesiol 2021; https://doi.org/10.1016/j.bjane.2021.12.002.
[51] Obara S, Morimoto I, Iseki Y, et al. The Effect of Obesity on Dose of Dexmedetomidine When Administered with Fentanyl during Postoperative Mechanical Ventilation–Retrospective. Fukushima J Med Sci 2015;61(1):38–46.
[52] Xu B, Zhou D, Ren L, et al. Pharmacokinetic and pharmacodynamics of intravenous dexmedetomidine in morbidly obese patients undergoing laparoscopic surgery. J Anesth 2017;31(6):813–20.
[53] Cortinez LI, Anderson BJ, Holford NH, et al. Dexmedetomidine pharmacokinetics in the obese. Eur J Clin Pharmacol 2015;71(12):1501–8.
[54] Rolle A, Paredes S, Cortinez LI, et al. Dexmedetomidine metabolic clearance is not affected by fat mass in obese patients. Br J Anaesth 2018;120(5):969–77.
[55] Ingrande J, Lemmens HJ. Dose adjustment of anaesthetics in the morbidly obese. Br J Anaesth 2010;105(Suppl 1):i16–23.
[56] Corcuera-Flores JR, Silvestre-Rangil J, Cutando-Soriano A, et al. Current methods of sedation in dental patients - a systematic review of the literature. Med Oral Patol Oral Cir Bucal 2016;21(5):e579–86.
[57] Oriby ME. Comparison of Intranasal Dexmedetomidine and Oral Ketamine Versus Intranasal Midazolam Premedication for Children Undergoing Dental Rehabilitation. Anesth Pain Med 2019;9(1):e85227.
[58] Zanaty OM, El Metainy SA. A comparative evaluation of nebulized dexmedetomidine, nebulized ketamine, and their combination as premedication for outpatient pediatric dental surgery. Anesth Analg 2015;121(1):167–71.
[59] Mei B, Meng G, Xu G, et al. Intraoperative Sedation With Dexmedetomidine is Superior to Propofol for Elderly Patients Undergoing Hip Arthroplasty: A Prospective Randomized Controlled Study. Clin J Pain 2018;34(9):811–7.
[60] Wang Q, Li H, Wei S, et al. Dexmedetomidine Added to Ropivacaine for Ultrasound-guided Erector Spinae Plane Block Prolongs Analgesia Duration and Reduces Perioperative Opioid Consumption After Thoracotomy: A Randomized, Controlled Clinical Study. Clin J Pain 2021;38(1):8–14.
[61] Moshiri E, Modir H, Kamali A, et al. Comparative analgesic, hemodynamic, pain and duration of sensory and motor block effects of dexmedetomidine, granisetron, and nitroglycerin added to ropivacaine in intravenous anesthesia for forearm surgeries: a randomized clinical study. Med Gas Res 2022;12(3):77–82.
[62] Vorobeichik L, Brull R, Abdallah FW. Evidence basis for using perineural dexmedetomidine to enhance the quality of brachial plexus nerve blocks: a systematic review and meta-analysis of randomized controlled trials. Br J Anaesth 2017;118(2):167–81.
[63] Cai H, Fan X, Feng P, et al. Optimal dose of perineural dexmedetomidine to prolong analgesia after brachial plexus blockade: a systematic review and Meta-analysis of 57 randomized clinical trials. BMC Anesthesiol 2021;21(1):233.

[64] Duncan D, Sankar A, Beattie WS, et al. Alpha-2 adrenergic agonists for the prevention of cardiac complications among adults undergoing surgery. Cochrane Database Syst Rev 2018;3:CD004126.
[65] Gallego-Ligorit L, Vives M, Valles-Torres J, et al. Use of Dexmedetomidine in Cardiothoracic and Vascular Anesthesia. J Cardiothorac Vasc Anesth 2018;32(3):1426–38.
[66] Aono J, Ueda W, Mamiya K, et al. Greater incidence of delirium during recovery from sevoflurane anesthesia in preschool boys. Anesthesiology 1997;87(6):1298–300.
[67] Uezono S, Goto T, Terui K, et al. Emergence agitation after sevoflurane versus propofol in pediatric patients. Anesth Analg 2000;91(3):563–6.
[68] Przybylo HJ, Martini DR, Mazurek AJ, et al. Assessing behaviour in children emerging from anaesthesia: can we apply psychiatric diagnostic techniques? Paediatr Anaesth 2003;13(7):609–16.
[69] Vlajkovic GP, Sindjelic RP. Emergence delirium in children: many questions, few answers. Anesth Analg 2007;104(1):84–91.
[70] Wei B, Feng Y, Chen W, et al. Risk factors for emergence agitation in adults after general anesthesia: A systematic review and meta-analysis. Acta Anaesthesiol Scand 2021;65(6): 719–29.
[71] Mason KP. Paediatric emergence delirium: a comprehensive review and interpretation of the literature. Br J Anaesth 2017;118(3):335–43.
[72] Yang X, Hu Z, Peng F, et al. Effects of Dexmedetomidine on Emergence Agitation and Recovery Quality Among Children Undergoing Surgery Under General Anesthesia: A Meta-Analysis of Randomized Controlled Trials. Front Pediatr 2020;8:580226.
[73] Sun L, Guo R, Sun L. Dexmedetomidine for preventing sevoflurane-related emergence agitation in children: a meta-analysis of randomized controlled trials. Acta Anaesthesiol Scand 2014;58(6):642–50.
[74] Zhang YZ, Wang X, Wu JM, et al. Optimal Dexmedetomidine Dose to Prevent Emergence Agitation Under Sevoflurane and Remifentanil Anesthesia During Pediatric Tonsillectomy and Adenoidectomy. Front Pharmacol 2019;10:1091; https://doi.org/10.3389/fphar.2019.01091.
[75] Hauber JA, Davis PJ, Bendel LP, et al. Dexmedetomidine as a Rapid Bolus for Treatment and Prophylactic Prevention of Emergence Agitation in Anesthetized Children. Anesth Analg 2015;121(5):1308–15.
[76] Sun M, Peng T, Sun Y, et al. Intraoperative use of low-dose dexmedetomidine for the prevention of emergence agitation following general anaesthesia in elderly patients: a randomized controlled trial. Aging Clin Exp Res 2021; https://doi.org/10.1007/s40520-021-01984-y.
[77] Liu J, Wang Y, Ma W. Shivering prevention and treatment during cesarean delivery under neuraxial anesthesia: a systematic review. Minerva Anestesiol 2018;84(12):1393–405.
[78] Hoffman J, Hamner C. Effectiveness of dexmedetomidine use in general anesthesia to prevent postoperative shivering: a systematic review. JBI Database Syst Rev Implement Rep 2016;13(12):287–313.
[79] Wang YQ, Zhang XJ, Wang Y. Effect of intrathecal dexmedetomidine on cesarean section during spinal anesthesia: a meta-analysis of randomized trials. Drug Des Devel Ther 2019;13:2933–9.
[80] Wang J, Wang Z, Liu J, et al. Intravenous dexmedetomidine versus tramadol for treatment of shivering after spinal anesthesia: a meta-analysis of randomized controlled trials. BMC Anesthesiol 2020;20(1):104.
[81] Kim YS, Kim YI, Seo KH, et al. Optimal dose of prophylactic dexmedetomidine for preventing postoperative shivering. Int J Med Sci 2013;10(10):1327–32.
[82] Yu G, Jin S, Chen J, et al. The effects of novel alpha2-adrenoreceptor agonist dexmedetomidine on shivering in patients underwent caesarean section. Biosci Rep 2019;28(2):39; https://doi.org/10.1042/BSR20181847.

[83] West N, Görges M, Poznikoff A, et al. Association of dexmedetomidine with recovery room and hospital discharge times: A retrospective cohort analysis. Paediatr Anaesth 2021;31(11):1170–8.
[84] Ma H, Wachtendorf LJ, Santer P, et al. The effect of intraoperative dexmedetomidine administration on length of stay in the post-anesthesia care unit in ambulatory surgery: A hospital registry study. J Clin Anesth 2021;72:110284.
[85] Xu C, Zhang Y, Zhang T, et al. Efficacy and Safety of Intranasal Dexmedetomidine During Recovery From Sevoflurane Anesthesia in Children: A Systematic Review and Meta-analysis. Clin Neuropharmacol 2021;44(5):157–68.
[86] Sin JCK, Tabah A, MJJ Campher, et al. The Effect of Dexmedetomidine on Postanesthesia Care Unit Discharge and Recovery: A Systematic Review and Meta-Analysis. Anesth Analg 2022; https://doi.org/10.1213/ane.0000000000005843.
[87] FDA. Dexmedetomidine package insert. Available at: https://www.accessdata.fda.gov/drugsatfda_docs/label/2020/021038Orig1s035lbl.pdf. Accessed March 8 2022.
[88] Sperotto F, Mondardini MC, Dell'Oste C, et al. Efficacy and Safety of Dexmedetomidine for Prolonged Sedation in the PICU: A Prospective Multicenter Study (PROSDEX). Pediatr Crit Care Med 2020;21(7):625–36.
[89] Shutes BL, Gee SW, Sargel CL, et al. Dexmedetomidine as Single Continuous Sedative During Noninvasive Ventilation: Typical Usage, Hemodynamic Effects, and Withdrawal. Pediatr Crit Care Med 2018;19(4):287–97.
[90] Daverio M, Sperotto F, Zanetto L, et al. Dexmedetomidine for Prolonged Sedation in the PICU: A Systematic Review and Meta-Analysis. Pediatr Crit Care Med 2020;21(7): e467–74.
[91] Constantin JM, Momon A, Mantz J, et al. Efficacy and safety of sedation with dexmedetomidine in critical care patients: a meta-analysis of randomized controlled trials. Anaesth Crit Care Pain Med 2016;35(1):7–15.
[92] Cruickshank M, Henderson L, MacLennan G, et al. Alpha-2 agonists for sedation of mechanically ventilated adults in intensive care units: a systematic review. *Health Technol Assess* Mar 2016;20(25):1–117, v-xx.
[93] Chen K, Lu Z, Xin YC, et al. Alpha-2 agonists for long-term sedation during mechanical ventilation in critically ill patients. Cochrane Database Syst Rev 2015;1(1):Cd010269.
[94] Lewis K, Piticaru J, Chaudhuri D, et al. Safety and Efficacy of Dexmedetomidine in Acutely Ill Adults Requiring Noninvasive Ventilation: A Systematic Review and Meta-analysis of Randomized Trials. Chest 2021;159(6):2274–88.
[95] Bouajram RH, Bhatt K, Croci R, et al. Incidence of Dexmedetomidine Withdrawal in Adult Critically Ill Patients: A Pilot Study. Crit Care Explor 2019;1(8):e0035.
[96] Glaess SS, Attridge RL, Christina Gutierrez G. Clonidine as a strategy for discontinuing dexmedetomidine sedation in critically ill patients: A narrative review. Am J Health Syst Pharm 2020;77(7):515–22.
[97] Berrens ZJ, Sauro AL, Tillman EM. Prevention of Withdrawal in Pediatric Patients Receiving Long-term Dexmedetomidine Infusions. J Pediatr Pharmacol Ther 2021;26(1):81–6.
[98] Cioccari L, Luethi N, Bailey M, et al. The effect of dexmedetomidine on vasopressor requirements in patients with septic shock: a subgroup analysis of the Sedation Practice in Intensive Care Evaluation [SPICE III] Trial. Crit Care 2020;24(1):441.
[99] Morelli A, Sanfilippo F, Arnemann P, et al. The Effect of Propofol and Dexmedetomidine Sedation on Norepinephrine Requirements in Septic Shock Patients: A Crossover Trial. Crit Care Med 2019;47(2):e89–95.
[100] Wu M, Liang Y, Dai Z, et al. Perioperative dexmedetomidine reduces delirium after cardiac surgery: A meta-analysis of randomized controlled trials. J Clin Anesth 2018;50: 33–42.
[101] Pereira JV, Sanjanwala RM, Mohammed MK, et al. Dexmedetomidine versus propofol sedation in reducing delirium among older adults in the ICU: A systematic review and meta-analysis. Eur J Anaesthesiol 2020;37(2):121–31.

[102] Soltani F, Tabatabaei S, Jannatmakan F, et al. Comparison of the Effects of Haloperidol and Dexmedetomidine on Delirium and Agitation in Patients with a Traumatic Brain Injury Admitted to the Intensive Care Unit. Anesth Pain Med 2021;11(3):e113802.
[103] Skrobik Y, Duprey MS, Hill NS, et al. Low-Dose Nocturnal Dexmedetomidine Prevents ICU Delirium. A Randomized, Placebo-controlled Trial. Am J Respir Crit Care Med 2018;197(9):1147–56.
[104] Deiner S, Luo X, Lin HM, et al. Intraoperative Infusion of Dexmedetomidine for Prevention of Postoperative Delirium and Cognitive Dysfunction in Elderly Patients Undergoing Major Elective Noncardiac Surgery: A Randomized Clinical Trial. JAMA Surg 2017;152(8):e171505.
[105] Dixit D, Endicott J, Burry L, et al. Management of Acute Alcohol Withdrawal Syndrome in Critically Ill Patients. Pharmacotherapy 2016;36(7):797–822.
[106] Hofherr ML, Abrahm JL, Rickerson E. Dexmedetomidine: A Novel Strategy for Patients with Intractable Pain, Opioid-Induced Hyperalgesia, or Delirium at the End of Life. J Palliat Med 2020;23(11):1515–7.
[107] Burns J, Jackson K, Sheehy KA, et al. The Use of Dexmedetomidine in Pediatric Palliative Care: A Preliminary Study. J Palliat Med 2017;20(7):779–83.
[108] Kent CD, Kaufman BS, Lowy J. Dexmedetomidine facilitates the withdrawal of ventilatory support in palliative care. Anesthesiology 2005;103(2):439–41.
[109] De Zen L, Della Paolera S, Del Rizzo I, et al. Home Intranasal Dexmedetomidine for Refractory Dystonia in Pediatric Palliative Care. J Pain Symptom Manage 2020;59(6):e3–5.
[110] Ferguson L, Wilson M. Intranasal dexmedetomidine: Procedural sedation in palliative care: A case report. Palliat Med 2021;35(8):1625–8.
[111] Laroche JP. Subcutaneous dexmedetomidine for baclofen withdrawal during palliative sedation. BMJ Support Palliat Care 2020;10(1):7–9.
[112] Thomas B, Lo WA, Nangati Z, et al. Dexmedetomidine for hyperactive delirium at the end of life: An open-label single arm pilot study with dose escalation in adult patients admitted to an inpatient palliative care unit. Palliat Med 2021;35(4):729–37.
[113] Mason KP, Zgleszewski S, Forman RE, et al. An exaggerated hypertensive response to glycopyrrolate therapy for bradycardia associated with high-dose dexmedetomidine. Anesth Analg 2009;108(3):906–8.
[114] Congdon JM, Marquez M, Niyom S, et al. Evaluation of the sedative and cardiovascular effects of intramuscular administration of dexmedetomidine with and without concurrent atropine administration in dogs. J Am Vet Med Assoc 2011;239(1):81–9.
[115] Subramanyam R, Cudilo EM, Hossain MM, et al. To Pretreat or Not to Pretreat: Prophylactic Anticholinergic Administration Before Dexmedetomidine in Pediatric Imaging. Anesth Analg 2015;121(2):479–85.
[116] Wu X, Hang LH, Wang H, et al. Intranasally Administered Adjunctive Dexmedetomidine Reduces Perioperative Anesthetic Requirements in General Anesthesia. Yonsei Med J 2016;57(4):998–1005.
[117] Naaz S, Bandey J, Ozair E, et al. Optimal Dose of Intrathecal Dexmedetomidine in Lower Abdominal Surgeries in Average Indian Adult. J Clin Diagn Res 2016;10(4):UC09–13.
[118] Gupta R, Bogra J, Verma R, et al. Dexmedetomidine as an intrathecal adjuvant for postoperative analgesia. Indian J Anaesth 2011;55(4):347–51.
[119] Abdel-Ghaffar HS, Mohamed SA, Fares KM, et al. Safety and Efficacy of Dexmedetomidine in Treating Post Spinal Anesthesia Shivering: A Randomized Clinically Controlled Dose-Finding Trial. Pain Physician 2016;19(4):243–53.

ELSEVIER MOSBY
Advances in Anesthesia 40 (2022) 131–147
ADVANCES IN ANESTHESIA

Anesthetic Management and Considerations for Electrophysiology Procedures

Yang Gu, MD[a], Heather L. Lander, MD[a], Ravie Abozaid, MD[a], Francis M. Chang, MD[a], Hugo S. Clifford, MD[a], Mehmet K. Aktas, MD[b], Brandon F. Lebow, MD[a], Kunal Panda, MD[a], Julie A. Wyrobek, MD[a,*]

[a]Department of Anesthesiology and Perioperative Medicine, University of Rochester School of Medicine & Dentistry, 601 Elmwood Avenue, Box 604, Rochester, NY 14642, USA; [b]Department of Medicine, Cardiology, University of Rochester School of Medicine & Dentistry, 601 Elmwood Ave, Floor G, Strong Ambulatory Care Facility, Rochester, NY 14642, USA

Keywords

• Electrophysiology laboratory • Anesthesiology • Catheter ablation • Cardioversion • Pacemaker • Implantable cardioverter-defibrillator (ICD) • ICD lead extraction

Key points

- The electrophysiology laboratory is a unique procedural area with specialized equipment and features, which create a potentially challenging work environment for the anesthesiologist.
- Heart failure, obstructive sleep apnea, and advanced age are common non-arrhythmia comorbidities encountered during electrophysiology procedures.
- Cardiac ablations, electrical cardioversions, insertion of cardiac implantable electronic devices, and lead extractions are all procedures that an anesthesiologist should understand to safely care for patients in the electrophysiology laboratory.

INTRODUCTION

In the cardiac electrophysiology (EP) laboratory, electrophysiologists treat cardiac arrythmias with ablation, high-voltage energy, and device implantation. Major advances in the early and mid-twentieth century led to the first

*Corresponding author. *E-mail address:* Julie_Wyrobek@urmc.rochester.edu

https://doi.org/10.1016/j.aan.2022.06.004

successful pacemaker implantation in 1960 and the first catheter-based ablation in 1981 [1–3]. Since then, the number of patients presenting for non-pharmacological treatment of arrythmias has dramatically increased worldwide [4–7]. These patients often present with significant comorbidities that are best cared by an anesthesiology team that understands the procedure, potential complications, and anesthetic implications [8,9]. This review describes the common procedures performed in the EP laboratory and addresses the associated anesthetic considerations.

GENERAL ANESTHETIC CONSIDERATIONS IN ELECTROPHYSIOLOGY

Staffing and location

Anesthesiology staffing models should be customized to fit the institution's policies and needs. A specialized, dedicated team is ideal as this builds familiarity with the procedures performed and improves communication with the EP team. All anesthesiology team members should be aware of the potential need for fluoroscopy and use methods to minimize radiation exposure. Although the exact risk to the anesthesia team is unknown, a recent report estimated that EP physicians have two to three times higher radiation exposure per year than diagnostic radiologists and develop a significant additional cancer risk [10]. Distance from the main operating rooms can be a barrier in providing optimal patient care and should be considered when assigning coverage [8,11]. As with other nonoperating room anesthesia suites, there must be immediate access to emergency medications, airway equipment, and additional staffing resources.

Environment

The EP laboratory contains specialized equipment and features that pose unique challenges for the anesthesiology team, as shown in Fig. 1. The C-arm fluoroscopy machine, which is invaluable to the electrophysiologist, often impedes access to the patient's airway [9,12]. This can prove especially challenging if there is unexpected respiratory decompensation. Similarly, appropriate intravenous and arterial access should be secured before the procedure. Staying abreast of intraprocedural steps can be difficult, as often the fluoroscopy screen and procedural sites are out of view of the anesthesia team [13]. Radiation exposure necessitates lead gowns, specialized eye wear, and lead screens which can further hamper mobility and safety [12]. Training, repetition, and consistency in procedural steps will aid the anesthesia team in developing familiarity in how best to overcome these challenges.

Anesthesiology equipment and monitoring

Anesthesiology equipment and monitoring requirements for the EP laboratory fall under the same standards as the operating room for sedation and general anesthesia cases [14]. An arterial line is prudent for higher risk procedures when arrhythmias may be poorly tolerated. End-tidal carbon dioxide monitoring should be used for any sedation case that requires at least moderate

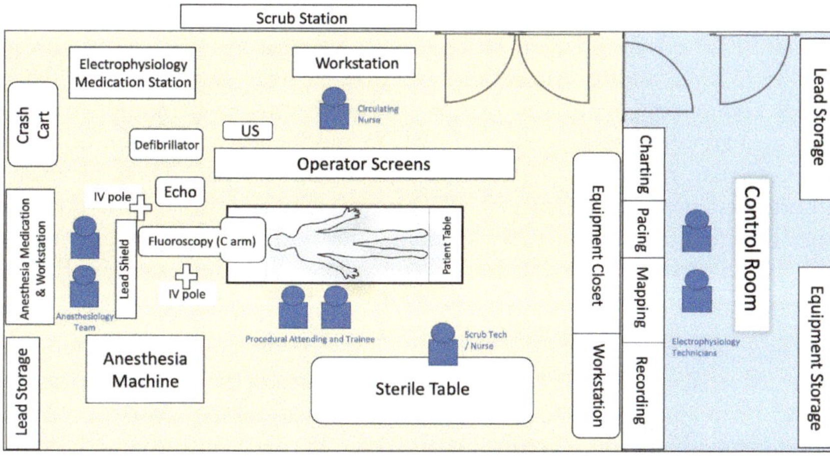

Fig. 1. An example of room layout for the electrophysiology laboratory. IV pole, intravenous pole, Echo, transesophageal echocardiography machine, US, ultrasound.

sedation (which is defined as a purposeful response to verbal or light tactile stimulation) [15]. Defibrillator pads should be attached to a biphasic external defibrillator with a backup defibrillator immediately available [16]. Many EP procedures require continuous infusions, such as isoproterenol or heparin, which necessitates the availability of infusion pumps. An esophageal temperature monitor is used during atrial ablation procedures to mitigate the risk of thermal complications such as atrio-esophageal perforation. It is essential that advanced emergency airway equipment be immediately available in an easy to access location, given the previously described physical barriers. A malignant hyperthermia kit is essential at locations where triggering anesthetics are administered. Furthermore, in EP laboratories that use a stereotactic magnetic navigation system, the use of magnets mandates that compatible anesthesia monitors be used.

Patient comorbidities

Given the nature and indication of procedures, it is not surprising that the EP laboratory presents anesthesiologists with challenging and sometimes moribund patients. The authors highlight three key comorbidities that are encountered frequently.

Heart failure

Heart failure (HF) is perhaps the most common pathology encountered in the EP laboratory. Hypoventilation, apnea, bleeding, and arrhythmias are all poorly tolerated. When timing permits, preprocedural optimization with the patient's cardiologist should take place before scheduling the EP procedure. Respiratory adjuncts such as high-flow nasal cannula (HFNC) or noninvasive ventilation (NIV) should be strongly considered in patients with marginal pulmonary status when undergoing monitored anesthesia care. HFNC creates a small PEEP effect and reduces dead-space ventilation. NIV can reduce pulmonary edema and afterload and increase cardiac output. These devices reduce respiratory acidosis to prevent right HF causing hemodynamic instability and arrythmias. The effect of NIV or mechanical ventilation on pulmonary vascular resistance (PVR) in HF is complex. The direct increase in intrathoracic pressure increases PVR. However, in patients with hypoventilation and atelectasis induced by sedation, the positive pressure can increase lung recruitment and ventilation, thereby mitigating increases in PVR or even reducing it [17].

Obstructive sleep apnea

Obstructive sleep apnea (OSA) is a common cause of atrial arrhythmias. Untreated sleep apnea leads to periods of hypoxemia and hypercarbia, which increase sympathetic tone, predispose to right HF, and can cause arrhythmias. Patients with OSA have a two- to three-fold increased risk of cardiopulmonary complications perioperatively [18]. Patients should be screened for sleep apnea using the STOP-BANG questionnaire, which should generate appropriate referrals for a pre-procedure sleep study [19].

Geriatric patients

Heart rhythm and conduction abnormalities occur at an increased frequency in older patients. These patients are more susceptible to delirium and postoperative cognitive dysfunction. Doses of anesthetic drugs should be lowered 20% to 50% as per recommendations in the geriatric anesthesiology literature to minimize side effects [20].

Medications

Anesthetic drugs

Many anesthetic drugs reduce resting adrenergic tone in a dose-dependent manner and directly affect the conduction system. Inhaled anesthetics reduce sinoatrial node discharge [21,22]. Sevoflurane, desflurane, and isoflurane prolong the action potential duration and may increase the QT interval, whereas propofol does not [23,24]. Propofol exhibits ion-channel inhibition that suppresses the autonomic nervous system, which can suppress ventricular arrhythmias. Propofol has minimal effect on the conduction system and has been used at high doses without affecting atrial tachyarrhythmias [24]. Opioids can raise the threshold for ventricular arrhythmias [24]. Benzodiazepines seem to have minimal effects on normal atrioventricular nodal or accessory pathway conduction and serve as a useful adjunct during sedation for EP studies [22,24]. Midazolam did not result in any autonomic suppression in a study that directly measured sympathetic ganglion nerve activity [25]. Owing to the sympathomimetic effects of ketamine, it can increase heart rate and shorten the action potential duration, making it suitable for use during EP studies. On the other hand, dexmedetomidine activates alpha-2A receptors leading to decrease in norepinephrine release, reducing inducibility of supraventricular tachycardia

(SVT) and ventricular tachycardia (VT) [24], and significantly suppressing sympathetic nerve activity [25]. Compared with propofol, dexmedetomidine has been associated with a lower incidence of VT post-cardiac surgery [26].

Considering the complex effects of anesthetic drugs can have on the conduction system, ongoing dialogue with the electrophysiologist is necessary to determine the appropriate depth of sedation.

Drugs requested during the procedure

- *Isoproterenol*, a beta-agonist, is frequently infused to facilitate induction and maintenance of arrhythmias such as SVT so that electro-anatomic mapping can be performed. Isoproterenol may also be used after ablation to assure non-inducibility of the treated arrhythmias.
- *Heparin* is commonly used during ablation procedures to prevent thrombus formation on catheters, especially those that require transseptal puncture for mapping and ablation in the left atrium or left ventricle. Activated clotting time (ACT) monitoring is required with a target range and frequency depending on the procedure and institutional practice.
- *Protamine* is used to reverse heparin at the discretion of the electrophysiologist. There are various institutional practices concerning its administration to detect and avoid protamine reactions; many include a small test dose followed by slow administration.

CARDIAC ABLATION PROCEDURES

Catheter ablation is an effective alternative to pharmacologic therapy in patients with atrial and ventricular tachyarrhythmias. The technique involves the percutaneous introduction of catheters into the heart under fluoroscopic guidance to record intracardiac signals [9]. Three-dimensional (3D) mapping systems are often used to recreate cardiac anatomy and allow electro-anatomic mapping which can facilitate identification of sites for ablation. For patients presenting in sinus rhythm, isoproterenol may be infused to induce tachycardia. Once the mechanism and site of origin of the arrhythmia is identified, radiofrequency (RF) ablation is delivered to create a localized scar that disrupts the arrhythmia. RF ablation is usually well tolerated but ablation in certain areas such as in the posterior wall of the left atrium may induce pain due to its proximity to the esophagus. Cryoablation as an alternative energy source is used to treat atrial fibrillation, and pulse field ablation is being developed as another alternative to treat arrhythmias.

During cardiac ablations, the venous system is commonly approached via the femoral veins. Less commonly, the internal jugular or subclavian vein approach may also be used. Diagnostic catheters are inserted to allow pacing, stimulation, and signal recording in the right atrium, right ventricle (apex or right ventricular outflow tract), the bundle of His, or the coronary sinus. The left heart can be accessed through a transseptal puncture from the right atrium into the left atrium or a retrograde aortic approach [27]. Complications associated with catheter ablation include death, myocardial ischemia, heart block, cardiac tamponade, thromboembolic complications, peripheral vascular injury, phrenic nerve injury, pulmonary vein stenosis, mitral valve injury, acute lung injury, heart block, endocarditis, and atrial-esophageal fistulae [28,29].

Atrial fibrillation and flutter ablation

Atrial fibrillation is the most common arrhythmia, with a worldwide incidence of up to 1%, whereas atrial flutter has an incidence of up to 0.1% in the United States [30,31]. Atrial fibrillation is often initiated by pulmonary vein triggers and random reentry in the pulmonary vein ostia leading to irregular atrial activation. In contrast, atrial flutter is a reentrant circuit and most often activates in a "typical" pattern that involves the cavotricuspid isthmus [32].

RF catheter ablation for atrial fibrillation aims to electrically isolate the pulmonary veins [33]. During catheter ablation, point-by-point RF ablation lesions are delivered to the pulmonary vein antrum to isolate each vein [32]. Cryoablation involves freezing the ostium of the pulmonary veins to achieve electrical isolation. Cryoballoon ablation involves inserting a catheter-delivered inflatable balloon into each pulmonary vein and inflating it with nitrous oxide (Fig. 2). The Fire and Ice trial demonstrated this to be non-inferior to RF ablation, with shorter procedure times [34].

General anesthesia is often preferred for ablation of atrial fibrillation. As this arrhythmia does not need to be induced, the suppressive effects of anesthetic drugs are less relevant, and general anesthesia offers increased patient comfort for long procedures. Further, catheter ablation requires good contact between the catheter tip and tissue. Patient movement and irregular respiration can make catheter-tissue contact more difficult and can limit the reliability of 3D mapping systems used during the ablation case. General anesthesia has been shown to lead to lower arrhythmia recurrence, lower rates of pulmonary vein reconnection, and shorter fluoroscopy times than conscious sedation [35]. Although patient movement is undesirable; neuromuscular blockade is often avoided. Monitoring of the phrenic nerve can help avoid injury during

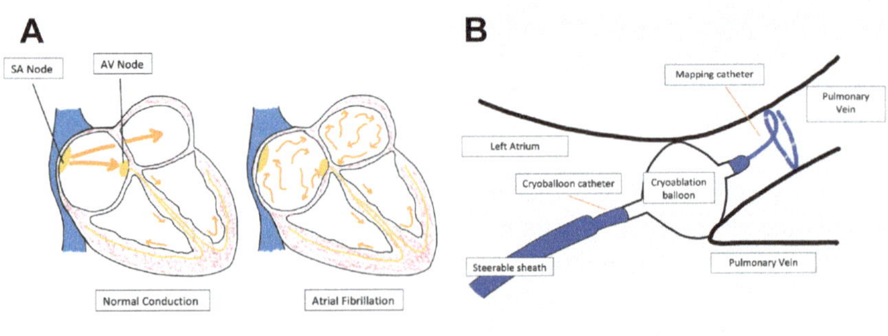

Fig. 2. (*A*) The electrical current pathway during normal conduction and in atrial fibrillation. (*B*) The cryoablation balloon is inserted directly into the pulmonary vein during the procedure.

ablation of the right pulmonary veins [36]. High-frequency jet ventilation can also be helpful in reducing movement due to respiration [37].

The reported major complications rates within 30 days of atrial fibrillation ablation ranges from 2.9% to 5.6% of cases, with lower complication rates observed in modern patient cohorts [38–40]. Major complications include pericardial effusion, tamponade, pulmonary vein stenosis, phrenic and vagal nerve injury, atrioesophageal fistula formation, esophageal injuries, bleeding, and thromboembolic events [41]. Balancing the risk of bleeding events with thromboembolism remains a challenge. Continuing warfarin therapy periprocedurally, as opposed to bridging with heparin, has been shown to reduce the risk of thromboembolism without increasing bleeding risk [42]. Intraprocedural heparin administration to maintain an ACT range of 300 to 400 reduces the risk of thrombus formation [41].

Supraventricular tachycardia ablation

SVT is a general term describing a group of arrhythmias originating at or above the atrioventricular node. SVT is caused by one of three mechanisms: reentry, increased automaticity, or triggered activity [43]. The incidence of SVT is approximately 35 cases per 100,000 patients with a prevalence of 2.25 cases per 1000 in the general population [43]. Catheter ablation using RF or cryothermal energy is now considered the first-line therapy for most supraventricular arrhythmias types [44]. SVT can be cured by catheter ablation with high success rates (95%–99%) with low complication rates (<1%). Guidelines recommend ablation for patients with recurrent SVT despite treatment or poorly tolerated SVT, although recommendations vary based on the SVT mechanism, site of origin, and known success rates [43].

Propofol has minimal effects on the QT interval and conduction system and thus is a commonly used sedative. Ketamine shortens the atrial conduction time, increases the heart rate, and induces arrhythmias; this may facilitate electrophysiological studies and ablations [45]. No significant difference in induction rates was noted between propofol and ketamine [8]. As for volatile anesthetics, although sevoflurane has been shown to reduce the sinoatrial conduction time and atrial–His (AH) interval time, this effect of sevoflurane has not been demonstrated in clinical practice [8].

Ventricular tachycardia ablation

VT or ventricular fibrillation (VF) is often the result of coronary artery disease and dilated or hypertrophic cardiomyopathy. Anesthesia considerations for VT ablation should focus on preoperative optimization, as candidates often have coronary stenosis, severely reduced left ventricular function, and other organ dysfunction including pulmonary, kidney, or liver failure. An in-depth review of current medications is also important. Amiodarone is of concern with its long elimination half-life and potential side effects of hypothyroidism and pulmonary toxicity. Both alpha-adrenergic and beta-adrenergic properties of amiodarone may lead to hypotension and atropine-resistant bradycardia during anesthesia. Anti-arrhythmic drugs are often held the day of the procedure or longer to enhance the induction of ventricular arrhythmias during the procedure.

Anesthesia selection for ventricular ablations is usually directed by the patient's underlying physical status. The decision for preinduction or a postinduction arterial line depends on the patients' baseline functional status, degree of cardiomyopathy, and arrhythmia burden. Intra-arterial access is necessary to allow beat-to-beat monitoring for dramatic hemodynamic changes. This will also allow for easier titration of vasopressor and inotropic medications. Equipment for rapid cardioversion–defibrillation should be readily available during the induction period and at the time of central venous access placement. The ectopy produced by the wire used during central venous catheter placement may precipitate the patient's underlying arrythmia. The use of volatile anesthetic versus IV anesthetics has shown little to no impact on the inducibility of VT [46].

Recently, mechanical circulatory support (MCS) devices have been used to support patients who exhibit hemodynamic instability during ventricular arrhythmia. These include intra-aortic balloon pumps, percutaneously implanted left ventricular assist devices such as Impella (Danvers, MA), and extracorporeal membrane oxygenation (ECMO) [47–50]. It is still unclear which device is optimal for support during ventricular ablation. ECMO offers the highest degree of cardiac output augmentation, but it also carries the highest risk for complications. A common cannulation strategy is shown in Fig. 3. With peripheral VA-ECMO, there is anterograde blood being ejected from the left ventricle and retrograde flow of blood from the iliac artery toward the aortic root. Depending on the strength of the native left ventricular ejection, the location of the mixing cloud can be anywhere from the aortic root to the distal descending aorta. By placing the arterial line and pulse oximeter on the right upper extremity, Harlequin syndrome or North–South syndrome can be avoided by ensuring blood in the coronary, and cerebral circulation

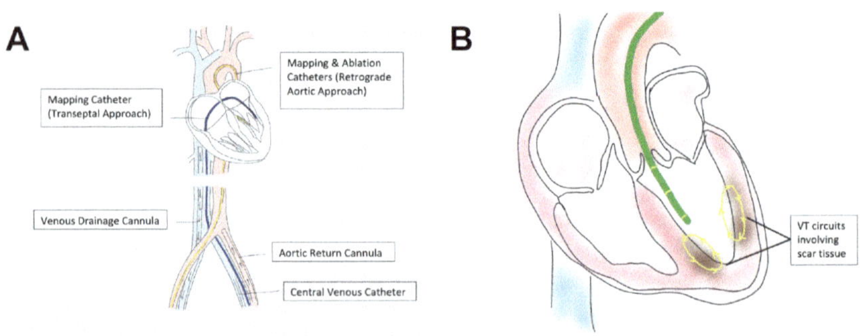

Fig. 3. (*A*) A common cannulation strategy to VA-ECMO-assisted VT ablation. The aortic return cannula and venous drainage cannula are inserted via the femoral artery and vein. Mapping and ablation catheters are inserted either via a transseptal approach through the femoral vein or via the femoral artery (*B*) in a retrograde approach.

is adequately oxygenated. Hemodynamic management relies on a balance of native cardiac output and ECMO augmentation. Increasing the dose of inotropic agent can increase risk for VT, and vasopressors can increase systemic vascular resistance (SVR) and lower cardiac output. Solely increasing ECMO flows will increase the effective afterload, making aortic valve opening and left ventricular ejection more difficult, which can lead to left ventricular dilation. Vascular injury and distal limb ischemia are also significant complications that can occur with use of MCS devices [51].

ELECTRICAL CARDIOVERSION

Electrical cardioversion for arrhythmias was first performed in the 1950s to successfully terminate VF and is currently also commonly performed in patients with atrial arrhythmias [52,53]. Although the procedure is brief, it can be very painful for the patient. An ideal anesthetic would result in rapid and only brief loss of consciousness, not accumulate with repeat dosing, and have minimal adverse effects on hemodynamics and respiration. Both propofol and etomidate have been used successfully for cardioversion procedures [53,54]. They can be easily titrated to achieve a deep plane of sedation and allow for expedited recovery. Midazolam and fentanyl have also been used but they tend to have significantly longer induction and recovery times [53]. Patients who have been in atrial fibrillation or flutter for more than 48 hours have a high risk of thromboembolism after cardioversion [55]. This risk can be reduced by maintaining therapeutic anticoagulation for 3 weeks before cardioversion or alternatively transesophageal echocardiography (TEE) to rule out left atrial appendage thrombus before cardioversion can be performed [56]. The decision to continue oral anticoagulation following cardioversion is often based on the patient's CHA_2DS_2–VASc score [57].

Pacemaker and implantable cardioverter-defibrillator insertion

The placement of cardiovascular implantable electronic devices (CIEDs) is another commonly performed procedure in the EP laboratory. CIEDs include permanent pacemakers (PPMs) and implantable cardioverter-defibrillators (ICDs). The indications for PPM and ICD placement are described in Table 1 [58–60].

For both PPM and ICD implantation, the left infraclavicular region is preferred. After positioning, local anesthetic is injected at the access site. Venous access is obtained either percutaneously or after a small incision is made to expose the subclavian/axillary vein. Often venography is performed to identify vein patency. Once venous access and guidewire placement are confirmed with fluoroscopy, a sheath is placed through and a lead with a rigid stylet is inserted. For CIEDs with more than a single lead, the right ventricular lead is placed first. The right ventricular lead is most commonly secured into the right ventricle (RV) apical and septal wall, and the right atrial lead is secured in the right atrial appendage. For biventricular pacing, the left ventricle (LV) lead is placed into the coronary sinus [61]. Conduction system pacing

Table 1
Indications for permanent pacemaker and implantable cardioverter defibrillator

Indications	
PPM	ICD
Symptomatic bradycardia due to disease or dysfunction of: • Sinus node • Atrioventricular node	Symptomatic ventricular tachycardia and ventricular fibrillation Long QT syndrome Brugada syndrome* Infiltrative cardiomyopathy* Hypertrophic cardiomyopathy* Ischemic cardiomyopathy with left ventricular ejection fraction (LVEF) <40% and inducible nonsustained ventricular tachycardia (NSVT) in EP study Primary prevention/prophylaxis • Ischemic cardiomyopathy ○ LVEF <30% and New York Heart Association (NYHA) class I symptoms ○ LVEF <35% and NYHA class II/III symptoms • Nonischemic cardiomyopathy ○ LVEF ≤35% and NYHA class II/III symptoms Arrhythmogenic right ventricular dysplasia* *if ≥ 1 risk factor for sudden cardiac death

such as His-bundle pacing or left bundle pacing, which requires implant of a lead into the His-bundle region or into the deep basal RV septum, respectively, may be performed in patients with HF. Once placement is confirmed, tests are performed to determine sensing and pacing thresholds and lead impedance. A deeper level of sedation may be required during defibrillation threshold testing which requires the induction of VF.

The implantation of both PPM and ICDs are minimally stimulating and can often be safely performed under local and monitored anesthesia care with mild–moderate sedation [8,62]. Comorbidities such as morbid obesity, severe OSA, high aspiration risk, the inability to lie flat, advanced pulmonary disease, volume overload, or severe dementia warrant consideration of general anesthesia. There have been successful CIED implants performed under regional anesthesia, specifically a unilateral pectoralis plane block [63]. This may be considered in high-risk patients in whom even light sedation is undesirable due to poor cardiopulmonary reserve.

Although traditional CIEDs have been primarily implanted transvenously, technological advances have resulted in alternatives such as leadless pacemakers (Micra-Medtronic) and subcutaneously implanted ICDs (s-ICD) [64,65]. Leadless pacemakers are a single-chamber pacemaker implanted into the right ventricle via a femoral vein delivery system. It is imperative to understand that the leadless pacemakers do not have a magnet mode and require reprogramming if asynchronous ventricular pacing is desired. The s-ICD, on the other hand, is a larger device implanted in the left lateral chest region that avoids the need for vascular access.

Insertion of an s-ICD can be stimulating and often requires general anesthesia as it includes a sizable left lateral chest wall incision, tunneling of the lead, intermuscular device placement, and defibrillation threshold testing.

LEAD EXTRACTION

Complications resulting from a rising rate of CIED implantations have resulted in an increased rate of lead extractions [66]. The decision to proceed with lead removal must weigh clinical need against the associated patient and procedure-related risks of complications. The most common indication for extraction is infection, which is associated with a higher risk of complications than noninfectious indications [67]. Management includes removal of infectious material, antibiotic therapy, and appropriate delay to reimplantation if CIED is still required.

The Heart Rhythm Society (HRS) published an expert consensus guideline for lead removal [68,69].

- *Elimination of infection:* definitive CIED infection, lead, or valvular endocarditis; sepsis with suspected CIED infection; pocket abscess, erosion, or chronic draining sinus; and persistent occult gram-positive bacteremia
- *Prevention of repeat thromboembolic events:* associated with lead thrombus pulmonary embolism (PE)
- *Venous stenosis management:* superior vena cava (SVC) stenosis or occlusion with limiting symptoms; planned venous stent deployment to prevent lead entrapment; and SVC or subclavian vein occlusion preventing implantation of a needed lead
- *Urgent treatment of other conditions:* leads causing life-threatening arrhythmias and conferring risk of impending perforation

CIED lead removal can be classified as either explant or extraction. Lead explant refers to the removal of leads implanted within 1 year using a simple traction technique [66,70]. Lead extraction is when specialized techniques are required to safely remove the lead, either when fibrosis becomes significant (implant duration > 1 year) or when other factors complicate removal. Transvenous lead extraction is most commonly performed from the site of implantation (subclavian/axillary vein) after the device and leads are exposed and prepared.

Despite the complexity involved in lead extractions, the reported risk of major complications is relatively low, between 0.19% and 1.8%. Major complications include cardiac tamponade, severe tricuspid regurgitation, vascular avulsion or tear, pulmonary embolism, stroke, and death [66,68,70]. When major complications occur, the risk of procedure-related mortality is significantly increased, from 0.4% for extractions overall to 24% [66].

Several factors have been identified which predict a higher risk of major complications during lead extraction, as shown in Table 2 [66,68,70,71].

The duration of the oldest implanted lead is one of the most significant risk factors. According to a risk-stratification scheme developed by the Mayo clinic, risks associated with age of oldest lead were:

Low risk: All leads less than 1 year.

Table 2
Risk factors for complications during implantable cardioverter-defibrillator lead extraction

Patient-Related Risk Factors	Device/Procedure-Related Risk Factors
• Low body mass index (<25 kg/m2) • Advanced age > 68 y • Female gender • Complex venous anatomy (small, tortuous, presence of shunting) • PM or ICD dependency due to underlying rhythm • Low LV function (<15% EF) • NYHA Class III and IV CHF • Severe pulmonary hypertension • Renal failure • Cerebrovascular disease, history of cerebrovascular accident (Hx CVA) • Coagulopathy • Presence of device infection, especially large and friable vegetations	• Implant duration > 1 y, rising with longer duration • Greater number of leads (>3) • Presence of ICD leads, especially with dual coils, or larger, more complex coils • Coronary sinus lead extraction • Inexperienced practitioners or centers

Moderate risk: Age 1 to 5 years for ICD leads, 1 to 10 years for PM leads.

High risk: greater than 5 years ICD leads, greater than 10 years PM leads.

Their data for major complications by this scheme demonstrated rates of 0% in low risk, 1.2% in moderate risk, and 5.3% in high-risk patients [66]. HRS suggests that minimum initial operator training should include 40 supervised lead extractions, with a minimum annual volume of 20. Institutional policies regarding access to an available cardiac surgery operating room should also be considered. Many institutions prefer to use "hybrid" ORs that are designed to accommodate routine and emergent circumstances during high-risk lead extractions.

To quickly detect hemodynamic changes, arterial access contralateral to the side of extraction prevents erroneous reading from movement of the ipsilateral subclavian artery during traction on the vein [66]. Femoral access is helpful in the case of trauma to upper extremity veins. Some centers routinely perform TEE to screen for complications such as tamponade. Descriptions of useful imaging views and associated findings are available for review [72]. The rationale for TEE monitoring during high-risk lead extraction include:

- *Early diagnosis and classifying severity of complications to guide management* (new pericardial effusion, tricuspid valve injury, cardiac avulsion, and hypovolemia)
- *Monitoring of rescue therapies* (guiding cardiopulmonary bypass [CPB] cannula placement, pericardial drainage)
- *Prevention of complications* (identification of large vegetations, large interatrial communications, or significant traction on SVC or myocardium during extraction)

- *Confirmation of lead removal* (assisting fluoroscopy), though fibrin sheaths referred to as "lead casts" may remain after extraction.

SUMMARY

EP is a rapidly expanding and evolving field with newer devices and techniques being performed every year. To safely perform anesthesia for patients undergoing procedures in the EP laboratory, a thorough understanding of the potential interactions between the patient's comorbidities, procedure being performed, and implications of anesthetic management is imperative. This knowledge will aid the anesthesiology team in reducing the risk of patient morbidity and increasing the likelihood of a successful procedural outcome.

CLINICS CARE POINTS

-An arterial line is recommended when the induction of arrhythmias during the procedure has the potential to lead to hemodynamic instability. -Defibrillator pads should be placed on the patient and attached to an external defibrillator prior to the initiation of any case in the EP laboratory. -An esophageal temperature monitor should be placed during atrial ablation procedures to mitigate the risk of an atrio-esophageal perforation. -During atrial ablation procedures, neuromuscular blockade is often avoided to facilitate monitoring of the phrenic nerve. -For geriatric patients, doses of anesthetic medications should be lowered according to geriatric anesthesiology literature to minimize side effects. -During VA-ECMO supported VT ablation, the pulse oximeter and/or arterial line should be placed in the right upper extremity to monitor for North-South syndrome. -Insertion of a subcutaneous ICD often requires general anesthesia as it involves a sizeable left lateral chest wall incision, lead tunneling, intermuscular device placement and threshold testing. -During high-risk lead extraction procedures, atrial access contralateral to the site of extraction is recommended to prevent erroneous reading from movement of the ipsilateral subclavian artery.

DISCLOSURE

The authors have nothing to disclose.

References

[1] Scheinman MM, Morady F, Hess DS, et al. Catheter-induced ablation of the atrioventricular junction to control refractory supraventricular arrhythmias. JAMA 1982;248(7):851–5.
[2] Luderitz B. Historical perspectives of cardiac electrophysiology. Hellenic J Cardiol 2009;50(1):3–16.
[3] Beck H, Boden WE, Patibandla S, et al. 50th Anniversary of the first successful permanent pacemaker implantation in the United States: historical review and future directions. Am J Cardiol 2010;106(6):810–8.
[4] Kumar S, Walters TE, Halloran K, et al. Ten-year trends in the use of catheter ablation for treatment of atrial fibrillation vs. the use of coronary intervention for the treatment of ischaemic heart disease in Australia. Europace : Eur pacing, arrhythmias, Card Electrophysiol : J

working groups Card pacing, arrhythmias, Card Cell Electrophysiol Eur Soc Cardiol 2013;15(12):1702–9.
[5] Kneeland PP, Fang MC. Trends in catheter ablation for atrial fibrillation in the United States. J Hosp Med 2009;4(7):E1–5.
[6] Eckardt L, Frommeyer G, Sommer P, et al. Updated Survey on Interventional Electrophysiology: 5-Year Follow-Up of Infrastructure, Procedures, and Training Positions in Germany. JACC Clin Electrophysiol 2018;4(6):820–7.
[7] Molitor N, Yalcinkaya E, Auricchio A, et al. Swiss National Registry on Catheter Ablation Procedures: Changing Trends over the Last 20 Years. J Clin Med 2021;10(14).
[8] Yildiz M, Yilmaz Ak H, Oksen D, et al. Anesthetic Management In Electrophysiology Laboratory: A Multidisciplinary review. J Atr Fibrillation 2018;10(5):1775.
[9] Cheruku S, Boud TJ, Kulkarni N, et al. Demystifying the EP Laboratory: Anesthetic Considerations for Electrophysiology Procedures. Int Anesthesiol Clin 2018;56(4):98–119.
[10] Picano E, Piccaluga E, Padovani R. Antonio Traino C, Grazia Andreassi M, Guagliumi G. Risks Related To Fluoroscopy Radiation Associated With Electrophysiology Procedures. J Atr Fibrillation 2014;7(2):1044.
[11] Anderson R, Harukuni I, Sera V. Anesthetic considerations for electrophysiologic procedures. Anesthesiol Clin 2013;31(2):479–89.
[12] Kwak J. Anesthesia for electrophysiology studies and catheter ablations. Semin Cardiothorac Vasc Anesth 2013;17(3):195–202.
[13] Aaij R, Abellan Beteta C, Adeva B, et al. First observation of the decay B(c)+–> J/psipi(+) pi- pi+. Phys Rev Lett 2012;108(25):251802.
[14] Standards for Basic Anesthetic Monitoring. In: Anesthesiologists ASo, ed 2020:1–3. Available at: https://www.asahq.org/standards-and-guidelines/standards-for-basic-anesthetic-monitoring.
[15] Practice Guidelines for Moderate Procedural Sedation and Analgesia 2018: A Report by the American Society of Anesthesiologists Task Force on Moderate Procedural Sedation and Analgesia, the American Association of Oral and Maxillofacial Surgeons, American College of Radiology, American Dental Association, American Society of Dentist Anesthesiologists, and Society of Interventional Radiology. Anesthesiology. 2018;128(3):437–79.
[16] Haines DE, Beheiry S, Akar JG, et al. Heart Rhythm Society expert consensus statement on electrophysiology laboratory standards: process, protocols, equipment, personnel, and safety. Heart Rhythm. 2014;11(8):e9–51.
[17] Kato T, Suda S, Kasai T. Positive airway pressure therapy for heart failure. World J Cardiol 2014;6(11):1175–91.
[18] Subramani Y, Singh M, Wong J, et al. Understanding Phenotypes of Obstructive Sleep Apnea: Applications in Anesthesia, Surgery, and Perioperative Medicine. Anesth Analg 2017;124(1):179–91.
[19] Chung F, Abdullah HR, Liao P. STOP-Bang Questionnaire: A Practical Approach to Screen for Obstructive Sleep Apnea. Chest. 2016;149(3):631–8.
[20] Andres TM, McGrane T, McEvoy MD, et al. Geriatric Pharmacology: An Update. Anesthesiol Clin 2019;37(3):475–92.
[21] Plunkett JJ, Reeves JD, Ngo L, et al. Urine and plasma catecholamine and cortisol concentrations after myocardial revascularization. Modulation by continuous sedation. Multicenter Study of Perioperative Ischemia (McSPI) Research Group, and the Ischemia Research and Education Foundation (IREF). Anesthesiology. 1997;86(4):785–96.
[22] Vladinov G, Fermin L, Longini R, et al. Choosing the anesthetic and sedative drugs for supraventricular tachycardia ablations: A focused review. Pacing Clin Electrophysiol 2018;41(11):1555–63.
[23] Kleinsasser A, Loeckinger A, Lindner KH, et al. Reversing sevoflurane-associated Q-Tc prolongation by changing to propofol. Anaesthesia 2001;56(3):248–50.
[24] Mittnacht AJ, Dukkipati S, Mahajan A. Ventricular tachycardia ablation: a comprehensive review for anesthesiologists. Anesth Analg 2015;120(4):737–48.

[25] Liu X, Rabin PL, Yuan Y, et al. Effects of anesthetic and sedative agents on sympathetic nerve activity. Heart Rhythm. 2019;16(12):1875–82.
[26] Herr DL, Sum-Ping ST, England M. ICU sedation after coronary artery bypass graft surgery: dexmedetomidine-based versus propofol-based sedation regimens. J Cardiothorac Vasc Anesth 2003;17(5):576–84.
[27] Bohora S, Tharakan J. Internal jugular/subclavian venous access in electrophysiology study and ablation. Indian Pacing Electrophysiol J 2009;9(4):190–4.
[28] Aldhoon A, Kautzner J. Complications of catheter ablation for atrial fibrillation. In. Cor et Vasa. Sci Direct 2012;54:e414–20.
[29] Aldhoon B, Wichterle D, Peichl P, et al. Complications of catheter ablation for atrial fibrillation in a high-volume centre with the use of intracardiac echocardiography. Europace. 2013;15(1):24–32.
[30] Granada J, Uribe W, Chyou PH, et al. Incidence and predictors of atrial flutter in the general population. J Am Coll Cardiol 2000;36(7):2242–6.
[31] Chugh SS, Havmoeller R, Narayanan K, et al. Worldwide epidemiology of atrial fibrillation: a Global Burden of Disease 2010 Study. Circulation 2014;129(8):837–47.
[32] Fujii S, Zhou JR, Dhir A. Anesthesia for Cardiac Ablation. J Cardiothorac Vasc Anesth 2018;32(4):1892–910.
[33] Haissaguerre M, Jais P, Shah DC, et al. Spontaneous initiation of atrial fibrillation by ectopic beats originating in the pulmonary veins. N Engl J Med 1998;339(10):659–66.
[34] Kuck KH, Brugada J, Furnkranz A, et al. Cryoballoon or Radiofrequency Ablation for Paroxysmal Atrial Fibrillation. N Engl J Med 2016;374(23):2235–45.
[35] Di Biase L, Conti S, Mohanty P, et al. General anesthesia reduces the prevalence of pulmonary vein reconnection during repeat ablation when compared with conscious sedation: results from a randomized study. Heart Rhythm. 2011;8(3):368–72.
[36] Bunch TJ, Bruce GK, Mahapatra S, et al. Mechanisms of phrenic nerve injury during radiofrequency ablation at the pulmonary vein orifice. J Cardiovasc Electrophysiol 2005;16(12): 1318–25.
[37] Hutchinson MD, Garcia FC, Mandel JE, et al. Efforts to enhance catheter stability improve atrial fibrillation ablation outcome. Heart Rhythm. 2013;10(3):347–53.
[38] Ngo L, Ali A, Ganesan A, et al. Institutional Variation in 30-Day Complications Following Catheter Ablation of Atrial Fibrillation. J Am Heart Assoc 2022;11(4):e022009.
[39] Gupta A, Perera T, Ganesan A, et al. Complications of catheter ablation of atrial fibrillation: a systematic review. Circ Arrhythm Electrophysiol 2013;6(6):1082–8.
[40] Muthalaly RG, John RM, Schaeffer B, et al. Temporal trends in safety and complication rates of catheter ablation for atrial fibrillation. J Cardiovasc Electrophysiol 2018;29(6):854–60.
[41] Calkins H, Kuck KH, Cappato R, et al. 2012 HRS/EHRA/ECAS expert consensus statement on catheter and surgical ablation of atrial fibrillation: recommendations for patient selection, procedural techniques, patient management and follow-up, definitions, endpoints, and research trial design. J Interv Card Electrophysiol 2012;33(2):171–257.
[42] Briceno DF, Madan N, Villablanca PA, et al. Periprocedural Anticoagulation for Catheter Ablation of Atrial Fibrillation: Practical Implications for Perioperative Management. J Cardiothorac Vasc Anesth 2017;31(4):1519–26.
[43] Sohinki D, Obel OA. Current trends in supraventricular tachycardia management. Ochsner J 2014;14(4):586–95.
[44] Calkins H, Kumar VK, Francis J. Radiofrequency catheter ablation of supraventricular tachycardia. Indian Pacing Electrophysiol J 2002;2(2):45–9.
[45] Wutzler A, Huemer M, Boldt LH, et al. Effects of deep sedation on cardiac electrophysiology in patients undergoing radiofrequency ablation of supraventricular tachycardia: impact of propofol and ketamine. Europace : Eur pacing, arrhythmias, Card Electrophysiol : J working groups Card pacing, arrhythmias, Card Cell Electrophysiol Eur Soc Cardiol 2013;15(7): 1019–24.

[46] Yoon J, Baik J, Cho MS, et al. Arrhythmia incidence and associated factors during volatile induction of general anesthesia with sevoflurane: a retrospective analysis of 950 adult patients. Anaesth Crit Care Pain Med 2021;40(3):100878.
[47] Monaco F, Ajello S, Calabrò MG, et al. Left Ventricular Unloading With an IABP in Patients Undergoing Ventricular Tachycardia Ablation With ECMO Support. J Cardiothorac Vasc Anesth 2021;35(9):2686–93.
[48] Craner RC, Carvajal T, Villablanca PA, et al. The Increasing Importance of Percutaneous Mechanical Circulatory Support in High-Risk Transcatheter Coronary Interventions: An Evidence-Based Analysis. J Cardiothorac Vasc Anesth 2018;32(3):1507–24.
[49] Bunch TJ, Mahapatra S, Madhu Reddy Y, et al. The role of percutaneous left ventricular assist devices during ventricular tachycardia ablation. Europace : Eur pacing, arrhythmias, Card Electrophysiol : J working groups Card pacing, arrhythmias, Card Cell Electrophysiol Eur Soc Cardiol 2012;14, Suppl 2:ii26-ii32.
[50] Vallabhajosyula S, Vaidya VR, Patlolla SH, et al. Venoarterial Extracorporeal Membrane Oxygenation Support for Ventricular Tachycardia Ablation: A Systematic Review. ASAIO J 2020;66(9):980–5.
[51] Schaefer AK, Distelmaier K, Riebandt J, et al. Access site complications of postcardiotomy extracorporeal life support. J Thorac Cardiovasc Surg 2021 S0022–5223–7.
[52] Sucu M, Davutoglu V, Ozer O. Electrical cardioversion. Ann Saudi Med 2009;29(3): 201–6.
[53] Cardioversion. In: Kaplan J, Cronin B, Maus T, editors. Kaplan's essentials of cardiac anesthesia for Noncardiac surgery. Elsevier; 2019.
[54] Stoneham MD. Anaesthesia for cardioversion. Anaesthesia 1996;51(6):565–70.
[55] Airaksinen KE, Grönberg T, Nuotio I, et al. Thromboembolic complications after cardioversion of acute atrial fibrillation: the FinCV (Finnish CardioVersion) study. J Am Coll Cardiol 2013;62(13):1187–92.
[56] January CT, Wann LS, Calkins H, et al. 2019 AHA/ACC/HRS Focused Update of the 2014 AHA/ACC/HRS Guideline for the Management of Patients With Atrial Fibrillation: A Report of the American College of Cardiology/American Heart Association Task Force on Clinical Practice Guidelines and the Heart Rhythm Society. J Am Coll Cardiol 2019;74(1):104–32.
[57] Olesen JB, Torp-Pedersen C, Hansen ML, et al. The value of the CHA2DS2-VASc score for refining stroke risk stratification in patients with atrial fibrillation with a CHADS2 score 0-1: a nationwide cohort study. Thromb Haemost 2012;107(6):1172–9.
[58] Epstein AE, DiMarco JP, Ellenbogen KA, et al. 2012 ACCF/AHA/HRS focused update incorporated into the ACCF/AHA/HRS 2008 guidelines for device-based therapy of cardiac rhythm abnormalities: a report of the American College of Cardiology Foundation/ American Heart Association Task Force on Practice Guidelines and the Heart Rhythm Society. J Am Coll Cardiol 2013;61(3):e6–75.
[59] Auricchio A, Stellbrink C, Sack S, et al. The Pacing Therapies for Congestive Heart Failure (PATH-CHF) study: rationale, design, and endpoints of a prospective randomized multicenter study. Am J Cardiol 1999;83(5B):130D–5D.
[60] Bristow MR, Saxon LA, Boehmer J, et al. Cardiac-resynchronization therapy with or without an implantable defibrillator in advanced chronic heart failure. N Engl J Med 2004;350(21):2140–50.
[61] Siegrist KK, Fernandez Robles C, Kertai MD, et al. The Electrophysiology Laboratory: Anesthetic Considerations and Staffing Models. J Cardiothorac Vasc Anesth 2021;35(9): 2775–83.
[62] Pinosky ML, Reeves ST, Fishman RL, et al. Intravenous sedation for placement of automatic implantable cardioverter-defibrillators. J Cardiothorac Vasc Anesth 1996;10(6):764–6.
[63] Mavarez AC, Ripat CI, Suarez MR. Pectoralis Plane Block for Pacemaker Insertion: A Successful Primary Anesthetic. Front Surg 2019;6:64.

[64] Friedman DJ, Parzynski CS, Varosy PD, et al. Trends and In-Hospital Outcomes Associated With Adoption of the Subcutaneous Implantable Cardioverter Defibrillator in the United States. JAMA Cardiol 2016;1(8):900–11.
[65] Karuppiah S, Prielipp R, Banik RK. Anesthetic consideration for patients with micra leadless pacemaker. Ann Card Anaesth 2020;23(4):493–5.
[66] Sonny A, Wakefield BJ, Sale S, et al. Transvenous Lead Extraction: A Clinical Commentary for Anesthesiologists. J Cardiothorac Vasc Anesth 2018;32(3):1101–11.
[67] Black-Maier E, Pokorney S, Christian A, et al. Outcomes Following Lead Extraction According to Indication: Infection Versus Non-Infection. J Am Coll Cardiol 2016;67(13).
[68] Wilkoff BL, Love CJ, Byrd CL, et al. Transvenous lead extraction: Heart Rhythm Society expert consensus on facilities, training, indications, and patient management: this document was endorsed by the American Heart Association (AHA). Heart Rhythm. 2009;6(7):1085–104.
[69] Kusumoto FM, Schoenfeld MH, Wilkoff BL, et al. 2017 HRS expert consensus statement on cardiovascular implantable electronic device lead management and extraction. Heart Rhythm. 2017;14(12):e503–51.
[70] Wazni O, Tarakji KG, Wilkoff BL. Lead Removal and Extraction. Clin Card Pacing, Defibrillation Resynchronization Ther 2017;937–58.
[71] Bongiorni MG, Kennergren C, Butter C, et al. The European Lead Extraction ConTRolled (ELECTRa) study: a European Heart Rhythm Association (EHRA) Registry of Transvenous Lead Extraction Outcomes. Eur Heart J 2017;38(40):2995–3005.
[72] Shillcutt SK, Schulte TE. Echo rounds: transesophageal echocardiography findings associated with transvenous lead extraction. Anesth Analg 2012;115(6):1282–5.

Advances in Anesthesia 40 (2022) 149–166

ADVANCES IN ANESTHESIA

Opioid-Free Anesthesia

The Pros and Cons

Valeria Carcamo-Cavazos, MD[a,b,*], Maxime Cannesson, MD, PhD[a,b]

[a]Department of Anesthesiology & Perioperative Medicine, David Geffen School of Medicine at UCLA, Los Angeles, CA, USA; [b]Ronald Reagan UCLA Medical Center, 757 Westwood Plaza, Suite 3325, Los Angeles, CA 90095-7403, USA

Keywords

• Opioid-free anesthesia • Opiate-sparing analgesia
• Multimodal pain management • Multimodal analgesia
• Enhanced recovery after surgery
• Procedure-specific postoperative pain management • Acute pain management
• Opioids side effects

Key points

- Opioid-free anesthesia (OFA) refers to the intraoperative anesthesia where no opiates are used and is often a viable option that spares patients the side effects of opiates without negatively affecting postoperative pain control.
- Multimodal analgesia (MMA) with an opiate-sparing approach should be the perioperative analgesic strategy of choice, with the goal of an opiate-free analgesic strategy when feasible.
- MMA can be accomplished by the concurrent use of various pharmacologic and nonpharmacologic analgesic strategies.
- Multimodal opiate-sparing analgesia is the perioperative analgesia strategy in Enhanced Recovery After Surgery (ERAS) pathways given it provides improved pain control minimizing the side effects of opiates.

Continued

*Corresponding author. Ronald Reagan UCLA Medical Center, 757 Westwood Plaza, Suite 3325, Los Angeles, CA 90095-7403. *E-mail address:* VCarcamo@mednet.ucla.edu

https://doi.org/10.1016/j.aan.2022.07.003
0737-6146/22/

Continued

- Evidence-based guidelines exist for MMA for specific surgeries and can be found in ERAS and procedure-specific postoperative pain management guidelines. However, the evidence behind these MMA recommendations remains incomplete, the ideal minimum combination of analgesic interventions for specific procedures remains uncertain, and the contribution of each individual analgesic strategy to improve pain is unknown and difficult to study.

Introduction

The International Association for the Study of Pain has recently (July 2020) revised the definition of pain for the first time since 1979 as "An unpleasant sensory and emotional experience associated with, or resembling that associated with, actual or potential tissue damage" [1]. This new definition aimed to separate the idea that nociception and pain come together, one can exist without the other. Indeed, the definition of pain has changed over the centuries. The definition of pain has evolved as a merely sensory experience, to recognize the important contributions that society, culture, and emotions have on the perception of pain [2].

Along with the definition of pain, the treatment of pain has evolved as we continue to understand the natural history of pain, the different kinds of pain, and the efficacy of various treatment modalities. In the 1990s, concerns about undertreatment of pain, the advocacy of pain as the fifth vital sign, as well as strong and misleading marketing of opioids by pharmaceuticals fueled an increase in opioid prescription for chronic noncancer pain [2–4]. Since the 1990s until 2012, the prescription of opioids largely increased as well as their misuse, which has largely fueled our current opioid abuse crisis [5]. Since 2012, opioid prescriptions have declined but deaths due to opiate overdose continued to climb with the use of heroin and most recently fentanyl driving the increase in mortality [5]. The opioid abuse crisis has become a public health emergency in the United States that we should all attempt to ameliorate.

Opioids continue to be a central component for the treatment of acute postoperative pain. Surgery, with subsequent opioid prescriptions, increases the risk of persistent opioid use because 0.5% to 6% of opioid-naive patients will continue to use opiates 1 year after surgery [6,7]. Millions of surgeries are performed in the United States every year [8,9]. Given the large number of surgeries performed in the United States, and the proportion of patients that use opioids chronically after surgeries, it is imperative that opioids are used perioperatively only when absolutely necessary and when no equally effective nonopioid alternatives exist. Anesthesiologists are well positioned to improve the opioids abuse crisis by the anesthetic choices we make for our patients.

Pain after surgery is common and continues to be poorly managed across Europe and in the United States [10,11]. Postoperative pain can have deleterious effects in patients' recovery, including decreased mobility to promote healing, respiratory complications, increased stress response, patient dissatisfaction, and increased risk of delirium [10,12]. Long-term effects of acute postsurgical pain are the development of chronic pain, which can significantly affect the quality of life of patients [10,11]. Opioids are commonly used to treat pain but they come with untoward side effects [10]. Opioid adverse effects are well known, and include postoperative nausea and vomiting (PONV), itching, sedation, confusion, respiratory depression, constipation, delirium, and the future risk of cancer recurrence, opioids abuse, and dependence [10,12]. Many of these side effects can hinder recovery after surgery. Opioids are currently often used for surgical pain given their effectiveness [10] but due to their significant side effect profile, in the face of an opioid abuse epidemic, and an aging population [13] in whom the side effects of opiates are amplified [14], many providers are attempting to use the minimum opiates necessary. The adverse side effects of opiates, along with the desire to improve pain control during and after surgery has shifted our focus for pain control from one that heavily relies on opiates, to using an opiate-sparing multimodal approach for postsurgical pain, where sometimes no opioids are used.

Opioid-free anesthesia (OFA) refers to the intraoperative anesthesia where no opiates are administered [15]. Under general anesthesia (GA), patients are unconscious, and the psychological components of pain are absent [15]; therefore, patients under GA do not experience pain but nociception. In the anesthetized patient, nociception and its successful treatment is inferred largely based on imperfect surrogates to include hemodynamic changes, increased respiratory rate, and movement in the nonparalyzed patient [16]. There have been attempts to create objective measures of nociception for the anesthetized patient that look at brain signaling through electroencephalography, and infratentorial balance of the autonomic nervous system, where nociception leads to an increase in the sympathetic tone and decrease in vagal tone [16,17]. An increase in heart rate and heart rate variability, increased sweating (thus skin conductance) and pupillary dilatation, which correlate with increased sympathetic activity, have been used to infer nociception through commercially available devices; however, it remains unclear whether any of these devices truly measures nociception, and their clinical application is unproven [17]. It is possible to control intraoperative surrogates for nociception, such as tachycardia and hypertension, using nonopiate alternatives, limiting the exposure of patients to opiates and their adverse side effects. However, many wonder, is this the right approach to intraoperative treatment of nociception, or does avoiding intraoperative opiates lead to worse pain after surgery?

In this article, we explore the evidence behind the use of various approaches for pain management intraoperatively, and how they affect patient outcomes. Importantly, we address the benefits and shortcomings of opiate-free versus opiate-sparing anesthesia. The topic remains controversial with passionate advocates on both sides [18], so we present some key questions surrounding OFA as a pro/con debate.

IS OPIOID-FREE ANESTHESIA FEASIBLE?

The pro argument

Absolutely. The main argument for using intraoperative opioids is to avoid hemodynamic changes, to aid with patients' waking up comfortably, and to preemptively avoid pain to decrease the development of persistent postsurgical pain [12]. However, we have other agents that can effectively avoid hemodynamic changes, such as beta-blockers, without the adverse effects of opioids. Given hemodynamic changes are imperfect measures of pain, we may be overtreating patients' presumed pain or transient pain, by giving opioids for any tachycardia and hypertension we observe. In addition, preemptive versus preventive opiates do not seem to decrease immediate postoperative pain [19]. Opioids have many known side effects that can adversely affect patients' recovery, and in a review by Frauenknecht and colleagues [12], they showed that the use of intraoperative opiates compared with opioid-free anesthesia (OFA), increased the risk of nausea and vomiting postoperatively without any benefit in patients' pain management. PONV is distressing to the patient and increases medical costs [20]. PONV is an important outcome to avoid in the Post Anesthesia Care Unit (PACU), which can be better accomplished by eliminating unnecessary opiate use.

Severe pain is a known risk factor for the development of chronic pain after surgery [21]. The use of intraoperative opiates does not decrease the risk of severe postoperative pain but may actually increase pain after surgery through opioid-induced hyperalgesia and possibly acute opiate tolerance [12,21]. Intraoperative opioids do not seem to possess the hoped for benefits of hemodynamic stability and decreased postoperative and possibly persistent postsurgical pain.

OFA is not only feasible but should be the standard of care because the use of opiates intraoperatively is not beneficial in many surgeries, and it can instead result in adverse effects to include PONV, opioid-induced hyperalgesia, and acute opiate tolerance.

The con argument

The systematic review and meta-analysis by Frauenknecht and colleagues [12] shows that opioid-free and opioid-inclusive anesthesia results in no significant differences in pain postoperatively. However, 60% of the studies included in the meta-analysis used remifentanil, a short-acting opiate with a very high incidence of opioid-induced hyperalgesia. More studies are needed to determine whether the pain would be different if longer acting opiates, with a decreased incidence of hyperalgesia, were used. Moreover, there is no mention of intraoperative hemodynamic changes, which if significant can have adverse outcomes in patients with cardiovascular disease or advanced age. It is necessary to determine if hemodynamic control is better achieved with opioid-free versus opioid-inclusive analgesia, and the implications in patient outcomes outside pain control.

Although current data shows no benefit on the use of preemptive opiates [19], the evidence is limited to certain types of surgeries (ie, hysterectomies) and low-risk patients (ASA 1–2) without chronic pain or opioid use [19]. In addition, the nonopiate pain medications that can be used intraoperatively carry risks, such as increased risk of acute kidney injury (AKI) with nonsteroidal anti-inflammatory drugs (NSAIDs), increased sympathetic response with ketamine, hypotension and bradycardia with dexmedetomidine, among many. Small doses of opiates tend to be safe and might prevent the use of polypharmacy with many untoward side effects. OFA is doable but it should not be the standard of care because many patients would benefit from the use of appropriately titrated opiates intraoperatively [22]. Opiate-sparing, not the extreme of OFA, should be the standard of care.

WHAT ARE THE PHARMACOLOGIC TOOLS FOR CONDUCTING OPIOID-FREE ANESTHESIA?

The pro argument

Treating nociception intraoperatively can be accomplished with nonopiate alternatives, in a multimodal approach. Multimodal analgesia (MMA) is effective at improving perioperative pain control while minimizing or eliminating side effects of any one of the multimodal agents, especially opiates. MMA has become an essential component of enhanced recovery after surgery (ERAS) pathways due to its ability to improve pain control and decrease analgesic side effects [23–27]. Preemptive analgesia, meaning the administration of medications to prevent pain in anticipation of a painful stimulus, should be favored when using nonopiate pain medications to minimize central sensitization and inflammation that can lead to significant pain after surgery [26]. Below we describe the different agents that can be used intraoperatively to accomplish OFA, and those that are less useful, with both their benefits and limitations. In general, a combination of nonopiate pain medications can be used safely and effectively to achieve opioid free-anesthesia (OFA) without compromising appropriate pain control after surgery.

Nonsteroidal anti-inflammatory drugs

NSAIDs inhibit cyclooxygenase (COX), leading to a decreased synthesis of prostaglandins. Prostaglandins play a key role in inflammation, as well as other processes, which account for the anti-inflammatory clinical benefit and side effects of NSAIDs [28].

Inflammation is a major mechanism that leads to acute postsurgical pain; therefore, the use of anti-inflammatory medications plays a key role in reducing pain after surgery [29]. NSAIDs are effective at reducing inflammation and certain types of acute and chronic pain [29], and they have been shown to significantly reduce opiate consumption, reduce opiate side effects (namely nausea/vomiting), and improve patient satisfaction when used for postoperative pain management [29–31]. Furthermore, there seems to be a potential for presurgical NSAIDs in addition to postoperative NSAIDs to further reduce pain and morphine consumption after surgery compared with NSAIDs given only for postoperative pain control [32], although the evidence behind this is limited.

There is concern that the use of NSAIDs in the perioperative period can lead to complications including renal dysfunction, bleeding, gastrointestinal discomfort, colon anastomotic leak, bone malunion/nonhealing, and cardiac events; however, in a review by Chang and colleagues (2021) [33], they conclude that short-term use of NSAIDs in the perioperative period is safe when patients' characteristics and comorbidities are considered. Notable exceptions where the risk of preemptive NSAIDs might exceed the benefit are patients with preexisting kidney disease, where significant bleeding is a risk or for colorectal surgeries. Patients with chronic kidney disease might be at an increased risk of AKI with NSAIDs, and the bleeding risk, although overall small, might be increased when NSAIDs are used intraoperatively [33]. In addition, there might be an increased risk of anastomotic leak when NSAIDs are used for colorectal surgery with colonic/rectal resection and primary anastomosis [29].

In summary, NSAIDs decrease pain, opiate consumption, and opiate adverse effects [29], and they can be safely used for a short period and in the lowest effective dose for postoperative pain control [33]. Therefore, NSAIDs should be used preoperatively and intraoperatively as part of OFA, combined with acetaminophen when not contraindicated [34] and continued postoperatively.

Acetaminophen

Acetaminophen's mechanism of action remains incompletely understood but it might act as an indirect COX inhibitor or through modulation of the cannabinoid system [24,26]. Acetaminophen is less effective for postoperative pain control compared with NSAIDs [29]. However, compared with NSAIDs, acetaminophen's side effect profile is favorable, with the most concerning side effect being hepatotoxicity if given at higher doses than recommended [26]. Several randomized controlled trials (RCTs) have shown improved pain control with decreased opiate use when administering acetaminophen preoperatively or postoperatively compared with placebo in abdominal hysterectomies, pediatric tonsillectomies, open nephrectomies, and lower extremity surgeries [26]. In some RCTs, administration of acetaminophen preoperatively shows improved pain control compared to when acetaminophen is administered postoperatively but this is not always the case [26]. Given the potential benefit of preemptive acetaminophen to improve postoperative pain control and its low risk profile, acetaminophen should be an integral component of OFA and ideally administered preoperatively in an oral formulation [35]. It must be noted that a systematic review by Ong and colleagues [34] found that NSAIDs with acetaminophen provide better pain relief than either medication alone, so when possible, acetaminophen and NSAIDs should be combined as part of MMA.

Ketamine

Ketamine is an N-methyl-D-aspartate (NMDA) receptor antagonist that is effective at treating surgical pain, and reduces opiate use during and after invasive surgery [26,36–38]. Even at subanalgesic doses, ketamine has been shown to decrease acute opiate tolerance and hyperalgesia [26,39]. In addition, ketamine when given with magnesium, reduces hemodynamic variability intraoperatively [36]. The benefits of ketamine on the development of chronic pain remain controversial [21] but given its mechanism of action as an NMDA antagonist and its effectiveness at reducing pain [39], ketamine could reduce the development of persistent postsurgical pain [37]. When used for major surgeries or special populations at risk of severe pain or adverse effect from opiates (chronic pain, opiate tolerance, obstructive sleep apnea [OSA]), ketamine can be a valuable addition to the multimodal pain management approach [26,39,40].

Ketamine can have some untoward side effects, namely neuroexcitatory side effects including hallucinations but these are only present when patients are awake [39] and in most cases cease after discontinuation of subanesthetic infusions commonly used in ERAS pathways [26]. When used during OFA, ketamine's neuroexcitatory effects are not apparent to anesthetized patients, and the analgesic effects are significant. Ketamine is an essential tool to accomplish OFA in patients undergoing invasive surgeries and/or with chronic pain and opiate tolerance.

Beta-blockers

Hemodynamic changes, tachycardia and hypertension, are used as surrogates for nociception when patients are under GA. However, hemodynamic changes are imperfect surrogates for nociception in the unconscious patient. Esmolol and other beta-blockers have been used to treat intraoperative hemodynamic changes in place of opiates [41–44]. Three meta-analyses and one systematic literature review analyzed RCTs investigating the use of beta-blockers (largely esmolol) versus placebo and/or opiates for hemodynamic control intraoperatively [41–44]. These reviews show that beta-blockers, when used instead of opiates to minimize hemodynamics changes, can decrease postoperative opiate use and, in most instances also, postoperative pain [41,42,44], and this reduction sometimes extends up to 72 hours postoperatively [41].

The safety profile of the intraoperative use of esmolol is good, with hemodynamic stability being similar in patients receiving esmolol infusions versus the control group, and without clinically significant hypotension or bradycardia in the esmolol group [41,42,44]. Studies show a trend toward decreased PONV in the esmolol group [41–44], although this was only statistically significant in the meta-analysis by Watts and colleagues [44]. The included RCTs in the reviews largely looked at studies with minimally invasive surgeries, including many laparoscopic abdominal surgeries [41,42,44], so future research should assess the opiate-sparing benefits of esmolol during large and invasive surgeries.

Esmolol infusions can be a valuable and underused addition to OFA, to control hemodynamic changes intraoperatively in place of the opioid alternative, without compromising hemodynamics, and with an actual benefit in improved pain control after surgery.

Neuroleptics

Neuroleptics are antagonists of voltage-gated calcium channels mostly in the central nervous system, which results in decreased release of neuroexcitatory neurotransmitters [45,46]. Gabapentin and pregabalin are commonly used neuroleptics that are effective for neuropathic pain. Neuroleptics were an integral part of ERAS pathways before 2020 due to several meta-analyses showing improved pain control, lower opiate use, and decreased opiate side effects with their use [26]. However, neuroleptics come with a myriad of side effects including sedation, visual disturbances, and respiratory depression [26] that can be augmented in older patients and with coadministration of opioids [35]. In a recent meta-analysis by Verret and colleagues (2020, [47]), that included 281 trials, the authors found that although there was a reduction in pain up to 48 hours after surgery with the use of neuroleptics (gabapentin and pregabalin alike), the reduction was clinically insignificant and came with significant side effects of dizziness and visual disturbances. Given this new evidence, neuroleptics should only be given as part of OFA in patients who have a chronic neuroleptic prescription but should not be started in the perioperative period for patients who are "neuroleptic naive" [35].

Intravenous lidocaine

Lidocaine blocks voltage-gated sodium channels and is used in medical practice as an antiarrhythmic and a local anesthetic. Intravenous (IV) lidocaine when used as an infusion has been shown to reduce analgesic consumption, result in early return of bowel function, decrease length of stay and potentially decrease persistent postsurgical pain after surgery, although this was apparent in early studies [21,25,26]. Lidocaine interacts at multiple receptors in addition to voltage-gated sodium channels, such as voltage-gated potassium channels, and NMDA receptors, leading to decreased inflammation, decreased pain and opioid use, and decrease hyperalgesia and persistent postsurgical pain [23,24,26]. The effectiveness of IV lidocaine for analgesia and to improve postoperative outcomes came into scrutiny after a 2018 literature review that found no clear benefit of IV lidocaine for a number of surgeries [48]. However, a recent meta-analysis of RCTs found that IV lidocaine seems to be more effective in specific surgeries, including open or laparoscopic abdominal surgeries [24,26,49] but its effects on improved pain control might be limited to the first 24 hours after surgery [49].

Lidocaine infusions are overall safe when patients are appropriately monitored [50], with minimal side effects, and seem to confer improved pain and postoperative outcomes in select surgeries [26,49]. Patients on lidocaine infusions outside of the operating room should be placed on a monitored bed, with staff trained on the signs of local anesthetic systemic toxicity (LAST), intralipid must be readily available, and with close follow-up by an acute pain service with 24/7 availability [50]. IV lidocaine should be considered as part of OFA for laparoscopic abdominal surgeries when no regional block is indicated. When regional blocks are used perioperatively, lidocaine infusions can be used with caution postoperatively if enough time has elapsed since the placement of the regional block to avoid LAST [50].

Magnesium sulfate

Magnesium is an NMDA receptor antagonist [25] that has been studied for postoperative pain control. Two meta-analyses [51,52] showed magnesium to be effective to reduce postoperative pain and opioid use after surgery. In addition, certain side effects that may be caused by magnesium, including dizziness, headache, PONV, or cardiovascular changes (hypotension and bradycardia) did not occur at a high rate with the use of magnesium [51]. Common side effects of magnesium toxicity such as weakness, decreased deep tendon reflexes or electrocardiogram changes were not reported in the studies used for the meta-analysis [51] but they were likely clinically insignificant. As a bonus, in patients receiving magnesium, the incidence of shivering was reduced [51]. Magnesium use should be considered for pain management during and after surgery in patients undergoing GA, and therefore can be a useful adjunct in OFA that carries minimal side effects.

Dexamethasone

Dexamethasone is commonly used to decrease the risk of postoperative nausea and vomiting [26,53]. In addition, steroids have anti-inflammatory properties and have been shown to decrease postoperative pain [26,53,54]. The doses needed for dexamethasone's analgesic effects (>0.1 mg/kg) may be higher than those required for its antiemetic effects under GA [54], whereas 8 mg of IV dexamethasone seem to be sufficient to provide analgesia under spinal anesthesia [53]. When performing a regional block, both systemic and perineural dexamethasone improve block quality and duration, with a greater effect from perineural dexamethasone but only of a few hours (1–4 hours) [55–57], with an unclear clinical significance in the prolonged block duration.

Dexamethasone can lead to hyperglycemia and poor wound healing but patients receiving a single dose of dexamethasone do not have an increased risk of wound infection or poor wound healing according to 2 meta-analyses looking at the effect of a single dose of dexamethasone intraoperatively for postoperative pain [53,54].

Dexamethasone should be given IV when appropriate for PONV prophylaxis and its anti-inflammatory properties, with the additional benefit of prolonging peripheral nerve blocks (PNBs) duration, and potential systemic analgesic effects.

Alpha-2 agonists:clonidine and dexmedetomidine

Clonidine and dexmedetomidine, both alpha-2 agonists, have been found to have analgesic properties, and result in reduced opiate use and nausea in the immediate postoperative period [25,58]. Of the 2, dexmedetomidine seems to be overall more effective [25,58], likely due to dexmedetomidine being 8 times more specific to α2 versus α1 (1620:1 vs 200:1) [59]. In addition to IV dexmedetomidine, perineural dexmedetomidine has been used to prolong block duration and decrease opiate use but not to the extent of dexamethasone [60].

Alpha-2 agonists can have significant hemodynamic side effects, with clonidine leading to significant hypotension, and dexmedetomidine causing both hypotension and bradycardia; therefore, alpha-2 agonists must be used cautiously in surgeries where significant hemodynamic changes are expected or in patients with cardiovascular disease [26,60].

Alpha-2 agonists are safe and effective adjuncts to improve pain control and decreased opiate use in select patients and surgeries [26,60]; however, dexmedetomidine might be preferred given more recent evidence behind its use for analgesia and given it is more easily titratable.

The con argument

The aforementioned medications should be used as part of a multimodal opiate-sparing approach but selection should be carefully tailored to specific patients and the invasiveness of surgeries to avoid drug–drug interactions, delayed emergence, and unjustified costs. A significant problem with the application of MMA is that although various medications seem to have a margin of benefit in pain control and opiate-sparing properties, few studies exist to determine the optimal combination of nonopiate adjuncts and their individual contribution to analgesia [10], which begs the question as to which combination and number of nonopiate analgesics is safe and effective to accomplish OFA.

There is a lack of evidence on the additive benefit of administering multiple nonopiate analgesics in an effort to eliminate opiates intraoperatively altogether, with significant risks of side effects that accumulate with each additional medication. Opiate-sparing analgesia with properly titrated opiates should be the preferred approach to intraoperative pain control. The effectiveness and safety of properly titrated opiates is well established compared with the unproven use of "opiate-free analgesic cocktails" and their increasing number of "ingredients."

WHAT ARE THE TECHNIQUES THAT FACILITATE OPIOID-FREE ANESTHESIA?

The pro argument

The use of neuraxial techniques, PNBs by the anesthesia team, and wound infiltration and/or targeted injections by surgeons, should be used intraoperatively whenever indicated [24] because these are some of the most powerful tools that facilitate OFA.

Neuraxial analgesia

Neuraxial techniques can be used as the main anesthetic, such as when using spinal and lumbar epidurals during c-sections, or for intraoperative "pain" control, such as when using thoracic epidurals during open abdominal surgeries under GA.

Spinal anesthesia provides complete anesthesia for multiple types of surgeries including orthopedic procedures such as knee and hip arthroplasties, and pelvic surgeries such as prostatectomies, cystectomies, and c-sections; however, debate exists whether the use of neuraxial versus GA should be favored in specific surgeries [61]. Opiates should be unnecessary when spinal anesthesia is used because nearly all nociception is blocked, although long-acting opiates can be given intrathecally to improve pain control for up to 24 hours after surgery with the caveat of increased opiate side effects [24,27,62].

Thoracic epidural analgesia (TEA) is highly recommended by ERAS guidelines for use during open colorectal surgeries, open cystectomies, and open general gynecologic surgery to improve postoperative pain control, return of bowel function, and morbidity and mortality [23,24,26,27,61,63]. TEA is also the standard of care for thoracic surgeries to improve pain control and decrease cardiac and respiratory complications [23,26,27,61,63,64]. The benefit of epidural analgesia is less clear in patients undergoing minimally invasive procedures [27,61,62]. TEA is generally placed preoperatively and patients undergo the surgery under GA [61]. The epidural can be used intraoperatively for pain control by bolusing the epidural with a short-acting or long-acting local anesthetic, before incision, without the need for additional opiates.

Neuraxial techniques are complex procedures that carry significant risks, including epidural failure, hypotension due to a sympathectomy, pruritus, urinary retention, lower extremity weakness with low thoracic or lumbar epidurals, postdural puncture headache and the more rare and catastrophic complications of infection, bleeding, nerve injury, LAST, epidural hematoma, and epidural abscess [26,61,63,65]. In addition, the use of epidural analgesia postoperatively requires an acute pain service to ensure safety and optimize the analgesia afforded by the epidural [66], which comes at increased costs [61]. The benefit of epidural analgesia is realized and justifies the significant risks and costs, when epidurals are used for large open surgeries, patients with chronic pain or chronic opiate use, or in patients with significant cardiopulmonary comorbidities [61,63].

Regional anesthesia techniques

PNBs, which include extremity and facial plane blocks, can be placed preincision to help with intraoperative pain control, and given these blocks can last up to 24 hours when given as a single injection and multiple days when a catheter is placed, they can provide postoperative pain relief [26,27,61]. The type of block used for a particular surgery will determine the extent of analgesia [26]. In general, the use of nerve blocks improves analgesia, and decreases postoperative opiate use and their side effects such as PONV [61,67]. The effectiveness of nerve blocks is such that they have been advocated in place of epidural analgesia given their improved side effect profile [61]. When quantifying analgesic effect, most studies focus on the pain control specific regional blocks provide after surgery [26], and this is likely due to the inability to objectively quantify nociception intraoperatively in patients under GA or deep sedation. The intraoperative analgesic effect of PNBs under GA is expected to be at least similar to the postoperative period; therefore, nerve blocks contribute to intraoperative analgesia and often provide complete analgesia for the purpose of OFA when administered before incision.

PNBs do have risks because they are procedures of varying complexity. Complications of PNBs include bleeding, infection, nerve injury, intravascular injection, LAST, and injury to structures near to where the needle manipulation occurs [26,65]. These complications are uncommon but nonetheless the benefit/risk ratio of using any particular nerve block should be assessed when deciding if a regional technique is indicated and justified based on the expected pain during and after a particular surgery.

Local infiltration analgesia by the surgeon

Local infiltration analgesia (LIA) refers to the injection of local anesthetic and sometimes other adjuvants in or near a surgical wound and intra-articularly, to provide intraoperative and postoperative analgesia [68]. LIA can be performed as a single injection or a catheter, and is most often performed by the surgeon [68]. LIA has been shown to decrease postoperative pain in multiple surgeries, including c-sections, video-assisted thoracic surgery, knee replacement surgeries, and laparoscopic cholecystectomies [26,27,61,68,69], and is an overall safer, cheaper, and easier alternative to regional techniques [68,69]. Given the potential benefits of wound local anesthetic infiltration, and the ease of implementation compared with regional techniques, LIA has been proposed as a favored approach for postoperative pain management in select surgeries [10,61,66,68]. Skin infiltration before surgical incision is a useful technique to minimize intraoperative nociception and to replace the use of opiates, thus facilitating OFA.

Minimally invasive surgical techniques

With the advent of minimally invasive surgical techniques, the need for invasive pain control strategies, including neuraxial and regional anesthesia, is reduced and often eliminated altogether [10,61,63]. Surgical technique influences outcomes and postoperative pain. The advent of minimally invasive surgeries has facilitated the application of OFA.

The con argument

Regional techniques, including neuraxial and PNBs, have the potential to provide complete analgesia intraoperatively but they come with risks [26,63,65]. In addition, PNBs and neuraxial anesthesia come with increased costs and are not indicated for many small procedures [10]. It seems unwise to rely on invasive analgesic techniques to allow OFA, when MMA with small doses of opiates may provide a nearly equally effective, and more efficient and accessible analgesic at decreased costs and risks.

Regional techniques may be unavailable in many hospitals due to the lack of expertise and costs. PNBs are seldom used in outpatient surgery centers in the United States, with only about 3% of procedures between 2010 and 2015 amenable to regional techniques receiving blocks, and this is even in the face of significant benefits in terms of improved pain control, decrease complications, and decreased PACU stay [67]. To our knowledge, there are no studies assessing the utilization of PNBs for surgeries that require inpatient stay but one can assume a similar trend. It is unclear why there is an underutilization of PNBs when indicated [10,67] but the trend shows that regional is a seldom available means to provide OFA. One must then not shy away from using carefully titrated doses of opiates intraoperatively in place of regional techniques, when the risk of regional technique often does not outweigh the benefit, and the availability of regional techniques remains limited.

Local infiltration by the surgeon and minimally invasive surgeries should be used when possible, and would lead to decreased need for opiates, in that we can agree. However, whether they can completely eliminate opiates remains to be shown.

SHOULD OPIOID-FREE ANESTHESIA BE PART OF EVERY ENHANCE RECOVERY AFTER SURGERY PATHWAY?

The ERAS Society supports the use of MMA to include various pharmacologic agents that when used together reduce pain while minimizing side effects of each medication, namely opiates, as well as advocates for the use of regional techniques whenever possible [24]. The overarching goal of the ERAS protocols is to improve recovery after surgery, and appropriate perioperative pain control with MMA is an essential component [23–25]. Per ERAS Society on systemic analgesia: "Using combination of non-opiates medications and regional analgesia may allow clinicians to avoid or significantly reduce systemic opiate consumption altogether, reserving them as a last resort only" [24].

The pro argument

Yes, OFA should be included in most, if not all, ERAS pathways for certain patient populations and types of surgeries. The ERAS Society supports the use of MMA with opioids only being used "as a last resort" [24]. Given opioids are rarely necessary during GA and in accordance with the goals of the ERAS society, OFA should be the standard of care when devising ERAS pathways.

The con argument

No, completely OFA would not be possible in a large proportion of surgeries for which ERAS protocols are developed. The ERAS guidelines support opiate-sparing MMA, and the ultimate goal should be to avoid opiates altogether. However, this is an often unreachable standard, and the use of appropriately titrated opiates as part of the multimodal approach is often necessary while applying other ERAS principles. One should not force the hand of clinicians to avoid opiates at all costs, which could be a disservice to patients' recovery.

SUMMARY/DISCUSSION

Appropriate postoperative pain control is essential to improve recovery, allowing for early mobility, earlier discharge, and improved patient satisfaction [70]. Opiate-sparing MMA improves pain control and decreases side effects, particularly from opiates [24]. Opiate-sparing intraoperative and postoperative analgesia should be the standard of care, and opiate-free pain control perioperatively should be the ultimate goal. Admittedly so, opiate-free postoperative pain control might be nearly unattainable for specific patients and surgeries. However, there are many tools that make OFA feasible for many types of surgeries, without negatively affecting postoperative pain control or overall recovery. OFA should be the favored strategy but adoption has been slow and with hesitation to abandon old opiate-heavy ways.

One of the big challenges of applying OFA is that it is difficult to change clinical practice even in the face of compelling evidence of the benefit of OFA with few risks. For instance, even in the light of ample evidence to support MMA in ERAS guidelines, there is a lack of implementation of the ERAS MMA in practice [10,71,72].

Another important challenge is that there are many pharmacologic, nonpharmacologic, and regional techniques that can be used to accomplish the goal of OFA, and the optimal combination of these for any one procedure while not adding unnecessary risks, is unknown [10,61]. In addition, not all surgeries, or patients, are the same, and although procedure-specific MMA guidelines exist, there is a lack of patient-specific guidelines, and the evidence behind procedure-specific guidelines is incomplete [24,70]. An important question is how to use the least combinations of adjuncts that allow patients' hemodynamics and pain control to be as well or better controlled than when opiates are used. We do not yet know the answer to this. The ERAS society guidelines (https://erassociety.org/guidelines/, [24]) along with the procedure-specific postoperative pain management collaboration guidelines (http://www.postoppain.org/, [73]) on evidence-based opiate-sparing analgesia for specific procedures can be used as a starting point, with the limitation that the guidelines can be broad, they do not incorporate all pharmacological modalities (ie, beta-blockers), it is unknown what benefit each component of ERAS contributes, they might not be applicable in specific hospital settings and they do not address specific patient populations such as patients with cancer pain or chronic opiate use [24,61,70].

The development of OFA protocols, with subsequent studies to assess their effectiveness to improve patient outcomes would be essential to confirm the value of OFA and help anesthesiologists broadly apply this revolutionary yet controversial approach to intraoperative pain control. The OFA guidelines would ideally be surgery, hospital and patient specific, and may become an important component of ERAS pathways in the future. In the meantime, anesthesiologists should aim to use the tools offered in this article to provide an opiate-free anesthetic whenever possible and certainly always aim for opiate-sparing anesthesia.

CLINICS CARE POINTS

- The use of opiates should be minimized to the least effective dose necessary and for the shortes duration needed, to avoid adverse side effects as well as the risk of dependance, abuse and addiction. Whenever possible, non-opioid alternatives for pain management should be utilized.

Conflicts of interest

V. Carcamo-Cavazos has no conflicts of interest to declare. M. Cannesson is a consultant for Edwards Lifesciences (Irvine, CA, USA) and Masimo Corp. (Irvine, CA, USA), and has funded research from Edwards Lifesciences and Masimo Corp.

References

[1] Raja SN, Carr DB, Cohen M, et al. The revised International Association for the Study of Pain definition of pain: concepts, challenges, and compromises. Pain 2020;161(9):1976–82.
[2] Bernard SA, Chelminski PR, Ives TJ, et al. Management of Pain in the United States-A Brief History and Implications for the Opioid Epidemic. Health Serv Insights 2018;11; https://doi.org/10.1177/1178632918819440:1178632918819440.
[3] Lyden J, Binswanger IA. The United States opioid epidemic. Semin Perinatol 2019;43(3): 123–31.
[4] Neuman MD, Bateman BT, Wunsch H. Inappropriate opioid prescription after surgery. Lancet 2019;393(10180):1547–57.
[5] Kharasch ED, Clark JD, Adams JM. Opioids and public health: the prescription opioid ecosystem and need for improved management. Anesthesiology 2022;136(1):10–30.
[6] Soneji N, Clarke HA, Ko DT, et al. Risks of developing persistent opioid use after major surgery. JAMA Surg 2016;151(11):1083–4.
[7] Brummett CM, Waljee JF, Goesling J, et al. New Persistent Opioid Use After Minor and Major Surgical Procedures in US Adults. JAMA Surg 2017;152(6):e170504.
[8] Steiner CA, Karaca Z, Moore BJ, et al. Surgeries in hospital-based ambulatory surgery and hospital inpatient settings, 2014: Statistical Brief #223. In: Healthcare cost and utilization project (HCUP) statistical briefs. Rockville (MD): Agency for Healthcare Research and Quality (US); 2020. Available at: https://www.ncbi.nlm.nih.gov/books/NBK442035/.
[9] Owings M, Jean L. Ambulatory and Inpatient Procedures in the United States, 1996. Vital Health Stat 1998;13(139):1–119.
[10] Rawal N. Current issues in postoperative pain management. Eur J Anaesthesiol 2016;33(3):160–71.
[11] Small C, Laycock H. Acute postoperative pain management. Br J Surg 2020;107(2): e70–80.
[12] Frauenknecht J, Kirkham KR, Jacot-Guillarmod A, et al. Analgesic impact of intra-operative opioids vs. opioid-free anaesthesia: a systematic review and meta-analysis. Anaesthesia 2019;74(5):651–62.
[13] United States Census Bureau, Population Division, Washington, DC. Projected population for the United States by age group and alternative immigration scenario: 2020 to 2060 (NP2017-D). 2019. Available at: https://www.census.gov/data/tables/2017/demo/popproj/2017-alternative-summary-tables.html. Accessed February 12, 2022.
[14] Prostran M, Vujović KS, Vučković S, et al. Pharmacotherapy of pain in the older population: the place of opioids. Front Aging Neurosci 2016;8:144.
[15] Chia PA, Cannesson M, Bui CCM. Opioid free anesthesia: feasible? Curr Opin Anaesthesiol 2020;33(4):512–7.
[16] Daccache G, Jeanne M, Fletcher D. The analgesia nociception index: tailoring opioid administration. Anesth Analg 2017;125(1):15–7.
[17] Ledowski T. Objective monitoring of nociception: a review of current commercial solutions. Br J Anaesth 2019;123(2):e312–21.
[18] Kharasch ED, Clark JD. Opioid-free anesthesia: time to regain our balance. Anesthesiology 2021;134(4):509–14.
[19] Doleman B, Leonardi-Bee J, Heinink TP, et al. Pre-emptive and preventive opioids for postoperative pain in adults undergoing all types of surgery. Cochrane Database Syst Rev 2018;12(12):CD012624.

[20] Elvir-Lazo OL, White PF, Yumul R, et al. Management strategies for the treatment and prevention of postoperative/postdischarge nausea and vomiting: an updated review. F1000Res 2020;9:F1000; https://doi.org/10.12688/f1000research.21832.1, Faculty Rev-983. Published 2020 Aug 13.
[21] Richebé P, Capdevila X, Rivat C. Persistent postsurgical pain: pathophysiology and preventative pharmacologic considerations. Anesthesiology 2018;129(3):590–607.
[22] Kharasch ED, Avram MJ, Clark JD. Rational perioperative opioid management in the era of the opioid crisis. Anesthesiology 2020;132(4):603–5.
[23] Gelman D, Gelmanas A, Urbanaitė D, et al. Role of multimodal analgesia in the evolving enhanced recovery after surgery pathways. Medicina (Kaunas) 2018;54(2):20.
[24] Beverly A, Kaye AD, Ljungqvist O, et al. Essential elements of multimodal analgesia in enhanced recovery after surgery (ERAS) guidelines. Anesthesiol Clin 2017;35(2):e115–43.
[25] Mitra S, Carlyle D, Kodumudi G, et al. New advances in acute postoperative pain management. Curr Pain Headache Rep 2018;22(5):35.
[26] Gabriel RA, Swisher MW, Sztain JF, et al. State of the art opioid-sparing strategies for postoperative pain in adult surgical patients. Expert Opin Pharmacother 2019;20(8):949–61.
[27] Wick EC, Grant MC, Wu CL. Postoperative multimodal analgesia pain management with nonopioid analgesics and techniques: a review. JAMA Surg 2017;152(7):691–7.
[28] Solomon D. NSAIDs: Pharmacology and Mechanism of Action. UpToDate. 2022. Available at: https://www.uptodate.com/contents/nsaids-pharmacology-and-mechanism-of-action. Accessed March/30/2022.
[29] Gupta A, Bah M. NSAIDs in the treatment of postoperative pain. Curr Pain Headache Rep 2016;20(11):62.
[30] McDaid C, Maund E, Rice S, et al. Paracetamol and selective and non-selective non-steroidal anti-inflammatory drugs (NSAIDs) for the reduction of morphine-related side effects after major surgery: a systematic review. Health Technol Assess 2010;14(17):1–iv.
[31] Elia N, Lysakowski C, Tramèr MR. Does multimodal analgesia with acetaminophen, nonsteroidal antiinflammatory drugs, or selective cyclooxygenase-2 inhibitors and patient-controlled analgesia morphine offer advantages over morphine alone? Meta-analyses of randomized trials. Anesthesiology 2005;103(6):1296–304.
[32] Doleman B, Leonardi-Bee J, Heinink TP, et al. Pre-emptive and preventive NSAIDs for postoperative pain in adults undergoing all types of surgery. Cochrane Database Syst Rev 2021;6(6):CD012978.
[33] Chang RW, Tompkins DM, Cohn SM. Are NSAIDs Safe? Assessing the risk-benefit profile of nonsteroidal anti-inflammatory drug use in postoperative pain management. Am Surg 2021;87(6):872–9.
[34] Ong CK, Seymour RA, Lirk P, et al. Combining paracetamol (acetaminophen) with nonsteroidal antiinflammatory drugs: a qualitative systematic review of analgesic efficacy for acute postoperative pain. Anesth Analg 2010;110(4):1170–9.
[35] Mariano E, Fishman S, Crowley M. Management of acute perioperative pain. UpToDate. 2022. Available at: https://www.uptodate.com/contents/management-of-acute-perioperative-pain. Accessed March/22/2022.
[36] Barrett W, Buxhoeveden M, Dhillon S. Ketamine: a versatile tool for anesthesia and analgesia. Curr Opin Anaesthesiol 2020;33(5):633–8; https://doi.org/10.1097/ACO.0000000000000916.
[37] Peltoniemi MA, Hagelberg NM, Olkkola KT, et al. Ketamine: a review of clinical pharmacokinetics and pharmacodynamics in anesthesia and pain therapy. Clin Pharmacokinet 2016;55(9):1059–77.
[38] Laskowski K, Stirling A, McKay WP, et al. A systematic review of intravenous ketamine for postoperative analgesia. Can J Anaesth 2011;58(10):911–23.
[39] Moon TS, Smith KM. Ketamine use in the surgical patient: a literature review. Curr Pain Headache Rep 2021;25(3):17.

[40] Schwenk ES, Viscusi ER, Buvanendran A, et al. Consensus guidelines on the use of Intravenous ketamine infusions for acute pain management from the american society of regional anesthesia and pain medicine, the american academy of pain medicine, and the american society of anesthesiologists. Reg Anesth Pain Med 2018;43(5):456–66.
[41] Härkänen L, Halonen J, Selander T, et al. Beta-adrenergic antagonists during general anesthesia reduced postoperative pain: a systematic review and a meta-analysis of randomized controlled trials. J Anesth 2015;29(6):934–43.
[42] Gelineau AM, King MR, Ladha KS, et al. Intraoperative esmolol as an adjunct for perioperative opioid and postoperative pain reduction: a systematic review, meta-analysis, and meta-regression. Anesth Analg 2018;126(3):1035–49.
[43] Harless M, Depp C, Collins S, et al. Role of esmolol in perioperative analgesia and anesthesia: a literature review. AANA J 2015;83(3):167–77.
[44] Watts R, Thiruvenkatarajan V, Calvert M, et al. The effect of perioperative esmolol on early postoperative pain: A systematic review and meta-analysis. J Anaesthesiol Clin Pharmacol 2017;33(1):28–39.
[45] Gabapentin: Drug Information. UpToDate. Available at: https://www.uptodate.com/contents/gabapentin-drug-information. Accessed March/30/2022.
[46] Pregabalin: Drug Information. UpToDate. Available at: https://www.uptodate.com/contents/pregabalin-drug-information. Accessed 3/30/2022.
[47] Verret M, Lauzier F, Zarychanski R, et al. Perioperative use of gabapentinoids for the management of postoperative acute pain: a systematic review and meta-analysis. Anesthesiology 2020;133(2):265–79 [published correction appears in Anesthesiology. 2020 Aug 21;:null].
[48] Weibel S, Jelting Y, Pace NL, et al. Continuous intravenous perioperative lidocaine infusion for postoperative pain and recovery in adults. Cochrane Database Syst Rev 2018;6(6): CD009642.
[49] Rollins KE, Javanmard-Emamghissi H, Scott MJ, et al. The impact of peri-operative intravenous lidocaine on postoperative outcome after elective colorectal surgery: a meta-analysis of randomised controlled trials. Eur J Anaesthesiol 2020;37(8):659–70.
[50] Foo I, Macfarlane AJR, Srivastava D, et al. The use of intravenous lidocaine for postoperative pain and recovery: international consensus statement on efficacy and safety. Anaesthesia 2021;76(2):238–50.
[51] De Oliveira GS Jr, Castro-Alves LJ, Khan JH, et al. Perioperative systemic magnesium to minimize postoperative pain: a meta-analysis of randomized controlled trials. Anesthesiology 2013;119(1):178–90.
[52] Murphy JD, Paskaradevan J, Eisler LL, et al. Analgesic efficacy of continuous intravenous magnesium infusion as an adjuvant to morphine for postoperative analgesia: a systematic review and meta-analysis. Middle East J Anaesthesiol 2013;22(1):11–20.
[53] Heesen M, Rijs K, Hilber N, et al. Effect of intravenous dexamethasone on postoperative pain after spinal anaesthesia - a systematic review with meta-analysis and trial sequential analysis. Anaesthesia 2019;74(8):1047–56.
[54] De Oliveira GS Jr, Almeida MD, Benzon HT, et al. Perioperative single dose systemic dexamethasone for postoperative pain: a meta-analysis of randomized controlled trials. Anesthesiology 2011;115(3):575–88.
[55] Baeriswyl M, Kirkham KR, Jacot-Guillarmod A, et al. Efficacy of perineural vs systemic dexamethasone to prolong analgesia after peripheral nerve block: a systematic review and meta-analysis. Br J Anaesth 2017;119(2):183–91.
[56] Heesen M, Klimek M, Imberger G, et al. Co-administration of dexamethasone with peripheral nerve block: intravenous vs perineural application: systematic review, meta-analysis, meta-regression and trial-sequential analysis. Br J Anaesth 2018;120(2):212–27.
[57] Zorrilla-Vaca A, Li J. Dexamethasone injected perineurally is more effective than administered intravenously for peripheral nerve blocks: a meta-analysis of randomized controlled trials. Clin J Pain 2018;34(3):276–84.

[58] Blaudszun G, Lysakowski C, Elia N, et al. Effect of perioperative systemic α2 agonists on postoperative morphine consumption and pain intensity: systematic review and meta-analysis of randomized controlled trials. Anesthesiology 2012;116(6):1312–22.
[59] Afonso J, Reis F. Dexmedetomidine: current role in anesthesia and intensive care. Rev Bras Anestesiol 2012;62(1):118–33.
[60] Kaye AD, Chernobylsky DJ, Thakur P, et al. Dexmedetomidine in Enhanced Recovery After Surgery (ERAS) Protocols for Postoperative Pain. Curr Pain Headache Rep 2020;24(5):21.
[61] Rawal N. Epidural technique for postoperative pain: gold standard no more? Reg Anesth Pain Med 2012;37(3):310–7.
[62] Simpson JC, Bao X, Agarwala A. Pain management in enhanced recovery after surgery (ERAS) protocols. Clin Colon Rectal Surg 2019;32(2):121–8.
[63] Bos EME, Hollmann MW, Lirk P. Safety and efficacy of epidural analgesia. Curr Opin Anaesthesiol 2017;30(6):736–42.
[64] Park SK, Yoon S, Kim BR, et al. Pre-emptive epidural analgesia for acute and chronic post-thoracotomy pain in adults: a systematic review and meta-analysis. Reg Anesth Pain Med 2020;45(12):1006–16.
[65] Neal JM, Barrington MJ, Brull R, et al. The second ASRA practice advisory on neurologic complications associated with regional anesthesia and pain medicine: executive summary 2015. Reg Anesth Pain Med 2015;40(5):401–30.
[66] Chou R, Gordon DB, de Leon-Casasola OA, et al. Management of postoperative pain: a clinical practice guideline from the american pain society, the american society of regional anesthesia and pain medicine, and the american society of anesthesiologists' committee on regional anesthesia, executive committee, and administrative council. J Pain 2016;17(2): 131–157[published correction appears in J Pain. 2016 Apr;17(4):508-510. Dosage error in article text].
[67] Gabriel RA, Ilfeld BM. Use of regional anesthesia for outpatient surgery within the united states: a prevalence study using a nationwide database. Anesth Analg 2018;126(6): 2078–84.
[68] Stamenkovic DM, Bezmarevic M, Bojic S, et al. Updates on wound infiltration use for postoperative pain management: a narrative review. J Clin Med 2021;10(20):4659.
[69] Ganapathy S, Brookes J, Bourne R. Local infiltration analgesia. Anesthesiol Clin 2011;29(2):329–42.
[70] Joshi GP, Kehlet H. Postoperative pain management in the era of ERAS: an overview. Best Pract Res Clin Anaesthesiol 2019;33(3):259–67.
[71] Kehlet H, Joshi GP. Enhanced recovery after surgery: current controversies and concerns. Anesth Analg 2017;125(6):2154–5.
[72] Berian JR, Ban KA, Liu JB, et al. Adherence to enhanced recovery protocols in NSQIP and association with colectomy outcomes. Ann Surg 2019;269(3):486–93.
[73] Procedure specific postoperative pain management (PROSPECT). Available at: http://www.postoppain.org/. Accessed March/20/2022.

Advances in Anesthesia 40 (2022) 167–183

ADVANCES IN ANESTHESIA

ELSEVIER
MOSBY

Anesthesia Machine and New Modes of Ventilation

Aditi Balakrishna, MD*, Lucille Brunker, MD,
Christopher G. Hughes, MD, MS, FCCM

Vanderbilt University School of Medicine, 1211 21st Avenue South, 422MAB, Nashville, TN 37212, USA

Keywords

• Anesthesia machine • Intraoperative ventilation • Lung-protective ventilation • Jet ventilation • Advanced lung monitoring

Key points

- The modern anesthesia machine has broad functionality as a mechanical ventilator; there are specific design features that provide safety and confer limitations.
- Lung-protective ventilation can be achieved in the operating room and is considered standard of practice.
- Specific patient and anesthetic conditions demand a tailored approach to choosing ventilatory parameters.
- Intraoperative scenarios may require the use of both standard and nonstandard (ie, jet ventilation) approaches to ventilation.
- Advanced monitoring tools exist that can help tailor ventilation strategy to the individual patient's lungs.

INTRODUCTION

Ventilating patients appropriately in the operating room (OR) setting requires an understanding of the anesthesia machine as well as how patient and anesthetic scenarios impact ventilation and oxygenation strategies, including the use of nonstandard ventilation strategies and advanced monitoring tools. This article provides an overview of these important topics.

Anesthesia machine overview

The anesthesia machine allows for oxygenation and positive pressure ventilation of patients under general anesthesia, as well as the delivery of inhaled

*Corresponding author. *E-mail address:* aditi.balakrishna@vumc.org

https://doi.org/10.1016/j.aan.2022.07.008
0737-6146/22/

anesthetics and the scavenging of waste gasses. Anesthesia machines have undergone significant development in the last several decades, and current models rely on advanced computer technology for both central and safety functions.

Unlike other ventilators, an anesthesia machine allows patients to rebreathe gasses to preserve those inhaled anesthetics and prevent pollution. However, carbon dioxide must be filtered out before gasses are rebreathed. The setup that allows this is called a circle system, which includes one-way valves, a carbon dioxide absorber, a reservoir bag that allows the provider to assist ventilation if needed and otherwise visualize spontaneous efforts, an adjustable pressure limiting valve to control the pressure in the system, and a Y-piece adaptor to connect the circuit to the patient. Anesthesia machines also incorporate scavenging systems to ensure that volatile anesthetics remain at safe concentrations in the OR environment [1].

The coronavirus disease-2019 (COVID-19) pandemic saw the use of anesthesia machines in the intensive care unit (ICU) setting during times of ventilator shortages. This highlighted the differences between ventilators used for longer durations of mechanical ventilation and those that are used in the OR.

Warming and humidification of gasses

ICU ventilators incorporate active warming and humidification or passive humidification (ie, heat and moisture exchanger [HME]), as fresh gas flow is constantly delivered from a non-humidified, compressed fresh gas source. Because anesthesia machines allow for rebreathing, and because carbon dioxide (CO_2) scavenging produces heat, gasses are heated and humidified within the circuit. When these machines are used for long periods of time, preventing the exhaustion of the CO_2 absorber and the accumulation of water in the circuit is important. It was recommended that fresh gas flow be at least equal to minute ventilation to prevent the accumulation of water.

Resistance and dead space considerations

Accumulated water can lead to increased resistance to gas flow, and it can be a nidus for infection. HME filters are still required to ensure appropriate humidity during long-term ventilation, and they also help to filter viral particles to avoid contamination of the machine. But these filters add a resistance point--particularly when clogged with secretions or water--and add additional dead space (approximately 30 cc).

Ability to deliver desired fraction of inspired oxygen

When fresh gas flow allows rebreathing, inspired oxygen can be lower than expected, depending on the level of oxygen consumption. Conversely, it may be impossible to provide high enough fraction of inspired oxygen (FiO_2) if the fresh gas flow exceeds the maximal flow of oxygen that the ventilator can provide (ie, if 20 L of fresh gas flow/minute is required, and only 12 L/min is possible on the anesthesia machine, 8 L/min of air must be added). This is not a concern with ICU ventilators, as they do not allow rebreathing [2,3].

There are other safety issues relating to monitoring of the machine and the use of volatile agents for sedation that also require consideration when anesthesia machines are used for longer-term ventilation. Given these differences from ICU ventilators and the relative lack of practical experience using anesthesia machines in this context, it may be unsurprising that patient outcomes were noted to be worse when these machines were used. An analysis of 89 mechanically ventilated patients with COVID-19 in Italy found significantly higher 60-day mortality among the 17 patients ventilated by anesthesia machine [4]. Several issues were attributed to the difficulty with humidification regulation.

Principles of lung-protective ventilation in the operating room

Mechanical ventilation results in non-physiologic stress and strain on lung tissue, which can cause injury. Strategies for minimizing ventilator-induced lung injury (VILI) have been well-studied in the ICU setting [5,6]. We will outline these principles and then discuss their application in the OR setting.

Lung-protective ventilation aims to reduce the footprint the ventilator has on the lung to prevent iatrogenic injury. Controlling the following parameters has been shown to limit VILI in the acute respiratory distress syndrome (ARDS) populations, and these findings are extrapolated to the OR population [7].

Tidal volume

Airflow will proceed down the path of least resistance, most commonly the healthy non-diseased lung spaces. Limiting tidal volumes to 6 cc/kg of ideal body weight (IBW) minimizes the risk of overdistension of normal lung tissue [5]. Excessive stretching of the collagen fibers that scaffold the parenchyma can result in inflammatory activation and injury, known as volutrauma [8].

Plateau pressure

Exposing the alveoli to high pressures can also be injurious, as it can overwhelm the elastic capacity of the lung parenchyma. Resultant damage is called barotrauma. At its extreme, barotrauma manifests as airway rupture, causing pneumothorax or pneumomediastinum. Maintaining the plateau pressure (Pplat) below 30 cm of water has been shown to decrease mortality in ARDS [5].

Pplat is determined by applying a hold maneuver at the end of inspiration and then measuring the pressure in the system (Fig. 1). With this maneuver, the pressure across the system can equilibrate, such that the measured pressure represents what the alveoli and small airways are being exposed to. The Pplat required to generate a given tidal volume provides information about lung compliance.

This stands in contrast to the peak pressure, which is influenced by the resistance of the whole system, including the large airways, the endotracheal tube, the ventilator circuit, and any associated filters. Anesthesia machines can be programmed to alarm and/or limit ventilation at a prespecified peak pressure as a safety mechanism.

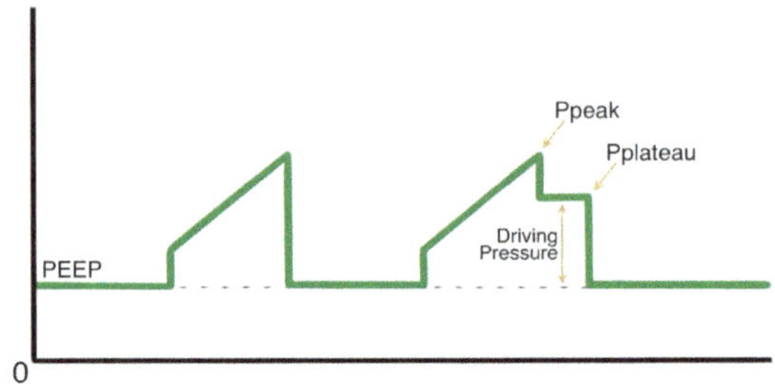

Fig. 1. Schematic of pressure vs time in a volume-controlled ventilation mode, showing the peak pressure (Ppeak) vs plateau pressure (Pplateau) and the driving pressure. (*Courtesy of* Phoebe Fraser.)

Driving pressure

The pressure exerted on the lungs while the ventilator achieves a given tidal volume is the driving pressure; it is equal to the Pplat minus the positive end-expiratory pressure (PEEP). In the ARDS population, it has been shown that maneuvers that decrease driving pressure increase survival rates when other lung-protective settings are already in place [6]. In this population, a driving pressure over 15 was associated with a higher risk of mortality.

Positive end-expiratory pressure

PEEP is used to maintain lung recruitment to minimize atelectasis and prevent atelectrauma, which is damage caused by repeated opening and closing of lung units. The appropriate amount of PEEP necessary in both the ICU population and the OR population remains a subject of debate and ongoing research. To date, there has not been proof that an arbitrarily high or low PEEP confers a benefit. Individualizing PEEP to the patient and clinical situation, however, may have benefits [9].

Although targeting these parameters has robust data in the ARDS population, the data have not been as uniform in the OR population.

Randomized controlled trials to examine the impact of lung-protective ventilation in the perioperative setting have used either markers of inflammation and other nonclinical factors as primary outcomes, or they have measured postop pulmonary complications, which can vary in scale or degree depending on the trial [7].

The heterogeneity of the outcome measures, patient populations, and relatively small trial size have rendered definitive conclusions lacking [7]. Where trial results have shown an impact of lung-protective ventilation, they have shown decreased inflammatory markers and postoperative pulmonary complications, and improved postoperative pulmonary function [10,11]. Accordingly, these principles are increasingly adopted in the clinical setting.

Standard modes of ventilation

Modern anesthesia machines can deliver ventilation via several standard ventilation modes, which differ in terms of which parameters are set by the provider and how the ventilator delivers airflow to the patient's lung. These parameters, in turn, influence the pressures and volumes targeted as outlined above. This article discusses volume control, pressure control, pressure regulated volume control, and pressure support [12]. Other modes, such as airway pressure release ventilation, proportional assist ventilation, and high frequency oscillatory or percussive ventilation are not frequently used in the OR, have limited data in the OR setting, and are out of the scope of this review.

Volume control, pressure control, and pressure-regulated volume control can all be exercised in 3 different ventilator strategies. In a controlled mandatory ventilation (CMV) strategy, all breaths are delivered by the ventilator without the incorporation of patient respiratory efforts. In an assist-control (AC) strategy, breaths are delivered at set intervals based on the specified respiratory rate, and patient respiratory efforts are supported with the same level of support as the mandatory breaths. In a synchronized intermittent mandatory ventilation (SIMV) strategy, the ventilator will synchronize the mandatory control breaths with the timing of patient effort (if applicable) and will provide pressure support to any additional breaths above the set mandatory control breaths [13,14].

Volume control

In volume-controlled modes, the clinician sets a tidal volume for the ventilator to deliver as well as a respiratory rate, PEEP, inspiratory-to-expiratory time (I:E) ratio, and Fio_2 (Fig. 2). The ventilator determines the amount of flow to deliver during the inspiratory segment of the respiratory cycle to produce the prespecified tidal volume; mathematically, the integral of flow over time is volume. The necessary flow rate is a result of both the other parameters set and the resistance points in the system. For example, an increase in respiratory rate will lead to increased flow and pressure to achieve the set tidal volume in the shorter inspiratory cycle. Ventilators will display the pressure in the respiratory cycle during the delivery of a breath; here, the pressure curve will be upsloping, and as previously described, an end-inspiratory hold will help differentiate between the peak pressure and Pplat to target lung-protective benchmarks.

The advantage of this mode is guaranteed tidal volumes, regardless of changes in patient position or condition that may impact airway resistance, allowing for consistent minute ventilation. The consequence may be changing pressures or higher peak inspiratory pressures that can contribute to barotrauma.

Pressure control

Pressure control modes require that the inspiratory pressure be set by the clinician (Fig. 3). Some ventilators have the user set the delta P or driving pressure, whereas others will have the user set peak inspiratory pressure. The provider also must set PEEP, respiratory rate, I:E ratio, and Fio_2. Depending on these settings and the compliance of the system, a tidal volume will be determined. Here, a constant pressure is delivered during the inspiratory time, and the

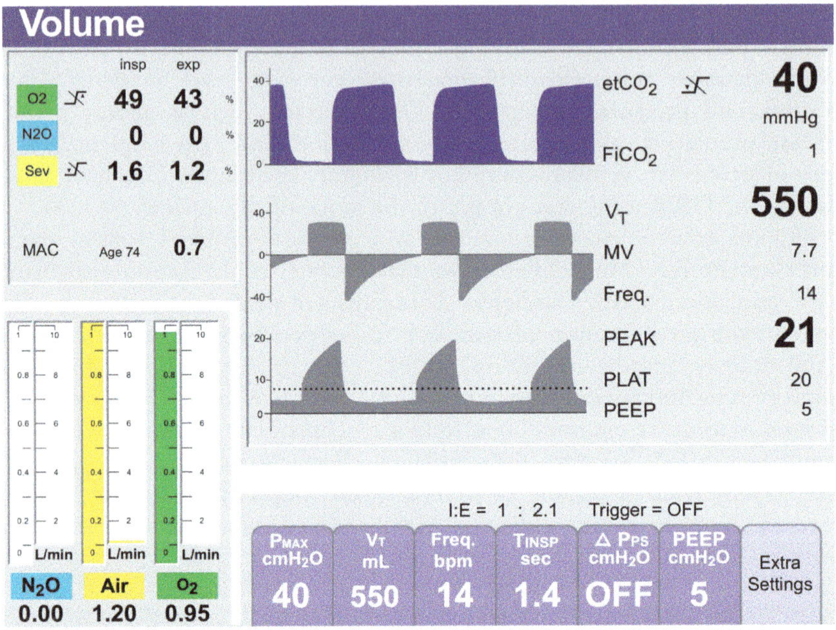

Fig. 2. Schematic of anesthesia machine in volume control mode. Note flat flow curve and upsloping pressure curve. Tidal volume, respiratory rate, inspiratory time (to modulate I:E), PEEP, and FiO_2 are set by the clinician. (*Courtesy of* Phoebe Fraser.)

flow rate (and resulting tidal volume) is a function of the resistance in system. A downsloping flow curve is the hallmark of this mode. Because changes in respiratory system compliance can change this flow curve, tidal volumes are not guaranteed. For example, reduced pulmonary compliance will lead to a lower tidal volume but also an increase in respiratory rate will lead to reduced time of driving pressure during inspiration and therefore a lower tidal volume. In the OR setting, variation in positioning, abdominal pressures, and other surgical conditions can exacerbate this variability, leading to inconsistent minute ventilation and the potential for hypoventilation, hyperventilation, or volutrauma. The advantage to this mode is that peak pressures are generally lower for a given desired tidal volume, and prespecifying peak pressures mean that barotrauma risk can be minimized or avoided.

Pressure-regulated volume control

PRVC, also known as Volume Auto Flow (Volume AF) or Pressure Control-Volume Guarantee, is a hybrid mode that allows the user to set a tidal volume and have breaths delivered via constant pressure, instead of a constant flow, during the inspiratory interval (Fig. 4). The ventilator adjusts the necessary pressure automatically based on the respiratory system compliance, thereby allowing the advantages of pressure control ventilation while maintaining constant tidal volume and minute ventilation.

Pressure support

This ventilator mode is a support mode for patient-initiated ventilation, although many ventilators have a built-in backup mode to ensure that the patient does not hypoventilate during the transition to spontaneous ventilation. The clinician sets an amount of additional pressure that the ventilator delivers during each patient-initiated breath, and the PEEP and FiO_2, but the respiratory rate and I:E is patient-driven (except for any backup settings the user chooses). Patient-initiated breaths are detected by the ventilator sensing negative inspiratory force by the patient. The user can specify the degree of effort--usually as a flow rate--required to initiate support to ensure that the ventilator is sensing patient inspiratory effort appropriately [12]. Over-sensing patient effort may confuse movement by the surgical team for the inspiratory effort, whereas under-sensing can lead to dyssynchrony or fatigue. Respiratory cycles are limited by the slowing of inspiratory flow. This mode is generally used when patients are breathing spontaneously during an anesthetic, either for the duration of the case or when the patient is nearing extubation. More clinician monitoring is required here than in other modes to ensure that the patient is meeting oxygenation and ventilation goals.

Patient conditions and impact on ventilation

Patients' comorbidities can significantly influence the ventilation strategy used to maintain lung-protective ventilation.

Healthy lungs

Initiating positive pressure ventilation for a patient with no medical comorbidities nonetheless changes that individual's respiratory mechanics. Their lungs will now require recruitment via some amount of PEEP to prevent atelectasis, which was previously prevented by negative pressure breathing. Lung compliance will likely be between 50 and 100 cc/cmH20, though supine positioning and surgical manipulation may decrease that value [15]. Ventilatory parameters should still adhere to lung-protective guidelines to prevent ventilator-associated lung injury of healthy lung, though the expected risk to this population is small.

Obstructive lung disease

Chronic obstructive pulmonary disease (COPD) and asthma cause limitation to exhalation during tidal breathing due to increased airway resistance. These factors impact what is seen on the anesthesia machine and how the anesthesia machine should be set and adjusted for patients with these comorbidities. Ensuring that patients can fully exhale at the end of each respiratory cycle is necessary to prevent gas trapping and the development of auto-PEEP. That in turn can lead to dynamic hyperinflation and cardiovascular compromise, and barotrauma. I:E ratios should be at least 1:2, and possibly longer, to allow completion of the respiratory cycle. Higher airway resistance may predispose airway collapse, leading to auto-PEEP at baseline. This must be considered when setting the patient's extrinsic PEEP to prevent overdistension [16]. Depending on the phenotype of COPD, the patient may also have decreased

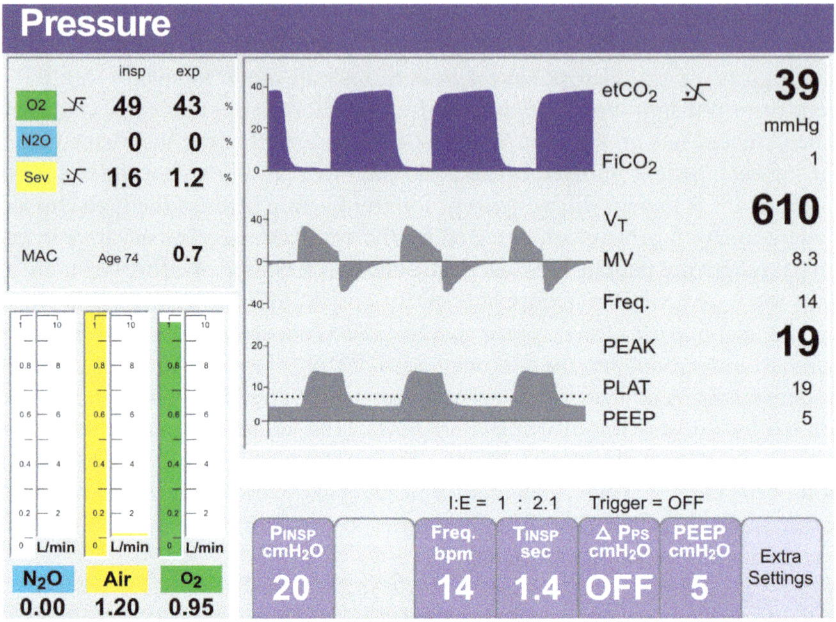

Fig. 3. Schematic of anesthesia machine in pressure control mode. Note flat pressure curve and downsloping flow curve. Driving pressure, respiratory rate, inspiratory time (to modulate I:E), PEEP, and FiO_2 are set by the clinician. (*Courtesy of* Phoebe Fraser.)

lung compliance, which may increase ventilatory pressures. These conditions also predispose patients to airway reactivity during intubation and mechanical ventilation, prompting bronchospasm and the need for treatment intraoperatively and postoperatively [17].

Restrictive lung disease

Restrictive lung disease leads to decreased lung compliance and poor lung recruitability. All lung volumes can be decreased on spirometry for these patients. Keeping tidal volumes small and respiratory rates somewhat higher is recommended to minimize barotrauma. Increasing inspiratory time in the I:E ratio and using pressure control or PRVC can also reduce the risk of high peak inspiratory pressures for these patients [18].

Obesity

Patients with elevated body mass index (BMI), particularly those with abdominal obesity, have a reduction in functional reserve capacity (FRC) and expiratory reserve volume because of the displacement of the diaphragm by abdominal fat. When supine, obese patients have an increase in airway resistance and development of expiratory flow limitation, which can lead to air trapping. This may be a function of the collapse of small airways due to elevated pleural pressures. Patients with Class III (BMI > 40) obesity have been shown

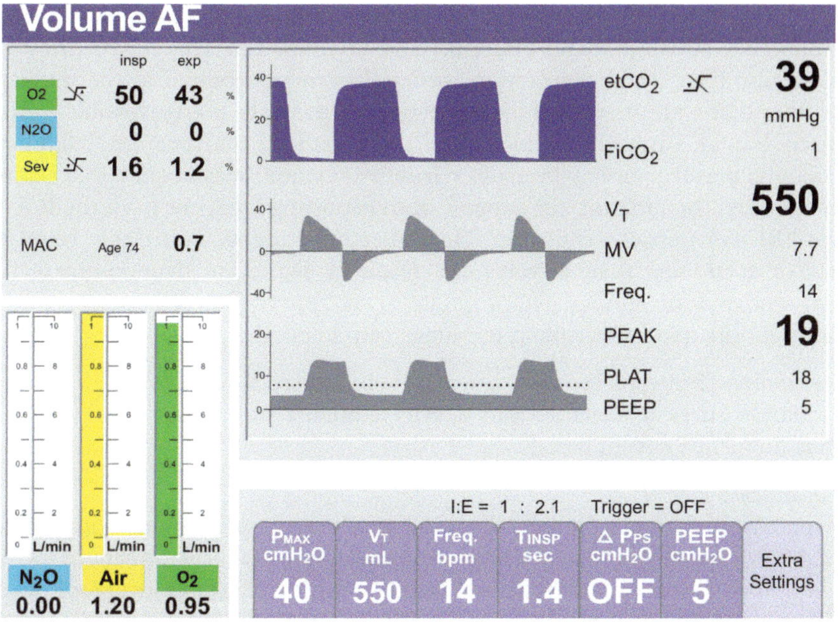

Fig. 4. Schematic of anesthesia machine in pressure control-volume guarantee (Volume AF) mode. Note flat pressure curve and downsloping flow curve. Tidal volume, respiratory rate, inspiratory time (to modulate I:E), PEEP, and FiO_2 are set by the clinician. (*Courtesy of* Phoebe Fraser.)

to need to generate significant intrathoracic pressure simply to initiate tidal breathing, which results in a significantly increased work of breathing at baseline [19]. When mechanical ventilation is instituted, these elevated pleural pressures predispose them to significant atelectasis—as transpulmonary pressures are likely to be negative unless appropriately balanced with elevated PEEP [20].

Elderly patients

Aging produces numerous changes to the respiratory system. Chest wall and spine degeneration leads to a restrictive physiology, which decreases compliance and increases work of breathing. Respiratory muscles also weaken over time. Forced expiratory volume (FEV1), vital capacity, and diffusion capacity for carbon monoxide (DLCO) decrease with age, whereas closing capacity, residual volume, and FRC increase. The collagen fibers that scaffold the parenchyma also weaken, creating "senile emphysema." These changes require adjustments to ventilation consistent with what was discussed for both obstructive and restrictive lung disease [21].

Intubated intensive care unit population

Patients in the ICU who are intubated for a primary pulmonary pathophysiology are likely to have reduced lung compliance compared with a patient with normal, healthy lungs. This can be from infectious processes but also from pulmonary edema, pleural effusions, and accumulating atelectasis. They will likely also have a higher secretion burden. In general, continuing the ventilator settings that were successful for the patient in the ICU is a reasonable starting place, though surgical conditions and the anesthesia machine capabilities (eg, ability to perform airway pressure release ventilation) may require that settings be adjusted. In addition, the process of transporting a patient from the ICU to the OR can impact ventilation. Disconnecting patients from their ventilator and/or suctioning their airways can result in significant de-recruitment that can render prior settings inappropriate or ineffective [22]. Minimizing disconnection time and re-recruiting the lungs can ameliorate this.

Ventilation strategies for different anesthetic/surgical conditions

Common surgical scenarios can heavily influence pulmonary mechanics and thus the plan for ventilation.

Laparoscopic surgery

Laparoscopic surgery requires the creation of pneumoperitoneum with pressurized CO_2. Insufflating the abdomen results in cephalad displacement of the diaphragm and mediastinum and reduces FRC. This can lead to increased pleural pressures, which exert collapsing force on alveoli. Atelectatic alveoli worsen lung compliance, leading to increased ventilatory pressures. Because of the upward diaphragmatic shift, patients are also at higher risk of endotracheal tube migration into a mainstem bronchus. Both problems are exacerbated by Trendelenburg positioning, which is common in many pelvic and lower abdominal laparoscopic procedures. The CO_2 used for insufflation can also be absorbed, thus requiring an increase in minute ventilation to compensate [23].

Prone positioning

Prone positioning is necessary for numerous surgical procedures. The major challenge relates to access to the airway and preventing disconnection, disruption, or occlusion of the endotracheal tube. Physiologically, the prone position is known to be beneficial for the respiratory system; indeed, it has a mortality benefit in the ICU setting in patients with severe ARDS [24]. As long as abdominal movement is not limited, FRC may actually increase, and chest wall and lung compliance do not change. There is also improved ventilation/perfusion (VQ) matching in this position [25].

One lung ventilation

Thoracic surgery frequently requires lung isolation for adequate surgical exposure. This can be achieved in several ways. Patients can be endobronchially intubated with either a traditional tube or an endobronchial tube; the latter has a smaller cuff, which allows for better positioning of the tube within a mainstem bronchus. Ventilation can then be provided only to the nonoperative lung. A bronchial blocker can be placed through a traditional endotracheal tube that occludes and vents the lung that needs to be deflated for the surgical procedure. Finally, a double lumen tube can be placed that allows for ventilation of one or both lungs; double lumen tubes also allow for suctioning and bronchoscopy of the individual lungs [26].

Ventilating the lungs in a differential manner confers significant physiologic consequences. When one lung ventilation commences, VQ matching is significantly worsened, and the shunt fraction increases. However, the degree of this change is modulated by compensatory mechanisms. Most thoracic surgeries take place in lateral decubitus position, with the nonoperative lung being dependent; this improves perfusion to the ventilated lung. Hypoxic pulmonary vasoconstriction (HPV) significantly decreases blood flow to the non-ventilated lung, reducing the expected change in PaO_2 by 40% to 50% [27]. The degree of HPV is increased with acidosis, hypercapnia, and hyperthermia, and it is attenuated by the opposite factors and increased left atrial pressure and using >1 MAC of a volatile anesthetic [28].

Depending on what the surgery is, vascular flow to the non-ventilated lung may be intentionally decreased (ie, the surgical team may clamp the flow to a lobe in preparation for resection) or simply obstructed during the course of tissue manipulation. Given that patients undergoing thoracic surgery often have baseline levels of lung vulnerability and that there exists a relatively higher incidence of acute lung injury after thoracic surgery, lung-protective strategies are used in this setting. Although some hypercapnia is permitted, tidal volumes are maintained at 4–6 cc/kg during one-lung ventilation to ensure that this does not become too severe. PEEP to the ventilated lung must be balanced with the risk of overdistension, particularly in patients with obstructive lung pathologies that are at risk for auto-PEEP, as this could worsen VQ mismatch.

Jet ventilation

There are multiple clinical scenarios and patient factors that demand a nonstandard approach to ventilation under general anesthesia. This section will discuss jet ventilation, which provides a means of ventilating and oxygenating patients during procedures that require a shared airway or a still chest for a prolonged period of time.

Jet ventilation was designed in the 1960s to provide continuous ventilation and continuous surgical access during rigid bronchoscopy. The first device connected the oxygen pipeline supply to the bronchoscope and allowed intermittent delivery of gas through a 0.035-in nozzle within the lumen of the bronchoscope via a hand-held pressure regulator with an on/off valve. The jet entrained air into the scope, producing a tidal volume, and exhalation was passive, as the bronchoscope was open to ambient air. Over the subsequent decades, new catheters and applications of this technology have found their way into the OR [29]. Of note, given that jet ventilation generally uses an open breathing system, CO_2 monitoring can be challenging and may require blood sampling.

Low-frequency jet ventilation

During laryngeal procedures, obscuring the larynx with an endotracheal tube can hinder surgical exposure. Accordingly, jet ventilation through a narrow bore catheter is useful. Jet continues to be used to allow simultaneous ventilation and surgical access during rigid bronchoscopy. Although specific catheters exist for these situations, jet can also be performed through airway exchange catheters or a cricothyroidotomy cannula should the clinical situation necessitate such a device.

In these scenarios, ventilation can be delivered at rates of 10 to 20 breaths per minute, and appropriate oxygenation and minute ventilation can be achieved by modulating the driving pressure, inspiratory time, respiratory rate, and FiO_2. Inhalation at this frequency is a result of convective flow from the jet and entrainment of the surrounding air, followed by passive exhalation. Jet ventilation can be delivered by a hand-held pressure regulator connected to a wall oxygen supply or via a dedicated jet ventilator, such as the Monsoon (Acutronic Medical Systems AG, Baar, Switzerland) [30,31].

High-frequency jet ventilation

High-frequency jet ventilation instills gas at a rate of 100 to 400 breaths per minute. Tidal volumes are significantly smaller than dead space volume, so convective or bulk flow is not responsible for gas exchange in this setting. Instead, laminar flow, mixing via Taylor dispersion, Pendelluft, molecular diffusion, and cardiogenic mixing occurs. Given this, driving pressure (not respiratory frequency) has the largest impact on ventilation efficacy.

This type of ventilation can predispose the patient to breath stacking and dynamic hyperinflation if there is insufficient air egress, which can cause barotrauma. The incidence of this problem is very low, and the mean and peak airway pressures end up being lower than during conventional ventilation in the vast majority of cases [32]. This makes it an attractive option for ventilation in the presence of bronchoplerual fistulae and tracheobronchial disruptions.

One significant advantage of this method is that it causes only minimal bronchial and mediastinal excursion. As a result, it has been used for pulmonary vein isolation and other electrophysiolgic procedures that benefit from eliminating respiratory movement that can affect ablation catheter position [33]. It has also been used to keep the diaphragm still so that ablations and biopsies in the liver or lung can be accomplished transcutaneously by interventional radiology [32].

Choosing fraction of inspired oxygen

Choosing an appropriate FiO_2 for intraoperative ventilation may require more consideration than simply targeting a normal oxygen saturation on pulse oximetry. Hyperoxia, or elevated tissue oxygen concentrations, can lead to the creation of reactive oxygen species (ROS). ROS can be both beneficial to immune defense systems and can be directly toxic to the tissue [34].

Hyperoxia has been investigated as a means of decreasing surgical site infections, particularly in abdominal surgery. Though early studies seemed to suggest a benefit to this strategy, the result was inconsistent, and the PROXI trial showed no significant difference in patients receiving 80% FiO_2 versus 30% FiO_2 in the perioperative period [35–40]. There remain some groups that advocate for higher FiO_2 given the variability in data [41].

Subsequent subgroup analyses of the PROXI trial attempted to identify whether there were measurable drawbacks to a high FiO_2 approach. High FiO_2 can result in absorption atelectasis, which could worsen postop pulmonary complications. One analysis investigated outcomes in the obese patient population, which is particularly vulnerable to atelectasis due to elevated baseline pleural pressures. They found no significant difference in both surgical site infections and postoperative pulmonary complications, although other means of addressing atelectasis in this population (eg, PEEP and recruitment) were not described in this paper [42].

Of concern, however, was the finding that long-term mortality may be worsened in patients with cancer treated with a high FiO_2 strategy. A follow-up of PROXI patients showed a hazard ratio of 1.45 for patients undergoing cancer surgery who were treated with 80% FiO_2 during the perioperative period at a 2.3-year follow-up [40]. The mortality difference, and a shorter cancer-free survival, was seen at a 4-year follow-up, but the incidence of new cancers was not different between groups [43].

Investigation has generally focused on these two quite disparate FiO_2 levels; subsequent study may still be required to elucidate whether there is an FiO_2 that balances risks and benefits of ROS creation in the surgical population.

There has also been an investigation into the idea that hyperoxia and its resulting increase in oxidative stress may contribute to neurocognitive dysfunction and other organ dysfunction, particularly post-cardiac surgery. Small studies have indicated that this may not be clinically significant, though there are larger studies planned to address this question [44,45].

Advanced monitoring tools

Esophageal balloon

The tenets of lung-protective ventilation provide guidance for minimizing ventilator-associated lung injury, but plateau and driving pressures comprise pressures from the whole respiratory system. They are a surrogate for the pressure exerted directly across an alveolus, as they are also affected by the chest wall. Measuring the transpulmonary pressure is more specific.

Transpulmonary pressure is defined as airway pressure minus pleural pressure. Measuring and acting upon transpulmonary pressure can help ensure that the patient's alveoli do not have net collapsing forces exerted on them, thus promoting atelectasis, and transpulmonary driving pressure and Pplat may give a clearer picture of the forces experienced by the alveoli, though the latter two are not used in clinical practice at this time.

Measuring pleural pressure directly in humans is prohibitive, but the pressure in the distal third of the esophagus provides a close approximation of the posterior pleural pressure, within ~3 cm H2O [46]. By approximating pleural pressure, an appropriate level of positive airway pressure can be set to keep the transpulmonary pressure zero or positive, which prevents a net trend toward atelectasis.

One caveat is that this tool does not provide robust information about heterogenous lung tissue, as it only measures the pressure in one part of the thorax, but it can provide important information to help with lung recruitment.

Electrical impedance tomography

Electrical impedance tomography (EIT) is a noninvasive, radiation-free imaging modality that maps a tissue dynamically by sending currents through an electrode belt placed around that area and creating a tomographic image based on the conductivity, permittivity, and impedance of that tissue.

This has been examined in several biological tissues, but thoracic imaging is a particularly useful application because lung tissue resistivity is multiple times higher than that of other thoracic soft tissues, creating a high contrast image. Moreover, resistivity varies significantly during a normal respiratory cycle, so EIT can create a dynamic map of aeration or lack thereof.

This can happen at the patient's bedside and is used more commonly in the ICU. There have been numerous research applications of EIT in the OR setting, including a recent study that examined the interaction of positioning, insufflation, and body habitus on ventilatory mechanics in robotic surgery [47].

SUMMARY DISCUSSION

The modern anesthesia machine can deliver high-quality ventilation in a number of common modes that each provide potential advantages and disadvantages to a patient. It also has limitations when compared with ventilators designed for long-term use, which became relevant at some points during the COVID-19 pandemic. Understanding the limitations of the equipment, and common ventilator strategies, is central to delivering safe, lung-protective ventilation. As patients get sicker and anesthetic scenarios become more complex, understanding how to use both standard and nonstandard modes of ventilation, knowing the benefits and harms of different oxygenation strategies, and being aware of advanced monitoring tools that can help further tailor their strategy will allow clinicians to take the best possible care of their patients.

CLINICS CARE POINTS

- Anesthesia machines are equipped with many of the features of ICU ventilators, but there are limitations to using them for long-term ventilation.
- Lung protective ventilation is considered standard of practice in the intraoperative setting, though there is not robust data to suggest it is necessary outside the ICU.
- Patient physiology and operative setting should be used to tailor ventilation strategy in the OR.

Acknowledgments
Figures created by Phoebe Fraser.

Conflicts of interest
Drs A. Balakrishna and L. Brunker have no conflicts of interest. Dr C.G. Hughes has received a research grant from Dr. Franz Kohler Chemie GMBH and is a consultant for Sedana Medical outside of the scope of this work.

References
[1] Pino RM, Bittner EA, Chitilian HV, et al. Massachusetts general hospital. Handbook of clinical anesthesia procedures of the Massachusetts general hospital. 10th edition. Philadelphia: Wolters Kluwer; 2022 cm.
[2] Loeb RL, Martin J. COVID-19: intensive care ventilation with anesthesia machines. In: Post TW, editor. UpToDate. Available at: https://www.uptodate.com/contents/covid-19-intensive-care-ventilation-with-anesthesia-machines. Accessed February 10, 2022. UpToDate; 2022.
[3] APSF/ASA guidance on purposing anesthesia machines as ICU ventilators. Available at: https://www.asahq.org/in-the-spotlight/coronavirus-covid-19-information/purposing-anesthesia-machines-for-ventilators. Accessed February 12, 2022.
[4] Bottiroli M, Calini A, Pinciroli R, et al. The repurposed use of anesthesia machines to ventilate critically ill patients with coronavirus disease 2019 (COVID-19). BMC Anesthesiol 2021;21(1):155.
[5] Acute Respiratory Distress Syndrome N, Brower RG, Matthay MA, et al. Ventilation with lower tidal volumes as compared with traditional tidal volumes for acute lung injury and the acute respiratory distress syndrome. N Engl J Med 2000;342(18):1301–8; https://doi.org/10.1056/NEJM200005043421801.
[6] Amato MB, Meade MO, Slutsky AS, et al. Driving pressure and survival in the acute respiratory distress syndrome. N Engl J Med 2015;372(8):747–55; https://doi.org/10.1056/NEJMsa1410639.
[7] Guldner A, Kiss T, Serpa Neto A, et al. Intraoperative protective mechanical ventilation for prevention of postoperative pulmonary complications: a comprehensive review of the role of tidal volume, positive end-expiratory pressure, and lung recruitment maneuvers. Anesthesiology 2015;123(3):692–713; https://doi.org/10.1097/ALN.0000000000000754.
[8] Gattinoni L, Quintel M, Marini JJ. Volutrauma and atelectrauma: which is worse? Crit Care 2018;22(1):264.
[9] Kacmarek RM, Villar J. Lung-protective Ventilation in the Operating Room: Individualized Positive End-expiratory Pressure Is Needed. Anesthesiology 2018;129(6):1057–9.
[10] Futier E, Constantin JM, Paugam-Burtz C, et al. A trial of intraoperative low-tidal-volume ventilation in abdominal surgery. N Engl J Med 2013;369(5):428–37; https://doi.org/10.1056/NEJMoa1301082.
[11] Severgnini P, Selmo G, Lanza C, et al. Protective mechanical ventilation during general anesthesia for open abdominal surgery improves postoperative pulmonary function. Anesthesiology 2013;118(6):1307–21.
[12] Hyzy RCJ, Shijing. Modes of mechanical ventilation. In: Post TW, editor. Available at: https://www.uptodate.com/contents/covid-19-intensive-care-ventilation-with-anesthesia-machines. Accessed February 10, 2022. UpToDate; 2022.
[13] Chatburn RL, El-Khatib M, Mireles-Cabodevila E. A taxonomy for mechanical ventilation: 10 fundamental maxims. Respir Care 2014;59(11):1747–63; https://doi.org/10.4187/respcare.03057.
[14] Pham T, Brochard LJ, Slutsky AS. Mechanical Ventilation: State of the Art. Mayo Clin Proc 2017;92(9):1382–400.

[15] Hess DR. Respiratory mechanics in mechanically ventilated patients. Respir Care 2014;59(11):1773–94.
[16] Reddy RM, Guntupalli KK. Review of ventilatory techniques to optimize mechanical ventilation in acute exacerbation of chronic obstructive pulmonary disease. Int J Chron Obstruct Pulmon Dis 2007;2(4):441–52.
[17] Stather DR, Stewart TE. Clinical review: Mechanical ventilation in severe asthma. Crit Care 2005;9(6):581–7.
[18] Baydur A. Mechanical ventilation in interstitial lung disease: which patients are likely to benefit? Chest 2008;133(5):1062–3; https://doi.org/10.1378/chest.07-2615.
[19] Florio G, De Santis Santiago RR, Fumagalli J, et al. Pleural Pressure Targeted Positive Airway Pressure Improves Cardiopulmonary Function in Spontaneously Breathing Patients With Obesity. Chest 2021;159(6):2373–83; https://doi.org/10.1016/j.chest.2021.01.055.
[20] Grassi L, Kacmarek R, Berra L. Ventilatory Mechanics in the Patient with Obesity. Anesthesiology 2020;132(5):1246–56; https://doi.org/10.1097/ALN.0000000000003154.
[21] Sharma G, Goodwin J. Effect of aging on respiratory system physiology and immunology. Clin Interv Aging 2006;1(3):253–60; https://doi.org/10.2147/ciia.2006.1.3.253.
[22] Bachmann MC, Morais C, Bugedo G, et al. Electrical impedance tomography in acute respiratory distress syndrome. Crit Care 2018;22(1):263; https://doi.org/10.1186/s13054-018-2195-6.
[23] Joshi GP. Anesthesia for laparoscopic and abdominal robotic surgery in adults. In: Post TW, editor. Available at: https://www.uptodate.com/contents/covid-19-intensive-care-ventilation-with-anesthesia-machines. Accessed February 10, 2022. UpToDate; 2022.
[24] Guerin C, Reignier J, Richard JC, et al. Prone positioning in severe acute respiratory distress syndrome. N Engl J Med 2013;368(23):2159–68; https://doi.org/10.1056/NEJMoa1214103.
[25] Feix B, Sturgess J. Anaesthesia in the prone position. Continuing Education Anaesth Crit Care Pain 2014;14(6):291–7; https://doi.org/10.1093/bjaceaccp/mku001.
[26] Ma MS, Peter D. One lung ventilation: general principles. In: Post TW, editor. Available at: https://www.uptodate.com/contents/covid-19-intensive-care-ventilation-with-anesthesia-machines. Accessed February 10, 2022. UpToDate; 2022.
[27] Sylvester JT, Shimoda LA, Aaronson PI, et al. Hypoxic pulmonary vasoconstriction. Physiol Rev 2012;92(1):367–520; https://doi.org/10.1152/physrev.00041.2010.
[28] Lohser J. Evidence-based management of one-lung ventilation. Anesthesiol Clin 2008;26(2):241–72; https://doi.org/10.1016/j.anclin.2008.01.011.
[29] Sanders R. Two ventilating attachments for bronchoscopes. Del Med J 1967;39:170.
[30] Evans E, Biro P, Bedforth N. Jet ventilation. Continuing Education Anaesth Crit Care Pain 2007;7(1):2–5; https://doi.org/10.1093/bjaceaccp/mkl061.
[31] Biro P. Jet ventilation for surgical interventions in the upper airway. Anesthesiol Clin 2010;28(3):397–409; https://doi.org/10.1016/j.anclin.2010.07.001.
[32] Galmen K, Harbut P, Freedman J, et al. The use of high-frequency ventilation during general anaesthesia: an update. F1000Res 2017;6:756.
[33] Elkassabany N, Garcia F, Tschabrunn C, et al. Anesthetic management of patients undergoing pulmonary vein isolation for treatment of atrial fibrillation using high-frequency jet ventilation. J Cardiothorac Vasc Anesth 2012;26(3):433–8.
[34] Singer M, Young PJ, Laffey JG, et al. Dangers of hyperoxia. Crit Care 2021;25(1):440.
[35] Greif R, Akca O, Horn EP, et al. Supplemental perioperative oxygen to reduce the incidence of surgical-wound infection. N Engl J Med 2000;342(3):161–7.
[36] Belda FJ, Aguilera L, Garcia de la Asuncion J, et al. Supplemental perioperative oxygen and the risk of surgical wound infection: a randomized controlled trial. JAMA 2005;294(16):2035–42.

[37] Pryor KO, Fahey TJ 3rd, Lien CA, et al. Surgical site infection and the routine use of perioperative hyperoxia in a general surgical population: a randomized controlled trial. JAMA 2004;291(1):79–87.
[38] Mayzler O, Weksler N, Domchik S, et al. Does supplemental perioperative oxygen administration reduce the incidence of wound infection in elective colorectal surgery? Minerva Anestesiol 2005;71(1–2):21–5.
[39] Gardella C, Goltra LB, Laschansky E, et al. High-concentration supplemental perioperative oxygen to reduce the incidence of postcesarean surgical site infection: a randomized controlled trial. Obstet Gynecol 2008;112(3):545–52; https://doi.org/10.1097/AOG.0b013e318182340c.
[40] Meyhoff CS, Jorgensen LN, Wetterslev J, et al. Increased long-term mortality after a high perioperative inspiratory oxygen fraction during abdominal surgery: follow-up of a randomized clinical trial. Anesth Analg 2012;115(4):849–54; https://doi.org/10.1213/ANE.0b013e3182652a51.
[41] Web Appendix 13a, Summary of the systematic review on perioperative oxygenation issued in 2016. Superseded by Appendix 13b and 13c. Global Guidelines for the Prevention of Surgical Site Infection World Health Organ. 2018. https://www.ncbi.nlm.nih.gov/books/NBK536427/. [Accessed 11 February 2022].
[42] Staehr AK, Meyhoff CS, Rasmussen LS, et al. Inspiratory oxygen fraction and postoperative complications in obese patients: a subgroup analysis of the PROXI trial. Anesthesiology 2011;114(6):1313–9; https://doi.org/10.1097/ALN.0b013e31821bdb82.
[43] Meyhoff CS, Jorgensen LN, Wetterslev J, et al. Risk of new or recurrent cancer after a high perioperative inspiratory oxygen fraction during abdominal surgery. Br J Anaesth 2014;113(Suppl 1):i74–81; https://doi.org/10.1093/bja/aeu110.
[44] Shaefi S, Shankar P, Mueller AL, et al. Intraoperative Oxygen Concentration and Neurocognition after Cardiac Surgery. Anesthesiology 2021;134(2):189–201; https://doi.org/10.1097/ALN.0000000000003650.
[45] Lopez MG, Pretorius M, Shotwell MS, et al. The Risk of Oxygen during Cardiac Surgery (ROCS) trial: study protocol for a randomized clinical trial. Trials 2017;18(1):295; https://doi.org/10.1186/s13063-017-2021-5.
[46] Mojoli F, Torriglia F, Orlando A, et al. Technical aspects of bedside respiratory monitoring of transpulmonary pressure. Ann Transl Med 2018;6(19):377; https://doi.org/10.21037/atm.2018.08.37.
[47] Tharp WG, Murphy S, Breidenstein MW, et al. Body Habitus and Dynamic Surgical Conditions Independently Impair Pulmonary Mechanics during Robotic-assisted Laparoscopic Surgery. Anesthesiology 2020;133(4):750–63.

Advances in Anesthesia 40 (2022) 185–200

ADVANCES IN ANESTHESIA

ELSEVIER
MOSBY

Anesthesia and Analgesia for the Obese Parturient

Mary Yurashevich, MD, MPH, Cameron R. Taylor, MD, Jennifer E. Dominguez, MD, MHS, Ashraf S. Habib, MBBCh, MSc, MHSc, FRCA*

Department of Anesthesiology, Division of Women's Anesthesia, Duke University School of Medicine, Durham, NC 27710, USA

Keywords

• Pregnancy • Obesity • Anesthesia • Analgesia • Labor • Cesarean delivery

Key points

- Obesity is a global health epidemic.
- Pregnant patients with obesity experience more obstetric and anesthetic complications during labor and delivery.
- Safe anesthesia management must consider the physiologic changes associated with both pregnancy and obesity.

The World Health Organization defines obesity as "abnormal or excessive fat accumulation that may impair health" and defines a body mass index (BMI) of $\geq$ 30 kg/m^2 as obese. It is further subdivided into class 1 obesity with a BMI of 30 to 34.9 kg/m^2, class 2 with a BMI of 35 to 39.9 kg/m^2, and class 3 with a BMI $\geq$ 40 kg/m^2; class 3 obesity is further divided into morbid obesity for a BMI 40 to 49.9 kg/m^2, super-obesity for a BMI 50 to 59.9 kg/m^2, and super-super obesity for a BMI $\geq$ 60 kg/m^2 [1–3]. Some groups have suggested using pregnancy-specific BMI cut-off values (5 kg/m^2 higher in each category at the time of delivery) to define obesity, but no formal classification exists [4]. In the United States, obesity has a prevalence of 40%, while more than one-third of women $\geq$ 20 years are obese [5,6]. It is associated with an increased risk of multiple morbidities, including diabetes, hypertension, and obstructive sleep apnea (OSA) in both pregnant and nonpregnant populations [7]. Obese

*Corresponding author. Department of Anesthesiology, Duke University Medical Center, Box 3094, Durham, NC 27710. *E-mail address:* ashraf.habib@duke.edu

https://doi.org/10.1016/j.aan.2022.07.004
0737-6146/22/

parturients experience higher rates of maternal, fetal, and obstetric complications compared with their nonobese counterparts during pregnancy, labor, and delivery (Box 1).

Furthermore, obesity is independently associated with a higher risk of maternal deaths. The 2021 Report on Mothers and Babies: Reducing Risk through Audits and Confidential Enquiries across the United Kingdom which examines maternal morbidity and mortality from 2017 to 2019 across the United Kingdom found that 23% of maternal deaths occurred in obese women [14]. Main and colleagues reviewed maternal deaths in California from 2002 to 2005 and found that deaths occurred more often in obese or morbidly obese women [15]. Over the past several decades, the anesthesia-related contribution to maternal mortality has decreased by a factor of 13, from 1.2:100,000 in 1976 to 1978 to 0.9:100,000 in 2013 to 2015 [16]. However, obesity has been implicated as a significant risk factor in anesthesia-related maternal deaths. Mhyre and colleagues reviewed anesthesia-related maternal mortality in Michigan between 1985 and 2003 and found that 6 out of the 8 women who died were obese [17]. In a study by Beckett and colleagues examining the incidence, management, and outcomes of cardiac arrest in pregnancy, 16 out of 66 arrests (24%) occurred solely as a consequence of obstetric anesthesia and 12 of the 16 women were obese [18].

The purpose of this review is to highlight the anesthetic considerations of caring for obese parturients in labor and delivery. These include predelivery

Box 1: Maternal, fetal, and obstetric complications in obese parturients [7–13]

Maternal complications

1. Obstructive sleep apnea
2. Diabetes mellitus
3. Hypertension
4. Pre-eclampsia

Fetal complications

1. Fetal macrosomia
2. Neural tube defects, orofacial, and limb reduction anomalies
3. Stillbirth delivery

Obstetric complications

1. Longer first stage of labor
2. Increased risk for cesarean delivery
3. Shoulder dystocia
4. Wound complications
5. Postpartum hemorrhage
6. Thromboembolic complications

planning, anesthetic considerations for labor analgesia and cesarean delivery, and aspects of postpartum care, such as analgesia and venous thromboembolism (VTE) prevention.

PREDELIVERY PLANNING

The American College of Obstetricians and Gynecologists (ACOG), as well as the Royal College of Obstetricians and Gynaecologists (RCOG), recommend a multidisciplinary approach to the care of obese parturients. Management of these patients should begin before pregnancy with preconception counseling and nutrition management. A formal anesthesia consultation is recommended during pregnancy for those with morbid obesity [19,20]. Compared with their nonobese counterparts, obese parturients are at increased risk of numerous complications as detailed in Box 1. A thorough history and physical examination should be performed at this consultation with special attention paid to comorbidities, such as hypertension, OSA, gestational diabetes, and pre-eclampsia. The physical examination should also include a thorough pulmonary, cardiovascular, and airway examination.

The anesthesia consultation is an opportunity to review and discuss the challenges that the obese parturient may have experienced previously, such as a history of difficult neuraxial, or difficult airway. It is also an opportunity to prepare patients for the anesthetic management options for their labor and delivery and should be conducted early enough in pregnancy to allow for optimization of maternal comorbidities. For example, they should be counseled that neuraxial catheter placement may be challenging and therefore early neuraxial analgesia may allow additional time to confirm the efficacy of the block and to decrease the need for general anesthesia in the event of an emergent cesarean delivery [2].

LABOR ANALGESIA

Neuraxial analgesia, including epidural, combined spinal epidural (CSE), and dural puncture epidural (DPE) techniques, is the preferred modality for laboring women with obesity. Labor epidural analgesia provides excellent pain relief and can be converted to a surgical anesthetic if a cesarean delivery becomes necessary, and therefore avoids general anesthesia with its associated risks in a patient population at higher risk for difficult intubation. Because of the increased likelihood of fetal macrosomia in obese parturients, a functional labor epidural can be particularly useful in the management of shoulder dystocia [8]. Vigilance is recommended in evaluating labor epidural blocks as those that require frequent top-ups may not be successfully converted to surgical anesthesia [21]. Therefore, labor epidural catheters that require frequent interventions to provide adequate analgesia should be replaced early to minimize the risk of failure of labor epidural conversions during an intrapartum cesarean delivery.

The CSE technique is an alternative to standard epidural for labor analgesia. CSEs provide a rapid onset of dense labor analgesia. Studies have shown that the epidural failure rate with CSE is lower than that of standard labor epidural because of confirmation that the epidural space is successfully reached when cerebrospinal fluid is obtained through the spinal needle [22,23]. The concern that the epidural catheter is "untested" until the spinal component of the CSE wears off, therefore delaying the recognition of an improperly placed or poorly functioning epidural catheter, has not been shown to be warranted in a study by Booth and colleagues [24].

DPE is another labor analgesia technique that may have advantages for obese parturients. Like CSE, this needle-through needle technique provides indirect confirmation that the epidural space has been successfully reached, though intrathecal medications are not given. Instead, all medications are given through the epidural catheter. One study reported several advantages of the DPE compared with epidural and CSE techniques, including less pruritus, hypotension, tachysystole, category II fetal heart tracings, as well as fewer requirements for epidural top-ups with DPE versus CSE or epidural and fewer asymmetric blocks with DPE versus epidural [25].

Given the technical challenges in identifying the epidural space in obese parturients, and the increased risk of "false loss of resistance" due to adipose tissue and hormonal softening of ligaments, CSE and DPE techniques may offer advantages over the standard epidural technique in this population. A recent small retrospective study reported fewer epidural catheter failures in super-obese parturients with CSE or DPE techniques compared with the standard epidural technique (9.2% versus 28.6%, $P < .001$) [26]. However, a recent prospective study reported no differences in the composite outcome of quality of labor analgesia or in its individual components (asymmetrical block, epidural top-ups, catheter adjustments, catheter replacement, and failed conversion to surgical anesthesia for cesarean delivery) between DPE and standard epidural techniques in obese parturients [27]. Most blocks in the prospective study were performed by experienced providers, whereas the majority of blocks in the retrospective study were performed by trainees with variable degrees of experience, which affects the failure rates. It is likely that the advantages of DPE compared with the standard epidural technique would be most apparent when the procedures are performed by inexperienced providers.

In the event of an inadvertent dural puncture, particularly in the context of challenging neuraxial block placement, continuous spinal labor analgesia may be considered in settings where safety protocols are in place and catheters can be managed directly by experienced providers. Intentional use of continuous spinal analgesia should not be routine due to the risk of post-dural puncture headache (PDPH) when performed using a 17- or 18-gauge Tuohy needle. The reported risk of PDPH in obese patients compared with nonobese women has been inconsistent in the literature. Miu and colleagues reported no difference in the incidence of PDPH between patients with BMI less than 30 kg/m^2 compared with those with greater than or equal to 30 kg/m^2 [28]. Peralta and colleagues, however, found that obese patients with BMI greater than 31.5 kg/m^2 were less likely to develop PDPH compared with those with lower

BMI after inadvertent dural puncture with a Tuohy needle [29]. Franz and colleagues found an increased risk of PDPH only in super-obese parturients, whereas there was no difference in the risk of PDPH in women with lower obesity classes compared with their nonobese counterparts [30]. It is important to note, that even when the risk of PDPH is reduced, it is still high at about 40% to 45%, therefore this technique should not be used routinely. Alternatively, continuous spinal anesthesia can be performed using a 22 to 24-gauge catheter advanced over a 27- or 29-gauge Quincke needle; however, this technique has not been specifically evaluated in obese parturients and has been reported to have a failure rate of up to 20% [31]. A continuous spinal catheter kit (Epimed Inc, Johnstown, NY) consisting of a flexible 23-gauge intrathecal cannula over a 27-gauge pencil-point spinal needle, is also available. This continuous spinal catheter has been evaluated by Tao and colleagues for use in labor analgesia as well as conversion to surgical anesthesia in 113 women; in 12 women (11%), the catheter was not successfully inserted or maintained in position, 2.6% of women developed PDPH in this study, the remaining 101 women had 83 spontaneous vaginal deliveries, 12 operative vaginal deliveries, and 18 cesarean deliveries. Of the 18 cesarean deliveries, 16 had continuous spinal catheter at the time of decision for cesarean and 15 were successfully converted to surgical anesthesia. However, this system was not specifically evaluated in obese women [32].

ANESTHESIA FOR CESAREAN DELIVERY

Anesthesia-related maternal mortality has steadily decreased over the last 4 decades [33,34]. The decline in the rates of general anesthesia for cesarean delivery has played an instrumental role in this decline as most anesthesia-related complications occurred under general anesthesia. Neuraxial anesthesia for cesarean delivery is the preferred method and general anesthesia should be reserved for emergencies or where neuraxial anesthesia is contraindicated. This is particularly relevant in this patient population with increased prevalence of OSA and increased risk for complications associated with general anesthesia, including airway-related complications.

Spinal Anesthesia

Single-shot spinal anesthesia produces a dense, reliable surgical anesthetic with quick onset [35]. Its primary limitation is the duration of the surgical block. In obese parturients, more time may be required to perform the cesarean delivery, therefore a continuous neuraxial technique, such as a CSE may be preferred [36]. A single-shot spinal anesthetic using a 25 to 27 gauge pencil point spinal needle may be technically challenging in obese parturients because of the excess adipose tissue relative to nonobese parturients. The use of the Tuohy needle for identification of the epidural space may be technically easier due to enhanced tactile feedback with the use of a larger gauge needle. Ross and colleagues randomized 44 morbidly obese parturients scheduled for elective cesarean delivery to either single-shot spinal anesthetic or

CSE technique and found that CSE may be accomplished with fewer attempts than single-shot spinal and was noninferior for the time of initiation of subarachnoid anesthesia [37].

Combined Spinal Epidural Anesthesia

A CSE is the preferred anesthetic technique for cesarean delivery for obese parturients. The CSE combines the dense block of a single-shot spinal with the ability to extend block duration using the epidural catheter [35]. Additionally, it is a useful technique in patients where a reduced spinal anesthetic dose may be desirable, such as those with cardiac disease to minimize hemodynamic instability, or in super-obese parturients.

Continuous Spinal Anesthesia

Continuous spinal anesthesia is another anesthetic option for cesarean delivery in obese parturients, although its use is limited by the risk of PDPH, as discussed earlier. Some providers advocate for the continuous spinal technique in morbidly obese patients as it provides a dense, reliable surgical block that can be titrated to the desired anesthetic level within minutes [38]. Its use could be helpful in emergent situations where a single-shot spinal technique or CSE may be difficult to perform quickly due to body habitus.

Double Catheter Technique

The double catheter technique for cesarean delivery has been described for anesthetic management of morbidly obese patients. McDonnell and colleagues described a case of a super-super obese parturient (BMI of 76 kg/m^2) with twin gestation undergoing elective cesarean delivery under lumbar CSE at the L3/L4 interspace and a thoracic epidural catheter at the T11/T12 interspace. A midline vertical incision extending above the umbilicus was utilized to deliver the twins. Surgical anesthesia was provided by the lumbar CSE while the thoracic epidural catheter was used for postoperative analgesia [39]. Polin and colleagues reported a case series of super-super obese parturients undergoing cesarean delivery with high vertical midline incision under a double catheter technique. The BMI of the parturients in this series ranged from 73 to 95 kg/m^2; a lumbar spinal catheter was titrated intraoperatively for surgical anesthesia and a thoracic epidural catheter was used for postoperative analgesia, although in one case, T6 surgical level could only be achieved after dosing the thoracic epidural catheter [40].

GENERAL ANESTHESIA FOR CESAREAN DELIVERY

Although not the preferred anesthetic modality for cesarean delivery, occasionally general anesthesia is necessary. In obese patients, general anesthesia presents unique challenges. Airway management can be more difficult due to increased adipose tissue within the pharyngeal structures, which can constrict the upper airway and may be associated with increased upper airway (retropalatal and retroglossal) collapsibility. Excess adipose tissue around the face, neck, and abdomen can complicate bag-mask ventilation and tracheal intubation [41]. Kheterpal and colleagues examined factors contributing to difficult mask ventilation and in over 22,000 mask ventilation attempts, BMI greater than 30 kg/m^2 was found to be an independent predictor of difficult mask ventilation [42]. Tracheal intubation can also be more difficult in obese patients with an incidence of up to 15.5% observed in one study, compared with 2.2% in nonobese counterparts [43].

Obesity contributes to decreased functional residual capacity (FRC), increased oxygen consumption, and increased airway resistance leading to rapid oxygen desaturation [44]. Pregnancy also decreases FRC because of the mechanical effects of the gravid uterus; FRC at term can be 15% to 20% below the nonpregnant state. Additionally, obese pregnant patients experience hypoxemia more frequently than nonobese parturients, as noted in arterial blood gas, which suggests a higher degree of venoarterial shunting [45]. Obese parturients also have increased work of breathing compared with nonobese counterparts due to excess chest wall weight–excess body weight increases oxygen consumption and CO_2 production [46]. For obese patients, supine positioning may cause FRC to fall below closing capacity, resulting in airway closure in the dependent lung regions and further shunting [47]. These physiologic changes, along with the further reduction in FRC expected during the induction of general anesthesia, make pregnant obese patients particularly at risk for rapid oxygen desaturation. Consequently, adequate preoxygenation is critical for obese parturients. This can be achieved with 3 minutes of tidal volume breathing or eight deep breaths in 1 minute with 100% oxygen [48]. Additionally, co-administration of high-flow nasal oxygen during preoxygenation and continued during rapid sequence induction can help to maintain oxygen saturation and prevent hypoxia during intubation [49].

In preparing for induction of general anesthesia and intubation, optimal positioning is critical. A head-up or the reverse-Trendelenburg position has been shown to increase the duration of apnea without desaturation compared with a supine position while simultaneously improving laryngeal exposure during direct laryngoscopy [50,51]. One study comparing the "sniff" and "ramped" positions for morbidly obese patients undergoing general anesthesia found that the "ramped" position obtained better laryngeal views when using a video Macintosh laryngoscope [52]. Troop elevation pillow (Bone Foam Inc., Corcoran, MN) and other commercially available positioning devices may help facilitate achieving the "ramped" position in morbidly obese parturients. Studies have also shown that video-assisted laryngoscopes provide earlier time to tracheal intubation, shorter apnea time, and better laryngoscopic views in obese patients when compared with direct Macintosh laryngoscopy [53,54]. Despite all of these considerations, some patients may remain difficult to intubate and/or mask ventilate, and ensuring the availability of extra personnel is important. Although a laryngeal mask airway cannot prevent aspiration of gastric contents, in situations of difficult airway, it may prove to be a lifesaving measure [38]. Providers should familiarize themselves with the guidelines developed by the Obstetric Anaesthetists Association and the Difficult

Airway Society for the management of difficult and failed intubations in obstetric patients [55].

Intravenous induction agents for obese patients should be dosed using ideal body weight rather than actual body weight [56]. Succinylcholine should be dosed based on total body weight, whereas rocuronium should be dosed based on ideal body weight [57,58]. Ideal dosing of reversal of neuromuscular blockage with sugammadex, a cyclodextrin, should be guided by neuromuscular monitoring and based on total body weight because of increased circulating plasma cholinesterase [3,59].

Emergence and extubation after general anesthesia require a safety plan; this may be a particularly vulnerable time for obese parturients as deaths due to hypoventilation and airway obstruction have been reported [17]. Therefore, particular vigilance is needed during emergence. Similar strategies that help to ensure safe induction and intubation, such as optimization of patient positioning (head elevated $> 30°$) and avoidance of upper airway obstruction after extubation should be employed [60]. Furthermore, patients should be fully awake, following commands with a complete reversal of neuromuscular blockade before extubation [61].

SPECIAL CONSIDERATIONS

Patient Positioning

Patients with elevated BMI are at increased risk of pressure sores and nerve injuries; so, care must be taken when positioning these patients during surgery [62]. Standard operating room tables have a maximum weight limit and the care team should be aware of these limitations. Transferring a laboring patient to the operating table for an intrapartum cesarean delivery can risk injury to both the patient and staff; therefore, the use of an air-inflated mat, such as the commercially available HoverMatt (HoverTech International, Allentown, PA), may be helpful, as well as ensuring that adequate numbers of experienced staff are involved in patient transfers [2]. Surgical visualization and exposure may necessitate retraction of the panniculus and/or angled suspension, but careful hemodynamic and respiratory monitoring is crucial as hypotension and desaturation have been observed with retraction of panniculus during cesarean delivery [63].

Blood Pressure Monitoring

Accurate blood pressure monitoring is imperative, yet can be challenging in obese patients [64]. Obese patients often have some degree of conicity to the shape of their arm which results in an irregular expansion of the rectangularly shaped standard noninvasive blood pressure cuff in the distal part of the arm leading to an inaccurate blood pressure reading [65]. Additionally, choosing an improperly sized cuff will also result in erroneous blood pressure readings with a cuff that is too small leading to inaccurately high blood pressure readings and one that is too large leading to inaccurately low blood pressure readings [66]. As a workaround, clinicians have sometimes placed noninvasive blood pressure cuffs on the forearm. One study reported a consistent correlation between noninvasive blood pressure and intra-arterial blood pressure monitoring for both systolic and diastolic blood pressure measurements (0.95 and 0.89, respectively) [67]. A conically shaped noninvasive blood pressure cuff for obese patients for the forearm has been developed and validated and should be considered for use in these patients [68]. For some patients, the use of intra-arterial blood pressure monitoring may be an alternative if noninvasive devices are not reliable or available. However, their use may be more limited to the intraoperative period, as well as the post-anesthesia care and intensive care units as their use may not be feasible elsewhere in the hospital [64].

Vascular Access

Obtaining peripheral intravenous (PIV) access can also be challenging in obese patients [69]. Multiple PIV attempts may be associated with an increased risk of infection and mechanical complications [70]. A systematic review and meta-analysis found that ultrasound guidance was associated with increased success rates compared with traditional techniques, but did not decrease the time to successful peripheral venous cannulation [71]. For the obese parturient with difficult PIV access, ultrasound should be considered early. Notably, standard length (up to 1.2 inches) and even extra-long (1.75–2.5 inches) peripheral venous cannulas may be associated with a risk of decannulation and extravasation of intravenous medications and fluids. A practical and useful alternative to consider when placing ultrasound-guided peripheral venous catheters is to use a standard 5.5 FR (15.5 Ga) pediatric central venous catheter (utilizing a Seldinger technique), which is 3.15 inches long, and provides the extra length required from the patients' skin to the lumen of the target peripheral vein. An additional advantage is that it is a double lumen catheter with 18- and 20-gauge lumens.

Neuraxial Needle Placement

The distance from the skin to the epidural space is increased with greater BMI due to a thicker subcutaneous layer [72]. However, the majority of obese parturients can still successfully receive neuraxial anesthesia using a standard length needle [38]. Longer-length spinal and epidural needles should be readily available but should only be used when the standard-length epidural needle is unable to reach the epidural space because longer needles might be more challenging to control.

Identification of the neuraxis in obese parturients can be challenging. Optimal positioning is crucial for successful block placement but can be limited by body habitus. Additional staffing may be necessary to ensure safe positioning during neuraxial block placement. Although both sitting and lateral positions may be utilized for block placement, the sitting position may achieve a higher likelihood of success as the flexed sitting position minimizes the distance between the skin and epidural space [72], and allows for easier identification of the midline compared with the lateral position. In a prospective observational study, obesity was associated with an increased likelihood of difficulty to palpate spinous processes and a reduced likelihood of adequate flexion positioning [73]. For patients with difficult block placement with standard palpation technique, the use of neuraxial ultrasound can help facilitate the identification of the midline and estimation of depth from skin to the epidural space. One randomized controlled study found that preprocedure ultrasound scanning increased the success rate and required fewer attempts for successful spinal placement in obese parturients undergoing cesarean delivery compared with a control group using anatomic landmarks ($P < .001$) [74]. Another study found that ultrasound use reduced the number of epidural needle redirections and the risk of failed epidural catheters in obese parturients [75]. An additional factor to consider is the increased risk of dislodging the epidural catheter in obese patients. In a study by Hamilton and colleagues, all patients who requested epidural anesthesia for labor or cesarean delivery were noted to have a clinically significant amount of epidural catheter movement (drawn inward) relative to the skin as they changed positions from sitting flexed to sitting upright to lateral decubitus; patients were grouped by BMI (<25, 25–30, and > 30 kg/m^2) with those patients in BMI greater than 30 kg/m^2 group noted to have the most catheter movement [76]. Therefore, it may be prudent to insert the epidural catheter at least 4 cm into the epidural space and have patients assume the sitting upright or lateral decubitus position before securing with tape to the skin to minimize catheter dislodgement.

Local Anesthetic Dosing

A reduced dose of intrathecal local anesthetic may be required in pregnant women versus nonpregnant women due to increased intrathecal spread of local anesthetics from epidural venous engorgement and the change in neural tissue permeability from the hormonal changes of pregnancy [77,78]. Obese parturients may require further dose reduction, although the literature does not support this for cesarean delivery, except perhaps for parturients with super obesity [79]. A few studies found no correlation between height, weight, BMI, and the height of surgical block achieved with spinal anesthesia using the standard 12 mg dose of bupivacaine; however, obese parturients were not specifically evaluated [80,81]. One study evaluated the ED50 and ED95 of intrathecal bupivacaine in morbidly obese parturients undergoing cesarean delivery and reported no significant differences compared with their nonobese counterparts [82]. Similarly, a retrospective study by Lamon and colleagues did not find an increased risk of higher sensory levels with a standard dose of spinal hyperbaric bupivacaine (10.5–12 mg) in obese compared with nonobese patients unless the BMI was greater than 50 kg/m^2 [79]. Those results were also confirmed in a prospective study by Ngaka and colleagues in parturients undergoing cesarean delivery with 10 mg of intrathecal bupivacaine co-administered with 10 mcg of intrathecal fentanyl. They found a higher block level by an average of 2 dermatomes at 25 minutes and a longer time to block regression in obese parturients with a mean BMI of 51 kg/m^2 compared with the nonobese group with a BMI of 27 kg/m^2; however, no significant differences in vasopressor requirements were observed [83]. Dosing of labor epidural catheters for obese parturients has similarly conflicting data. Panni and colleagues conducted an up-down sequential allocation study examining the minimum local analgesic concentration of bupivacaine in obese and nonobese pregnant women and found that bupivacaine requirements for initiation of analgesia were significantly reduced by a factor of 1.68 [95% confidence interval (CI) of 1.32–2.29] in the obese group, with a significantly higher initial level of block [84]. Other studies, however, found that body weight had minimal impact on the local anesthetic dose for labor epidural analgesia, although obese parturients were not specifically evaluated [85,86].

Thromboprophylaxis

Pregnant and postpartum women have a four-to-five-fold increased risk of VTE compared with nonpregnant women [87]. VTE remains a leading cause of maternal mortality worldwide [88]. Obesity is an independent risk factor for thromboembolism [89]. An analysis of 2,449,133 women with singleton pregnancies undergoing delivery hospitalization in California from 2008 to 2012 found an increasing prevalence of antepartum and postpartum VTE with increasing BMI; women with class III obesity had the highest risk of pregnancy-related VTE compared with women with normal BMI [90]. Despite this, recommendations for thromboprophylaxis vary among RCOG, ACOG, and the American College of Chest Physicians [87,91,92]. Because of this variability among governing bodies, most institutions have developed their own protocols for VTE prophylaxis in this patient population. Close communication and coordination of the timing of VTE prophylaxis and placement (and removal) of neuraxial catheters are essential to minimize the risk of central neuraxial hematoma [93,94].

SUMMARY

Obesity is a growing epidemic worldwide. Obese parturients are particularly vulnerable to increased maternal and fetal complications. Anesthesia for obese parturients can be uniquely challenging and must be tailored to take into consideration pharmacologic dosing and the physiologic changes associated with obesity and pregnancy in this patient population.

CLINICS CARE POINTS

- Neuraxial analgesia is the preferrred modality for pain relief laboring women with obesity.
- Neuraxial anesthesia with a catheter based technique is the preferred anesthetic modality for cesarean delivery for obese parturients.

- In cases where general anesthesia must be performed, careful planning of airway management is critical for safe care of obese parturients.

Disclosure

The authors have nothing to disclose.

References

[1] WHO. Available at: https://www.who.int/news-room/fact-sheets/detail/obesity-and-overweight. Accessed December 4, 2020.
[2] Taylor CR, Dominguez JE, Habib AS. Obesity And Obstetric Anesthesia: Current Insights. Local Reg Anesth 2019;12:111–24.
[3] Patel SD, Habib AS. Anaesthesia for the parturient with obesity. BJA Educ 2021;21(5): 180–6.
[4] Dennis AT, Lamb KE, Story D, et al. Associations between maternal size and health outcomes for women undergoing caesarean section: a multicentre prospective observational study (The MUM SIZE Study). BMJ Open 2017;7(6):e015630.
[5] Collaboration NCDRF. Worldwide trends in body-mass index, underweight, overweight, and obesity from 1975 to 2016: a pooled analysis of 2416 population-based measurement studies in 128.9 million children, adolescents, and adults. Lancet 2017;390(10113): 2627–42.
[6] Flegal KM, Carroll MD, Ogden CL, et al. Prevalence and trends in obesity among US adults, 1999-2008. JAMA 2010;303(3):235–41.
[7] Jensen MD, Ryan DH, Apovian CM, et al. 2013 AHA/ACC/TOS guideline for the management of overweight and obesity in adults: a report of the American College of Cardiology/ American Heart Association Task Force on Practice Guidelines and The Obesity Society. J Am Coll Cardiol 2014;63(25 Pt B):2985–3023.
[8] Tonidandel A, Booth J, D'Angelo R, et al. Anesthetic and obstetric outcomes in morbidly obese parturients: a 20-year follow-up retrospective cohort study. Int J Obstet Anesth 2014;23(4):357–64.
[9] Tabet M, Flick LH, Tuuli MG, et al. Prepregnancy body mass index in a first uncomplicated pregnancy and outcomes of a second pregnancy. Am J Obstet Gynecol 2015;213(4):548 e1–7.
[10] Dempsey JC, Ashiny Z, Qiu CF, et al. Maternal pre-pregnancy overweight status and obesity as risk factors for cesarean delivery. J Matern Fetal Neonatal Med 2005;17(3):179–85.
[11] Dietz PM, Callaghan WM, Morrow B, et al. Population-based assessment of the risk of primary cesarean delivery due to excess prepregnancy weight among nulliparous women delivering term infants. Matern Child Health J 2005;9(3):237–44.
[12] Stothard KJ, Tennant PW, Bell R, et al. Maternal overweight and obesity and the risk of congenital anomalies: a systematic review and meta-analysis. JAMA 2009;301(6): 636–50.
[13] Salihu HM, Dunlop AL, Hedayatzadeh M, et al. Extreme obesity and risk of stillbirth among black and white gravidas. Obstet Gynecol 2007;110(3):552–7.
[14] Saving Lives, Improving Mothers' CareLessons learned to inform maternity care from the UK and Ireland Confidential Enquiries into Maternal Deaths and Morbidity 2017-19. 2021.;
[15] Main EK, McCain CL, Morton CH, et al. Pregnancy-related mortality in California: causes, characteristics, and improvement opportunities. Obstet Gynecol 2015;125(4):938–47.
[16] Lucas DN, Bamber JH. UK Confidential Enquiry into Maternal Deaths - still learning to save mothers' lives. Anaesthesia 2018;73(4):416–20.
[17] Mhyre JM, Riesner MN, Polley LS, et al. A series of anesthesia-related maternal deaths in Michigan, 1985-2003. Anesthesiology 2007;106(6):1096–104.

[18] Beckett VA, Knight M, Sharpe P. The CAPS Study: incidence, management and outcomes of cardiac arrest in pregnancy in the UK: a prospective, descriptive study. BJOG 2017;124(9):1374–81.
[19] American College of Obstetricians and Gynecologists' Committee on Practice Bulletins-Obstetrics. Obesity in Pregnancy: ACOG Practice Bulletin, Number 230. Obstet Gynecol 2021;137(6):e128–44.
[20] Denison FC, Aedla NR, Keag O, et al. Care of Women with Obesity in Pregnancy: Green-top Guideline No. 72. BJOG 2019;126(3):e62–106.
[21] Bauer ME, Kountanis JA, Tsen LC, et al. Risk factors for failed conversion of labor epidural analgesia to cesarean delivery anesthesia: a systematic review and meta-analysis of observational trials. Int J Obstet Anesth 2012;21(4):294–309.
[22] Pan PH, Bogard TD, Owen MD. Incidence and characteristics of failures in obstetric neuraxial analgesia and anesthesia: a retrospective analysis of 19,259 deliveries. Int J Obstet Anesth 2004;13(4):227–33.
[23] Miro M, Guasch E, Gilsanz F. Comparison of epidural analgesia with combined spinal-epidural analgesia for labor: a retrospective study of 6497 cases. Int J Obstet Anesth 2008;17(1):15–9.
[24] Booth JM, Pan JC, Ross VH, et al. Combined Spinal Epidural Technique for Labor Analgesia Does Not Delay Recognition of Epidural Catheter Failures: A Single-center Retrospective Cohort Survival Analysis. Anesthesiology 2016;125(3):516–24.
[25] Chau A, Bibbo C, Huang CC, et al. Dural Puncture Epidural Technique Improves Labor Analgesia Quality With Fewer Side Effects Compared With Epidural and Combined Spinal Epidural Techniques: A Randomized Clinical Trial. Anesth Analg 2017;124(2):560–9.
[26] Arnolds D, Scavone B. Neuraxial labor analgesia failure rates in women with a body mass index >/=50kg/m(2): a single-center retrospective study. Int J Obstet Anesth 2021;48:103176.
[27] Tan HS, Reed SE, Mehdiratta JE, et al. Quality of Labor Analgesia with Dural Puncture Epidural versus Standard Epidural Technique in Obese Parturients: A Double-blind Randomized Controlled Study. Anesthesiology 2022; https://doi.org/10.1097/ALN.0000000000004137.
[28] Miu M, Paech MJ, Nathan E. The relationship between body mass index and post-dural puncture headache in obstetric patients. Int J Obstet Anesth 2014;23(4):371–5.
[29] Peralta F, Higgins N, Lange E, et al. The Relationship of Body Mass Index with the Incidence of Postdural Puncture Headache in Parturients. Anesth Analg 2015;121(2):451–6.
[30] Franz AM, Jia SY, Bahnson HT, et al. The effect of second-stage pushing and body mass index on postdural puncture headache. J Clin Anesth 2017;37:77–81.
[31] Alonso E, Gilsanz F, Gredilla E, et al. Observational study of continuous spinal anesthesia with the catheter-over-needle technique for cesarean delivery. Int J Obstet Anesth 2009;18(2):137–41.
[32] Tao W, Grant EN, Craig MG, et al. Continuous Spinal Analgesia for Labor and Delivery: An Observational Study with a 23-Gauge Spinal Catheter. Anesth Analg 2015;121(5):1290–4.
[33] Hawkins JL, Koonin LM, Palmer SK, et al. Anesthesia-related deaths during obstetric delivery in the United States, 1979-1990. Anesthesiology 1997;86(2):277–84.
[34] Hawkins JL, Chang J, Palmer SK, et al. Anesthesia-related maternal mortality in the United States: 1979-2002. Obstet Gynecol 2011;117(1):69–74.
[35] Riley ET, Cohen SE, Macario A, et al. Spinal versus epidural anesthesia for cesarean section: a comparison of time efficiency, costs, charges, and complications. Anesth Analg 1995;80(4):709–12.
[36] Butwick A, Carvalho B, Danial C, et al. Retrospective analysis of anesthetic interventions for obese patients undergoing elective cesarean delivery. J Clin Anesth 2010;22(7):519–26.
[37] Ross VH, Dean LS, Thomas JA, et al. A randomized controlled comparison between combined spinal-epidural and single-shot spinal techniques in morbidly obese parturients

undergoing cesarean delivery: time for initiation of anesthesia. Anesth Analg 2014;118(1):168–72.
[38] Soens MA, Birnbach DJ, Ranasinghe JS, et al. Obstetric anesthesia for the obese and morbidly obese patient: an ounce of prevention is worth more than a pound of treatment. Acta Anaesthesiol Scand 2008;52(1):6–19.
[39] McDonnell NJ, Paech MJ. The management of a super morbidly obese parturient delivering twins by caesarean section. Anaesth Intensive Care 2007;35(6):979–83.
[40] Polin CM, Hale B, Mauritz AA, et al. Anesthetic management of super-morbidly obese parturients for cesarean delivery with a double neuraxial catheter technique: a case series. Int J Obstet Anesth 2015;24(3):276–80.
[41] Yurashevich M, Habib AS. Anesthetic management for robotic hysterectomy in obese women. Curr Opin anaesthesiology 2021;34(3):238–45.
[42] Kheterpal S, Han R, Tremper KK, et al. Incidence and predictors of difficult and impossible mask ventilation. Anesthesiology 2006;105(5):885–91.
[43] Juvin P, Lavaut E, Dupont H, et al. Difficult tracheal intubation is more common in obese than in lean patients. Anesth Analg 2003;97(2):595–600, table of contents.
[44] Murphy C, Wong DT. Airway management and oxygenation in obese patients. Can J Anaesth = J canadien d'anesthesie 2013;60(9):929–45.
[45] Eng M, Butler J, Bonica JJ. Respiratory function in pregnant obese women. Am J Obstet Gynecol 1975;123(3):241–5.
[46] Dempsey JA, Reddan W, Rankin J, et al. Alveolar-arterial gas exchange during muscular work in obesity. J Appl Physiol 1966;21(6):1807–14.
[47] Oberg B, Poulsen TD. Obesity: an anaesthetic challenge. Acta Anaesthesiol Scand 1996;40(2):191–200.
[48] Chiron B, Laffon M, Ferrandiere M, et al. Standard preoxygenation technique versus two rapid techniques in pregnant patients. Int J Obstet Anesth 2004;13(1):11–4.
[49] Gleason JM, Christian BR, Barton ED. Nasal Cannula Apneic Oxygenation Prevents Desaturation During Endotracheal Intubation: An Integrative Literature Review. *West J Emerg Med* Mar 2018;19(2):403–11.
[50] Dixon BJ, Dixon JB, Carden JR, et al. Preoxygenation is more effective in the 25 degrees head-up position than in the supine position in severely obese patients: a randomized controlled study. Anesthesiology 2005;102(6):1110–5 [discussion: 5A].
[51] Levitan RM, Mechem CC, Ochroch EA, et al. Head-elevated laryngoscopy position: improving laryngeal exposure during laryngoscopy by increasing head elevation. Ann Emerg Med 2003;41(3):322–30.
[52] Collins JS, Lemmens HJ, Brodsky JB, et al. Laryngoscopy and morbid obesity: a comparison of the "sniff" and "ramped" positions. Obes Surg 2004;14(9):1171–5.
[53] Dhonneur G, Abdi W, Ndoko SK, et al. Video-assisted versus conventional tracheal intubation in morbidly obese patients. Obes Surg 2009;19(8):1096–101.
[54] Andersen LH, Rovsing L, Olsen KS. GlideScope videolaryngoscope vs. Macintosh direct laryngoscope for intubation of morbidly obese patients: a randomized trial. Acta Anaesthesiol Scand 2011;55(9):1090–7.
[55] Mushambi MC, Kinsella SM, Popat M, et al. Obstetric Anaesthetists' Association and Difficult Airway Society guidelines for the management of difficult and failed tracheal intubation in obstetrics. Anaesthesia 2015;70(11):1286–306.
[56] Ingrande J, Lemmens HJ. Dose adjustment of anaesthetics in the morbidly obese. Br J Anaesth 2010;105(Suppl 1):i16–23.
[57] Lemmens HJ, Brodsky JB. The dose of succinylcholine in morbid obesity. Anesth Analg 2006;102(2):438–42.
[58] Meyhoff CS, Lund J, Jenstrup MT, et al. Should dosing of rocuronium in obese patients be based on ideal or corrected body weight? Anesth Analg 2009;109(3):787–92.
[59] Tan HS, Habib AS. Obesity in women: anaesthetic implications for peri-operative and peripartum management. Anaesthesia 2021;76(Suppl 4):108–17.

[60] Young CC, Harris EM, Vacchiano C, et al. Lung-protective ventilation for the surgical patient: international expert panel-based consensus recommendations. Br J Anaesth 2019;123(6): 898–913.
[61] Benumof JL. Obesity, sleep apnea, the airway and anesthesia. Curr Opin anaesthesiology 2004;17(1):21–30.
[62] Burke WM, Gossner G, Goldman NA. Robotic surgery in the obese gynecologic patient. Clin Obstet Gynecol 2011;54(3):420–30.
[63] Whitty RJ, Maxwell CV, Carvalho JC. Complications of neuraxial anesthesia in an extreme morbidly obese patient for Cesarean section. Int J Obstet Anesth 2007;16(2):139–44.
[64] Eley VA, Christensen R, Guy L, et al. Perioperative Blood Pressure Monitoring in Patients With Obesity. Anesth Analg 2019;128(3):484–91.
[65] Bonso E, Saladini F, Zanier A, et al. Accuracy of a single rigid conical cuff with standard-size bladder coupled to an automatic oscillometric device over a wide range of arm circumferences. Hypertens Res 2010;33(11):1186–91.
[66] Manning DM, Kuchirka C, Kaminski J. Miscuffing: inappropriate blood pressure cuff application. Circulation 1983;68(4):763–6.
[67] Leblanc ME, Auclair A, Leclerc J, et al. Blood pressure measurment in severeky obese patients:validation of the forearm approach in different arm positions. Am J Hypertens 2019;32(2):175–85.
[68] Hersh LT, Sesing JC, Luczyk WJ, et al. Validation of a conical cuff on the forearm for estimating radial artery blood pressure. Blood Press Monit 2014;19(1):38–45.
[69] Sebbane M, Claret PG, Lefebvre S, et al. Predicting peripheral venous access difficulty in the emergency department using body mass index and a clinical evaluation of venous accessibility. J Emerg Med 2013;44(2):299–305.
[70] Zingg W, Pittet D. Peripheral venous catheters: an under-evaluated problem. Int J Antimicrob Agents 2009;34(Suppl 4):S38–42.
[71] Stolz LA, Stolz U, Howe C, et al. Ultrasound-guided peripheral venous access: a meta-analysis and systematic review. J Vasc Access 2015;16(4):321–6.
[72] D'Alonzo RC, White WD, Schultz JR, et al. Ethnicity and the distance to the epidural space in parturients. Reg Anesth pain Med 2008;33(1):24–9.
[73] Ellinas EH, Eastwood DC, Patel SN, et al. The effect of obesity on neuraxial technique difficulty in pregnant patients: a prospective, observational study. Anesth Analg 2009;109(4): 1225–31.
[74] Sahin T, Balaban O, Sahin L, et al. A randomized controlled trial of preinsertion ultrasound guidance for spinal anaesthesia in pregnancy: outcomes among obese and lean parturients: ultrasound for spinal anesthesia in pregnancy. J Anesth 2014;28(3):413–9.
[75] Balki M, Lee Y, Halpern S, et al. Ultrasound imaging of the lumbar spine in the transverse plane: the correlation between estimated and actual depth to the epidural space in obese parturients. Anesth Analg 2009;108(6):1876–81.
[76] Hamilton CL, Riley ET, Cohen SE. Changes in the position of epidural catheters associated with patient movement. Anesthesiology 1997;86(4):778–84 [discussion: 29A].
[77] Lee Y, Balki M, Parkes R, et al. Dose requirement of intrathecal bupivacaine for cesarean delivery is similar in obese and normal weight women. Revista brasileira de anestesiologia 2009;59(6):674–83.
[78] Saravanakumar K, Rao SG, Cooper GM. Obesity and obstetric anaesthesia. Anaesthesia 2006;61(1):36–48.
[79] Lamon AM, Einhorn LM, Cooter M, et al. The impact of body mass index on the risk of high spinal block in parturients undergoing cesarean delivery: a retrospective cohort study. J Anesth 2017;31(4):552–8.
[80] Hartwell BL, Aglio LS, Hauch MA, et al. Vertebral column length and spread of hyperbaric subarachnoid bupivacaine in the term parturient. Reg Anesth 1991;16(1):17–9.
[81] Norris MC. Height, weight, and the spread of subarachnoid hyperbaric bupivacaine in the term parturient. Anesth Analg 1988;67(6):555–8.

[82] 50) and ED(95) of intrathecal bupivacaine in morbidly obese patients undergoing cesarean delivery. In: Carvalho B, Collins J, Drover DR, et al, editors. Anesthesiology 2011;114(3): 529–35.
[83] Ngaka TC, Coetzee JF, Dyer RA. The Influence of Body Mass Index on Sensorimotor Block and Vasopressor Requirement During Spinal Anesthesia for Elective Cesarean Delivery. Anesth Analg 2016;123(6):1527–34.
[84] Panni MK, Columb MO. Obese parturients have lower epidural local anaesthetic requirements for analgesia in labour. Br J Anaesth 2006;96(1):106–10.
[85] Milligan KR, Cramp P, Schatz L, et al. The effect of patient position and obesity on the spread of epidural analgesia. Int J Obstet Anesth 1993;2(3):134–6.
[86] Duggan J, Bowler GM, McClure JH, et al. Extradural block with bupivacaine: influence of dose, volume, concentration and patient characteristics. Br J Anaesth 1988;61(3):324–31.
[87] American College of O, Gynecologists' Committee on Practice B-O. ACOG Practice Bulletin No. 196: Thromboembolism in Pregnancy. Obstet Gynecol 2018;132(1):e1–17.
[88] Say L, Chou D, Gemmill A, et al. Global causes of maternal death: a WHO systematic analysis. Lancet Glob Health 2014;2(6):e323–33.
[89] Rocha AT, de Vasconcellos AG, da Luz Neto ER, et al. Risk of venous thromboembolism and efficacy of thromboprophylaxis in hospitalized obese medical patients and in obese patients undergoing bariatric surgery. Obes Surg 2006;16(12):1645–55.
[90] Butwick AJ, Bentley J, Leonard SA, et al. Prepregnancy maternal body mass index and venous thromboembolism: a population-based cohort study. BJOG 2019;126(5):581–8.
[91] Bates SM, Greer IA, Middeldorp S, et al. VTE, thrombophilia, antithrombotic therapy, and pregnancy: Antithrombotic Therapy and Prevention of Thrombosis, 9th ed: American College of Chest Physicians Evidence-Based Clinical Practice Guidelines. Chest 2012;141(2 Suppl):e691S–736S.
[92] Palmerola KL, D'Alton ME, Brock CO, et al. A comparison of recommendations for pharmacologic thromboembolism prophylaxis after caesarean delivery from three major guidelines. BJOG 2016;123(13):2157–62.
[93] Leffert L, Butwick A, Carvalho B, et al. The Society for Obstetric Anesthesia and Perinatology Consensus Statement on the Anesthetic Management of Pregnant and Postpartum Women Receiving Thromboprophylaxis or Higher Dose Anticoagulants. Anesth Analg 2018;126(3):928–44.
[94] Horlocker TT, Vandermeuelen E, Kopp SL, et al. Regional Anesthesia in the Patient Receiving Antithrombotic or Thrombolytic Therapy: American Society of Regional Anesthesia and Pain Medicine Evidence-Based Guidelines (Fourth Edition). Reg Anesth Pain Med 2018;43(3): 263–309.

Advances in Anesthesia 40 (2022) 201–221

ADVANCES IN ANESTHESIA

Contemporary Anesthetic Evaluation and Management for Electroconvulsive Therapy

Francis V. Salinas, MD, FASA[a,b]

[a]Swedish Medical Center, Seattle and Issaquah, Washington, USA; [b]Medical Director of Anesthesia Services and Interventional Platform-Swedish Issaquah Hospital, Issaquah, Washington, USA

Keywords

• Electroconvulsive therapy • Intravenous anesthesia • Neuromuscular blockade

Key points

- Electroconvulsive therapy (ECT) is an effective treatment of severe major depression, bipolar disorder, severe schizophrenia, and catatonia.
- There are significant hemodynamic changes associated with the ECT procedure.
- Contemporary (modified) ECT with general anesthesia and neuromuscular blockade has a very low risk of severe major adverse cardiac complications.
- The anesthesiologist must be aware of the potential for the anesthetic agents to interfere with achieving a therapeutic seizure.
- Proper airway management, targeting hyperoxia and mild hypocapnia, optimizes both patient safety and therapeutic efficacy of ECT.

INTRODUCTION

Electroconvulsive therapy (ECT) is a medical treatment most often used in patients with severe major depression that has not responded to other treatments. ECT is also indicated for patients with other severe psychiatric conditions, including bipolar disorder, schizophrenia, schizoaffective disorders, catatonia, and neuroleptic malignant syndrome. ECT is typically indicated when other treatments, including multiple medications and psychotherapy, have failed [1]. ECT is also indicated when patients require rapid treatment response because of the severity of their ongoing condition, such as being at risk for suicide, or in the case of catatonia, can result in significant self-harm from severe malnutrition and dehydration [2].

E-mail address: fvsalinasmd@gmail.com

https://doi.org/10.1016/j.aan.2022.07.005

Historically, ECT was first described in 1938 by Italian physicians Ugo Cerletti and Luigi Bini and was performed for almost 30 years without anesthesia, and this is referred to as "unmodified ECT." ECT involves administering a brief electrical stimulus to the brain to induce a therapeutic generalized seizure. Unmodified ECT was performed from 1938 through 1968 with patients occasionally suffering fractures and joint dislocations along with considerable anticipatory fear and anxiety [3]. Contemporary "modified ECT" involves inducing general anesthesia with neuromuscular blockade before inducing the therapeutic seizure [2,3].

ECT is administered to an estimated 100,000 patients annually in the United States (~5000 ECT procedures are performed in the author's community hospitals annually) and an estimated 1,000,000 patients worldwide. ECT has established therapeutic efficacy and cost-effectiveness for treatment of severe depression [4–6] and schizophrenia [7]. More recently, the US Food and Drug Administration's redesignation of ECT devices from class III (high risk) to class II (moderate risk, requiring special precautions) for severe symptoms is analogous to "on-label" indications for use of drugs. This redesignation helps decrease the stigma associated with the procedure by acknowledging its safety and effectiveness [2,3,8]. Thus, the application of ECT is expected to increase. Because anesthesia is now an essential part of contemporary ECT, the anesthesiologist must have a thorough understanding of the physiologic effects of the induced seizure, the associated risks and complications, and the potential for the administered anesthetic agents to interfere with therapeutic efficacy of the ECT treatment [9,10]. The goal of this review is to combine an evidence-based update with the experience of the author's institution to provide a practical approach to anesthetic care for the patient undergoing ECT.

TECHNICAL AND PROCEDURAL ASPECTS OF ELECTROCONVULSIVE THERAPY

Procedural location and monitoring

The anesthesiologist should be knowledgeable about the technical aspects of the ECT procedure to optimize the collaboration and shared decision making with team members providing care for the patient: typically, a psychiatrist, anesthesiologist, and nursing teams in both the procedural and recovery areas. Depending on institutional guidelines or preferences, ECT may be performed in an operating room or nonoperating anesthesia location such as a preoperative procedural area, postanesthesia care unit (PACU), or a dedicated room for ECT. ECT may be performed on an inpatient basis, and in the author's practice, it is typically performed on an outpatient basis. Because ECT is performed under general anesthesia, standard American Society of Anesthesiologists (ASA) monitoring is required, and equipment to manage emergencies (difficult airway, cardiac arrest, and malignant hyperthermia) should be immediately available. Standard preparations should include anesthesia machine (if present) checkout, and preparation of routinely administered anesthetic agents, medications to treat the anticipated physiologic effects and possible side effects (headache, nausea and vomiting, postictal agitation [PIA], and myalgias), as well as equipment for advanced airway management. In addition, the ECT machine itself will have electroencephalography (EEG) monitoring not only to confirm that a seizure has occurred but also to enable the team to assess the duration and quality of the seizure. The EEG parameters are displayed with 2 channels from monitoring leads placed over the frontal and mastoid locations. Although monitoring of the motor component of the seizure may be assessed by electromyography, more commonly, a blood pressure cuff is placed around the right ankle and inflated (after the patient achieves adequate hypnosis) 20 to 30 mm Hg above the systolic blood pressure to prevent the neuromuscular blocking agent (NMBA) from entering the foot. After the electrical stimulus is applied, the team members observe the foot and record the duration of the tonic-clonic contractions. Last, a peripheral nerve stimulator should be used to confirm adequate depth of neuromuscular blockade before delivery of the electrical stimulus, and to precisely assess the return of adequate neuromuscular strength during the postictal recovery phase.

Stimulating electrode placement

Induction of the therapeutic seizure is achieved by briefly passing an electrical current across the brain via 2 electrodes (either disposable adhesive pads or metal disks) applied to the scalp, ensuring that there is adequate skin contact to minimize impedance at the electrode-scalp interface. There are 3 standard electrode positions in contemporary ECT practice:

- Bilateral (bitemporal): 1 electrode is applied over each temple. Bilateral stimulation has the greatest therapeutic efficacy and most rapid onset of response but may cause the most cognitive side effects (acute postictal confusion-agitation, memory impairment).
- Right unilateral: 1 electrode is applied over the right temple and the other is applied just to the right of the vertex. Right unilateral placement avoids initial stimulation of the dominant left cerebral hemisphere (controls language and mathematical abilities in the majority [95%] of the population). Unilateral stimulation results in slightly lower therapeutic efficacy, but generally causes fewer adverse cognitive side effects.
- Bifrontal: each electrode is placed on the forehead above the outer (lateral) canthus of each eye. Bifrontal may be as effective as bitemporal with similar frequency of adverse cognitive side effects to right unilateral.

In the author's practice, treatment typically starts with right unilateral stimulation, and patients who do not respond after 3 to 5 ECT treatments may be switched to the bitemporal approach at the discretion of the treating psychiatrist. In contrast, patients who develop unacceptable cognitive side effects with bitemporal stimulation may be switched to right unilateral stimulation.

Electrical stimulus

The type and intensity of delivered electrical stimulus affects both the therapeutic efficacy and adverse cognitive effects of ECT. The current standard is to deliver a brief (0.5–2.0 milliseconds) pulse square waveform. The dose of stimulus affects the therapeutic efficacy, speed of response, and adverse cognitive effects and can be quantified in either absolute units of electrical charge (millicoulombs) or multiples of seizure threshold. The seizure threshold refers to the minimal electrical stimulus charge required to induce an acceptable seizure (typically 15–70 seconds on the EEG recording); the minimal amount is typically determined at the first treatment session by initially delivering a predetermined minimal charge and incrementally increasing (if necessary) to induce an acceptable seizure, which establishes the initial seizure threshold. The typical bilateral stimulus dose is 1.5 to 2.5 times the seizure threshold, and typical unilateral stimulus dose is 6 times the seizure threshold. Heightened vigilance is especially important during the initial dose titration, especially if the stimulus does not result in a seizure. Direct electrical stimulation of the vagus nerve with a subconvulsive stimulus may produce a significant (and unopposed) parasympathetic response and result in severe bradycardia or even brief periods of asystole. If a seizure is not elicited, the patient is hyperventilated for 30 to 40 seconds, and a subsequent (increased) stimulus charge is administered. During these dose titration sessions, it is important to ensure adequate levels of hypnosis and neuromuscular blockade.

Seizure quality and duration

Most therapeutic seizures last 15 to 70 seconds as observed by EEG monitoring, which typically lasts 10% to 30% longer than the motor component. Additional EEG characteristics than can predict response to ECT include ictal amplitude measures and postictal suppression [11]. Seizures of less than 15 seconds duration may not be therapeutic and should be followed by an incrementally higher stimulus dose after a 60-second period of hyperventilation. A prolonged seizure (typically defined as one lasting longer than 3 minutes) is a potentially serious complication that can occur in approximately 2% of cases. Prolonged seizures increase the risk of postictal confusion, short-term memory impairment, and headache. In the author's practice, the seizure is terminated at 2 minutes by administering either a small dose of propofol (30–50 mg) or a benzodiazepine (BZD) (midazolam 1–2 mg) [12].

PHYSIOLOGICAL CHANGES DURING ELECTROCONVULSIVE THERAPY

The physiology of the patient changes rapidly and significantly during the brief course of an ECT session [13,14]. After delivery of the electrical stimulus and before the onset of seizure, direct stimulation of the vagal nuclei leads to a parasympathetic surge during the tonic phase leading to arrhythmias including bradycardia with or without hypotension, premature atrial and ventricular contractions, hypotension, and occasionally, a transient episode of asystole. Overall, poststimulation asystole usually resolves within 3 to 6 seconds without any clinically significant sequela. A recent review suggests that right unilateral electrode stimulation holds a greater risk for bradycardia and asystole compared with either bitemporal or bifrontal electrode placement [15]. A history of hypertension or preexisting ischemic changes on ECG did not predict asystole. In contrast, unstable cardiac conditions, age greater than 65 years, prestimulus hypoxia, and preprocedural use of beta-blockers or acetylcholinesterase inhibitors increase the risk of symptomatic bradycardia or asystole [16].

The clonic phase of the seizure then follows, characterized by sympathetic discharge that can cause tachycardia and hypertension [17]. During this period, the rate-pressure product (heart rate × blood pressure) can increase 2- to 4-fold with a 30% to 40% increase in systolic blood pressure and 20% increase in heart rate [17,18]. The duration of sympathetic stimulation typically correlates with the length of the seizure and usually resolves within 10 to 20 minutes of the end of the seizure. After termination of the seizure, there is a second parasympathetic surge than can also lead to asystole and more commonly occurs in well-conditioned patients with a low resting heart rate [19]. Cerebral blood flow, cerebral metabolic rate, cerebral metabolic oxygen consumption, and intracranial pressure increase temporarily during the clonic phase of the seizure and correlates with the degree of systemic blood pressure elevation [20,21].

PREANESTHETIC ASSESSMENT AND MANAGEMENT

ECT is generally considered a low-risk procedure, but psychiatrists often request a medical evaluation before beginning an ECT treatment course. The goal of the medical evaluation is to identify medical issues that place the patient at risk, to propose strategies to mitigate that risk, and to anticipate complications that may occur during and after the procedure [22,23]. Although no specific laboratory tests are required in the pre-ECT evaluation, it is appropriate to measure serum electrolytes for patients taking diuretics and those with a history of chronic renal disease or stable congestive heart failure. Institutional polices may dictate specific preprocedural testing for patients receiving general anesthesia. The history should focus on risk factors for cardiac ischemia or arrhythmia, heart failure, and the presence of intracranial pathology (masses, vascular malformations, increased intracranial pressure [ICP]).

Coexisting cardiac disease

Although not explicitly stated in the American Heart Asssociation-American College of Cardiology guidelines, ECT can be treated as a low-risk procedure because it is usually well tolerated, even in those with cardiac risk factors, because the duration of hemodynamic changes is brief and the mortality rate is low. The incidence of overall serious medical events [24,25] and more specifically, major adverse cardiac events (MACE), is infrequent [26,27]. The most frequently reported MACEs were acute heart failure, arrhythmia, and acute pulmonary edema with an incidence (95% confidence interval [CI]) of 24 (12.48–46.1), 25.8 (14.8–45), and 4.92 (0.85–28.6) per 1000 patients or 2.44 (1.27–4.69), 4.66 (2.15–10.1), and 1.5 (0.71–3.14) per 1000 ECT treatments within 30 days after ECT. All-cause mortality was 0.42 (0.11–1.52) deaths per 1000 patients and 0.06 (0.02–0.23) deaths per 1000 ECT treatments

[26]. Overall, in this one review, cardiac deaths accounted for 29% (23 of 79) of deaths within 30 days of treatment. In a nationwide cohort study with 1-year follow-up, the incidence of MACE was lower in the ECT-treated versus non-ECT group (1.4% vs 2.3%; hazard ratio, 0.65%; 95% CI, 0.49–0.85) [27]. Patients with a previous history of myocardial infarction, coronary artery disease, prior coronary revascularization (coronary artery bypass grafting, percutaneous coronary intervention), prior valvular repair or replacement, and cardiac implantable electronic device (CIED) such as a pacemaker or implantable cardiac defibrillator (ICD) should be evaluated by a cardiologist for risk assessment and recommendations for medical optimization.

The management of patients with CIED such as a pacemaker or ICD is like that for other surgical procedures wherein electromagnetic interference (EMI) is a concern [28]. Modern CIEDs are resistant to the effects of EMI but may become damaged or reprogrammed in certain circumstances. The most common source of interference during ECT comes from muscle movement due to fasciculations or inadequate muscle relaxation. If a patient is not pacemaker dependent, a magnet should be available, but does not need to be placed over the battery during ECT. In contrast, if the patient is pacemaker dependent and the risk for EMI is high, consultation with the cardiology or institutional CIED team is necessary to reprogram the device before (to asynchronous mode) and after the procedure. If a patient has an ICD, placing a magnet over the battery renders the therapy function inactive (will not deliver a therapeutic shock), but the device will continue to monitor and record the patient's rhythm. If a malignant arrhythmia is observed, prompt removal of the magnet is critical. From a practical perspective, it is important to have a backup form of external pacing and defibrillation in any patient with CIED undergoing ECT.

Coexisting neurologic disease

Patients with known or suspected pathology (masses, vascular lesions, ICP, prior cerebrovascular accident) should be evaluated by a neurologist and/or neurosurgeon [29–32]. Evaluation should consist of a detailed history and physical examination to assess and establish baseline neurologic function. Any concerning signs (abnormal motor examination or papilledema) or symptoms (suspicious headache) should prompt a further investigation, including neuroimaging. In patients with documented intracranial pathology, the decision to proceed with ECT should be made on a case-by-case basis with a team approach between the psychiatrist, neurologic consultants, and the anesthesiologist [30–32]. In the cases of poststroke depression, ECT has been found be safe and effective [33].

Deep brain stimulation (DBS) is increasingly being performed for Parkinson disease, essential tremor, and dystonia not adequately controlled by medications. An important safety concern when performing ECT in patients with DBS devices is that the electrical current conducted through an implanted DBS metal electrode could cause heating of the electrode, resulting in damage to electrode or brain tissue surrounding the electrode. This damage in turn could potentially cause loss of DBS treatment efficacy or neuronal injury. An additional concern is that passing an electrical current through the brain could lead to malfunctioning or reprogramming (of the specified stimulation parameters of the DBS) to an incorrect stimulation pattern. In the most recent and largest publication to date, 22 cases were reported with no adverse events (no evidence of brain tissue damage, no change in either device function or position of the DBS electrode position) related to the presence of DBS devices in patients undergoing ECT [34]. In each individual case, the choice of ECT electrode placement was based on routing the ECT stimulus current path away from the DBS electrodes and avoiding the burr holes (skull defects) through which the DBS electrodes were placed. However, the investigators cautioned that there are no prospective or large-scale published data assessing the safety of ECT in patients with DBS.

ECT is contraindicated in patients with cochlear implants based on the US Food and Drug Administration instructions from manufacturers [35]. However, a cadaveric human head model with cochlear implants did not demonstrate electrical injury to the device. In the most recent review, which includes the cadaveric study and 4 case reports, there was no evidence of harm to either the device or the patient related to ECT treatment [36]. The investigators recommend a multidisciplinary approach between the psychiatrist, anesthesiologist, and otologists, weighing the risks and benefits of ECT in patients with cochlear implants [36]. When possible, the investigators recommend unilateral electrode placement contralateral to the cochlear implant or bilateral temporal electrode placement if appropriate. Similar to ECT treatment in patients with DBS, the cochlear implant should be turned off and the external device removed. After the course of ECT is completed, the cochlear implant should be evaluated for any damage or malfunction by the manufacturer and otologist. As a corollary, the safety of cranial metallic objects (cMO) in 24 cases has been reviewed. The theoretic concerns included heating of brain tissue, bleeding from the clip or coil application sites because ECT is associated with a hyperdynamic cardiovascular state, as well as significant increases in cerebral blood flow and velocity [37]. The additional cMOs included cerebral aneurysm clips, cerebral coils, DBS devices, cochlear implants, and foreign bodies. There were no ECT-related complications.

Electroconvulsive therapy in pregnancy

The treatment of psychiatric conditions in the pregnant patient poses unique challenges, because psychotropic medications may have significant side effects in both the mother and fetus. ECT is thought to be safe in pregnant patients as published in a joint statement by American Psychiatric Association and the American College of Obstetricians and Gynecologists [38]. The multidisciplinary care team for pregnant patients undergoing ECT should include a psychiatrist (with experience in administering ECT to pregnant patients), an anesthesiologist (ideally experienced with both ECT and obstetric care), a maternal-fetal medicine specialist who can coordinate the plan for therapy, and an onsite obstetrician who can interpret periprocedural fetal heart rate (FHR) monitoring and provide treatment of obstetric-related complications or effect delivery if indicated. Potential risks can arise from anesthetic delivery, the provoked seizure, and the physiologic response to seizures. In a recent review that included 4 systemic reviews (884 cases), the most common adverse events associated with ECT are temporary, self-limited FHR changes, and contractions, which rarely progress to labor [39]. Another review reported on 32 cases of ECT treatment specifically during the first trimester of pregnancy [40]. Based on these 2 reviews, the rates of vaginal bleeding/placental abruption, prolonged FHR abnormalities, stillbirths, or preterm delivery do not appear to be increased in patients who undergo ECT during pregnancy compared with the general obstetric population. Owing to the expected physiologic changes associated with pregnancy, considerations for the increased risk of aspiration and the decision to intubate should be made on a case-by-case basis. Glycopyrrolate is preferred to prevent or treat bradycardia because it does not cross the placenta as easily as atropine. Administration of sodium citrate and intravenous (IV) famotidine 40 to 60 minutes before the procedure can mitigate the effects of aspiration if it occurs. Intubation is the least preferred option for managing the risk of aspiration because of its increased morbidity during pregnancy due to weight gain, edema, and hypervascularity, where even minor trauma can lead to significant bleeding. In addition, hyperventilation should be avoided, because it may lead to fetal hypoxia and acidosis due to a combination of decreased uteroplacental blood flow via vasoconstriction as well as a left shift of the maternal oxygenation curve [40,41]. After 23 weeks, continuous periprocedural FHR monitoring (and postprocedure nonstress test as indicated) should be performed, and the ECT procedure needs to be administered in a facility with resources for treating anesthetic and neonatal emergencies. In the scenario when the parturient has preeclampsia, continuous arterial blood pressure monitoring and esmolol and/or nicardipine should be readily available to monitor and rapidly treat the sympathetic surges related to ECT [41]. A recent review provides detailed recommendations for the multidisciplinary management of ECT in pregnant patients [42].

Management of anticoagulation during electroconvulsive therapy

There is a paucity of data on which to guide recommendations for the management of anticoagulation during ECT. The primary concern in a therapeutically anticoagulated patient is the potentially increased risk of intracerebral hemorrhage in the scenario of severe and prolonged hypertension during the sympathetic surge associated with the clonic phase of ECT. In contrast, discontinuation of anticoagulation places the patient at risk for a venous thromboembolism (VTE) event. In several small published case series, no major adverse bleeding or cerebrovascular events occurred in patients maintained on their respective therapeutic oral dose of anticoagulation [43–45]. In the absence of guiding data, an interdisciplinary approach should address the risks and benefits for each individual patient. The team should consider the risk and benefit of temporarily discontinuing anticoagulation (until the ECT course is completed) if the VTE is considered low. In contrast, if the VTE risk is considered high, continuing anticoagulation with attention to maintaining a therapeutic range is a reasonable approach. Prompt recognition and treatment of severe hypertension with esmolol-nicardipine and/or administering prophylactic doses of labetalol should be planned by the anesthesiologist and psychiatrist.

Management of chronically administered psychotropic medications

Because ECT is indicated for patients with severe treatment (medication)-resistant psychiatric conditions, it is common for them to present for treatment while still receiving these medications. Because psychotropic medications possess synergistic effects with ECT, they are often continued during the treatment period [46]. Several psychotropic medications may have potentially dangerous interactions with anesthetic agents routinely administered during ECT [47]. Common classes of antidepressant medications include selective serotonin reuptake inhibitors (SSRIs), serotonin-norepinephrine reuptake inhibitors (SNRIs), tricyclic antidepressants (TCAs), and monoamine oxidase inhibitors (MAOs). Additional common psychotropic medications include mood stabilizers (lithium, carbamazepine, valproate), antipsychotics (chlorpromazine, clozapine, quetiapine, olanzapine, risperidone, thioridazine, perphenazine, and haloperidol), and BDZs. The indications and choice of which agents to use rest primarily with the psychiatrists. However, the anesthesiologist should be aware of potentially important interactions of psychotropic medications with ECT.

- SSRIs include paroxetine, sertraline, and fluoxetine; common SNRIs include duloxetine and venlafaxine. Because their primary mechanism of action is blocking reuptake of serotonin at the presynaptic membrane (with minimal effects at adrenergic and cholinergic receptors), they are associated with few interactions with ECT medications. Patients taking SSRI and SNRI medications are at increased risk for serotonin syndrome characterized by clonus, hyperreflexia, agitation, and hyperthermia. Sertraline and fluoxetine are cholinesterase inhibitors and may potentially prolong the duration of action of succinylcholine.
- TCAs such as amitriptyline, nortriptyline, and imipramine also inhibit the presynaptic reuptake of serotonin and norepinephrine and can potentially potentiate the vasopressor effects of ephedrine, epinephrine, and norepinephrine. TCAs also possess antimuscarinic effects and can contribute to an elevated resting heart rate, postural hypotension, urinary retention, dry mouth, blurred vision, and sedation (which may contribute to delayed emergence from anesthesia).
- MAOs such as phenelzine and selegiline inhibit the enzymes responsible for the breakdown of amine neurotransmitters (norepinephrine and serotonin) and potentially exaggerate the vasopressor effects of ephedrine. Direct-acting inotropic (epinephrine and norepinephrine) and vasopressor agents (phenylephrine) may be safely used if titrated incrementally and at decreased doses.

Concomitant use of meperidine should be avoided, because combined use of these agents may precipitate serotonin syndrome.

- Mood stabilizers include lithium, the anticonvulsants carbamazepine and sodium valproate, and lamotrigine. Lithium can potentially increase the adverse cognitive effects of ECT and is typically held for 12 hours before treatment. Anticonvulsant mood stabilizers may impact seizure induction or duration and may be held the day before treatment. Carbamazepine is a potent inhibitor of the cytochrome P450 3A4 enzyme system and may potentially prolong the duration of action of succinylcholine. Lamictal may be associated with an increased risk of missed seizures and decreased seizure duration.
- Antipsychotic medications may enhance the effects of central nervous system depressants and may decrease anesthetic requirements. These medications may also affect the activity of the cytochrome P450 2D6 enzyme that metabolizes beta-blockers, potentially impacting their efficacy in treating the sympathetic surge associated with ECT. All antipsychotics are associated with an increased risk of extrapyramidal symptoms and importantly, the rare but life-threatening side effect of neuroleptic malignant syndrome (NMS). NMS is characterized by the classic tetrad of fever, muscle rigidity, autonomic instability, and severe mental status changes (agitation, confusion, coma) [48,49]. A high index of suspicion, confirmation with significant elevations (>4-fold above upper limit of normal) of creatine kinase, and negative workup for other possible causes (serotonin syndrome, malignant hyperthermia, and acute recreational drug intoxication) is key to prompt diagnosis and treatment.
- BDZs have the potential to inhibit induction of a therapeutic seizure, and in most circumstances, they are typically tapered and discontinued before ECT. In cases of malignant catatonia in which parenteral BDZs are acutely initiated (and followed by informed consent and medical consultation for ECT), they may be withheld 12 hours before ECT therapy if tolerated. In cases in which high doses of BDZs are required or they cannot be discontinued, reversal with IV flumazenil (0.5–1.0 mg administered immediately before treatment) may be required to elicit an adequate therapeutic seizure [50]. Flumazenil may also be used in BDZ-free patients with high seizure thresholds to facilitate induction of ECT seizures [51].

ANESTHETIC MANAGEMENT FOR THE ELECTROCONVULSIVE THERAPY PROCEDURE

The fundamental goals of general anesthesia for ECT are as follows:

1. Provide hypnosis (asleep and unaware) before inducing a therapeutic seizure, and more specifically before administration of neuromuscular blockade.
2. Provide comfort in the periprocedural session. Although the delivered shock during ECT itself does not cause significant postprocedural pain, similar to electrical cardioversion, the applied shock would be painful to an awake patient. Opioids are typically not required, although ECT may cause postprocedural headache, myalgias, and nausea, which can be treated or prevented by the anesthesiologist.
3. In conjunction with the psychiatrist, choose the appropriate anesthetic agents and doses and provide the optimal physiologic conditions (hyperoxia and mild hypocapnia) that optimize the quality and duration of the therapeutic seizures.

4. Keep the patient safe by anticipating, recognizing, and promptly treating the potentially significant hemodynamic changes of ECT.

Preanesthetic medications

Headache is the most common adverse effect of ECT, occurring with a weighted mean incidence of 32.8% [52,53]. In most patients who experience a headache, it will be transient, mild, and readily treated with over-the-counter oral acetaminophen or nonsteroidal anti-inflammatory agents. A prophylactic dose of IV ketorolac (15–30 mg IV) is an effective treatment for patients who report a history of severe postprocedural headaches. In patients with a history of migraines, therapeutic or prophylactic sumatriptan may be an effective agent when symptoms are compatible with a vascular headache. Postprocedural nausea occurs in approximately 25% of patients, and prophylaxis and/or treatment with IV ondansetron is a cost-effective and practical approach. Caffeine may also be administered in patients when seizure duration is deemed inadequate [54,55]. Caffeine, IV or oral, increases the seizure duration in a dose-dependent manner without affecting seizure threshold, and is associated with faster rate of recovery from depression and minimizes the need for higher stimulus dose to elicit seizure [56,57]. However, the caffeine dose may have to be increased with successive ECT sessions. In patients with a prior history of severe symptomatic bradycardia or prolonged asystole, as well as excessive oral secretions during ECT, premedication with either glycopyrrolate 0.2 mg or atropine 0.2 mg may be considered [58].

In the author's ECT practice, the patient is typically transported into the operating room (OR) by the perioperative team while the anesthesiologist transports the previously treated patient to the PACU and hands them off to the recovery room nurses specifically trained to provide phase 1 recovery after ECT. After the patient leaves the OR, the ECT nurse cleans the anesthesia station and changes the anesthetic circuit and suction equipment. The patient is transported to the OR by the ECT nurse once the anesthesiologist has completed charting wasted controlled substances (methohexital and BDZs) for the previous patient, and confirms the anesthesia workstation, anesthesia record, and medications are ready for the incoming patient. For patients with previous ECT sessions, the author's practice meets the patient in the OR and performs a brief interview to review conduct and recovery of the most recent ECT session. Forty minutes are reserved for the first (index) ECT session when they meet a patient for the first time. This duration allows a detailed review of their medication list, pertinent medical history, and medical consultations and laboratory data. At the initial ECT session, formal written consent is obtained (which in the author's institutional practice is then valid for 30 days), followed by thorough airway evaluation, including detailed examination for potential difficulties in mask ventilation and the presence of loose teeth. The additional time also facilitates closer observation by the ECT team in the PACU to assess for any signs of symptoms of PIA. Subsequent ECT sessions typically take 20 minutes from the time the patient enters the room until the next patient enters the room. Given the high volume of patients (24–27 patients/d), the rapid turnover, the ECT team (psychiatrist, anesthesiologist, ECT nurse, and PACU nurses) must have a high level of communication, teamwork, and experience to optimize the safety and efficacy for each patient undergoing an ECT session.

Stepwise technique for delivery of anesthesia and airway management for electroconvulsive therapy

In a stepwise coordinated fashion, the ECT team proceeds as follows:

1. The anesthesiologist places standard ASA monitors and briefly reviews issues related to the previous ECT session (headache, nausea, myalgias), while the ECT nurse places the EEG monitoring leads bilaterally at the frontal and mastoid positions (for 2-channel recording) and the right ankle blood pressure cuff. Simultaneously, the psychiatrist reviews the notes from the previous ECT and formulates a plan with the anesthesiologist for the choice and dose of anesthetic and any adjuvant medications, as well as the electrical charge parameters.
2. The patient is then preoxygenated (inspired concentration of 100%) for 1 minute and continuously encouraged to actively hyperventilate, by taking deep, maximum-capacity breaths (voluntary hyperventilation) [59]. After the initial vital signs are obtained (which determines the systolic blood pressure value to isolate the right foot), a safety pause is conducted confirming the anesthetic agents and adjuvants to be administered.
3. The IV hypnotic agent is administered, and once hypnosis is confirmed, perfusion of the right foot with NMBA is prevented by inflating the blood pressure cuff around the right ankle to 20% above the initial systolic blood pressure [60].
4. The NMBA is administered and followed by bag-mask ventilation of the patient (to achieve controlled hyperventilation and hyperoxia) until adequate neuromuscular blockade is achieved before the delivery of the electrical stimulus. The author typically uses a peripheral nerve stimulator to monitor evoked motor responses of the adductor pollicis to ensure complete skeletal muscle relaxation. Active hyperventilation to a target end-tidal CO_2 of 30 mm Hg with 100% oxygen is performed to achieve cerebral hypocapnia and hyperoxia, which together act synergistically to improve seizure quality and decrease the electrical charge needed to generate a therapeutic seizure [61,62]. Despite routine preoxygenation, the incidence of desaturation during ECT ranges from 17% to 29%. Risk factors for oxygen desaturation during ECT include obesity and seizure duration [63,64]. Morbidly obese patients are at particularly high risk for oxygen desaturation due to physiologic parameters and difficulties with mask ventilation. Strategies to prevent oxygen desaturation in morbidly obese patients during ECT include head up position, use of apneic oxygenation, high-flow nasal cannula, and use of supraglottic airway devices in cases of difficult mask ventilation. In addition, because muscle fasciculations induced by succinylcholine markedly increase oxygen consumption, a defasciculating dose of a nondepolarizing NMBA may be considered in morbidly obese patients during ECT [65].
5. Despite the administration of NMBAs, direct electrical stimulation of the temporalis, masseter, and pterygoid muscles causes forceful jaw clenching. Just before administering the electrical stimulus, the anesthesiologist places a soft bite block into the patient's mouth to protect the teeth, tongue, and oral soft tissues. Proper

technique is to ensure that the tongue is directed inferior and posterior, and that the chin is held firmly against the bite block.
6. The psychiatrist delivers the electrical stimulus with the predetermined electrode placement and parameters for total electrical charge.
7. The team then observes for the onset and duration of seizures (via EEG recording, observation of the motor contractions of the right foot). During both the tonic and subsequent clonic phase of the seizure, the heart rate, rhythm, and blood pressure are checked frequently to assess and promptly treat any significant prolonged cardiovascular response.
8. Once the seizure has spontaneously terminated, the anesthesiologist manually ventilates the patient until objective return of adequate neuromuscular strength has returned and continues to assist ventilation until the patient can maintain a patent upper airway. The anesthesiologist must be vigilant to maintain an adequate level of hypnosis until return of adequate spontaneous ventilation to prevent what can be a distressing sense of "air hunger" if the patient has regained consciousness while still having a significant degree of neuromuscular blockade.
9. Once the patient has regained the ability to maintain spontaneous ventilation-oxygenation, and stable cardiovascular parameters, they are then transported to PACU and handed off to the recovery room nurses.

Choice of induction anesthetic agent

The selected hypnotic anesthetic agent should have a rapid onset of action and ideally should have minimal interference with inducing an effective therapeutic seizure. The minimum effective dose should be administered because lower doses are associated with increased rates of response to ECT [66]. Because all anesthetic agents have the potential to interfere with the generation of a therapeutic seizure, the choice and dose of the anesthetic agent must be tailored to the individual needs of the patient during the course of their ECT sessions [9,67,68].

- Methohexital: Methohexital remains the induction agent of choice because it has a rapid onset of hypnotic action (20–30 seconds), short duration of action (6–8 minutes), and low cost with the generic formulation. A starting dose of 1 mg/kg of ideal body weight (IBW) is adjusted over the next several treatments based on the patient's responses with typical dose range varying from 0.6 mg/kg to 1.5 mg/kg IBW [69].
- Propofol: Propofol (doses of 1–1.5 mg/kg IBW) possesses a similarly rapid onset of action (20–30 seconds) and a duration of action of approximately 8 to 10 minutes. The advantages of propofol include a better quality of recovery in the PACU and significantly lower increases in blood pressure and heart rate with treatment. The disadvantages of propofol include increased seizure threshold (requiring increased electrical stimulus charge requirements) and shorter seizure duration [70–72]. Typical indications for choosing propofol include patients with lower seizure thresholds, history of prolonged seizures, severe and refractory postprocedural nausea/vomiting, and severe PIA. In patients with prior mild to moderate PIA, we typically administer propofol 0.5 mg/kg after EEG confirmation that the seizure has terminated [73].

- Etomidate: Etomidate (doses of 0.2–0.4 mg/kg IBW) has a slightly longer onset of action (30–45 seconds) but similar duration of hypnotic action as methohexital and propofol. Advantages of etomidate include minimal effect on seizure threshold, longer seizure duration, and increased safety profile in patients with compromised cardiac function [74,75]. Disadvantages include a higher incidence of postoperative nausea and vomiting, myoclonus, and a theoretic concern for adrenocortical suppression (especially for patients receiving multiple ECT treatments) [76].
- Ketamine: Ketamine is a dissociative anesthetic that when administered as an IV bolus of 1 mg/kg, results in a patient unresponsive to voice commands or painful stimuli within 60 to 90 seconds [77]. Although ketamine has been consistently shown to increase seizure duration and decrease electrical charge dose requirements, it has not been found to enhance improvement of depressive symptoms [78]. Ketamine possesses moderate sympathomimetic activity resulting in mild tachycardia and hypertension and may superimpose additional myocardial oxygen demand during the sympathetic phase of ECT or may mitigate the risk for bradycardia or asystole in patients with a low resting heart rate. In addition, ketamine increases salivation and glycopyrrolate is typically administered as a premedication when ketamine is chosen and may further contribute to tachycardia.
- Volatile inhalational agents: Although general anesthesia for ECT is almost always accomplished with IV anesthetics, there are unique circumstances when a volatile inhalational induction may be required: severe needle phobia, severe agitation preventing placement of an IV catheter, or intolerance to IV induction [79,80]. Sevoflurane is the agent of choice for inhalational induction because of its rapid onset and lower incidence of airway irritation. Data on sevoflurane for induction of anesthesia suggest that it is safe but may be associated with a shorter motor duration compared with methohexital, but a longer duration compared with propofol. Sevoflurane could also be useful in the final trimester of pregnancy because it may inhibit ECT-induced uterine contractions [42]. Importantly, undesired effects of sevoflurane on seizure duration and the hemodynamic response to ECT can be attenuated by discontinuing its administration after induction.

Depth of anesthesia

As noted previously, the minimum effective dose of anesthetic should be administered because lower doses are associated with increased rates of response to ECT [66]. The patient should have an adequate level of hypnosis (rendered asleep and unaware) before administration of an NMBA to prevent the patient from experiencing a sensation of being awake but paralyzed, as well as to prevent awareness during the delivery of the electrical stimulus (analogous to desiring a level of sedation before the delivery of electrical cardioversion for arrhythmias). Clinically, an appropriate level of hypnosis is confirmed noting loss of response to verbal commands in conjunction with noting the predicted onset of anesthesia for the different IV anesthetic agents. Processed EEG monitoring with bispectral index (BIS) or Narcotrend (MonitorTechnik, Hanover Germany) may be a useful tool to assist in determining the optimal time for seizure induction. Studies have observed increased seizure duration and improved seizure quality with higher preictal values (within the targeted range of values from 40 to 60) [81,82]. Despite these observations, the use of BIS monitoring has not yet been proposed widely to provide helpful benefits, including reducing the number of ECT sessions to achieve satisfactory clinical response, and subsequent time to recover from an individual ECT session. Thus, in their clinical practice, the author's institution does not find routine BIS monitoring for ECT to be clinically advantageous or cost effective.

Neuromuscular blocking agents

Succinylcholine remains the NMBA of choice for ECT due to its rapid onset and short duration of action, and subsequent rapid recovery from neuromuscular blockade. The goal of providing neuromuscular blockade for ECT is to minimize the potential risk of physical trauma associated with uncontrolled tetanic muscle contractions balanced by the desire to allow for the prompt recovery of both diaphragmatic and upper airway muscle strength to regain adequate unassisted spontaneous ventilation. The minimum effective dose of succinylcholine to prevent injury is 1.06 mg/kg (with a 95% CI of 1.0–1.27 mg/kg) in 90% of patients [83]. However, there is significant variability in the clinical response to succinylcholine [69,84]. In a large retrospective study, after the administration of the initial dose of 1 mg/kg and observation of the clinical response, there was a significant range of dose requirements (minimum dose required was 0.29 mg/kg, whereas the maximum dose required was 2.1 mg/kg). After the initial treatment, 36% of patients required a dose adjustment. In addition, 4.6% of patients required doses that were more than 2 SD above the initial mean dose, and 1.2% required doses that were more than 2 SD below the initial mean dose [84]. For those patients with contraindications to succinylcholine, rocuronium at a dose of 0.3 to 0.6 mg/kg should be used. The applied electrical stimulation should only be administered when maximal neuromuscular blockade (twitch suppression of >90% with quantitative neuromuscular monitoring or absence of twitch response with qualitative monitoring) has been achieved. The time to reach optimal neuromuscular conditions for succinylcholine (at a dose of 1 mg/kg) is 84 ± 30 seconds, and for rocuronium (at a dose of 0.6 mg/kg) it is 222 ± 60 seconds. The time to achieve 90% recovery of twitch height after a dose of succinylcholine is 9.37 + 3.2 minutes [83]. In contrast, after appropriate timing and dosage of neostigmine reversal of rocuronium, the time to achieve greater than 90% recovery of twitch height is 19.5 ± 5.7 minutes. Thus, the major disadvantage of rocuronium is a longer time from injection to complete muscle relaxation, as well as a significantly longer time to recovery when neostigmine is used for reversal. In the author's practice, when rocuronium (at a dose of 0. 6 mg/kg) is used, sugammadex is administered for reversal after termination of the seizure; typically 8 mg/kg total body weight of sugammadex is used to produce equally rapid recovery from rocuronium muscular relaxation compared with spontaneous recovery from 1 mg/kg succinylcholine [85].

Management of hemodynamic response during electroconvulsive therapy

Bradycardia and/or asystole is self-limited in most patients undergoing ECT. In some cases, it is necessary to administer either atropine or glycopyrrolate to treat severe symptomatic bradycardia or asystole. In patients who have had prior episodes of severe bradycardia or prolonged asystole, typically a prophylactic dose of either atropine 0.2 mg or glycopyrrolate 0.2 mg is administered at the author's institution. In addition, plans should be in place for immediate application and administration of transcutaneous pacing.

Anticipation, preparation, and close monitoring to treat significant or prolonged responses to the sympathetic stimulation are critical to minimize adverse cardiovascular or cerebrovascular complications. The decision to treat should be based on severity and duration of the hypertension and/or tachycardia in conjunction with the patient's individual risk of cardiovascular complications. The author's practice typically administers esmolol (0.5–1.0 mg/kg) for either prophylaxis or treatment of hypertension and tachycardia. Labetalol is an alternative agent but has a slower onset of action and longer duration of action compared with esmolol. Alternative agents with a rapid onset of action that more specifically target hypertension include bolus doses of either nicardipine (100–200 μg) or nitroglycerin (0.2–0.3 μg/kg).

Management of postictal agitation

PIA is an acute confusional state characterized by disorientation, restlessness, and poor response to verbal communication that may last 1 to 60 minutes after ECT. The reported incidence (10%–40%) varies widely based on the criteria used for diagnosis [73,86,87]. Factors associated with an increased risk for PIA include male gender, increased body mass index, active substance abuse, increased seizure duration, and prolonged time to emergence. The patient typically has no recollection of the time period. PIA is mostly self-limiting. Mild cases can be easily managed with supportive measures and repeated reassurance and reorientation by the ECT team. More severe or prolonged cases can increase the risk of injury to the patient or PACU staff and may require acute treatment with midazolam (1–2 mg), propofol (30–50 mg), or haloperidol (1–2 mg). In patients with a prior history of PIA, the author's group typically administers midazolam (1–2 mg) and/or propofol (30 mg) once the seizure has terminated [70].

SUMMARY

ECT is an effective medical treatment of severe psychiatric conditions. ECT is associated with a well-recognized physiologic bimodal response to the electrical stimulus characterized by an initial parasympathetic predominance, followed by a period of significant sympathetic response. Proper anesthetic preparation and management is an essential component of contemporary ECT and consists of general anesthesia with neuromuscular blockade, and skilled airway management to optimize the safety and therapeutic efficacy. Choice and dosage of the anesthetic agents should be made based on the individual patient's comorbidities, potential for the agents to decrease therapeutic efficacy, and response to therapy over the course of the ECT series of sessions.

DISCLOSURE

The author has nothing to disclose.

References

[1] Gaynes BN. Benefits of electroconvulsive therapy for patients with major depressive disorder. JAMA Netw Open 2021;4(7):e2116674.
[2] Espinoza RT, Kellner CH. Electroconvulsive therapy. N Engl J Med 2022;387(7):667–72.
[3] Lava-Parmele S, Lava C, Parmele JB. The historical struggles of modified electroconvulsive therapy: how anesthesia came to the rescue. J Anesth Hist 2021;7(2):17–25.
[4] Rönnqvist I, Nilsson FK, Nordenskõjld. Electroconvulsive therapy and risk of suicide in hospitalized patients with major depressive disorder. JAMA Netw Open 2021;4(7): e2116589.
[5] Slade EP, Jahn DR, Regenold WT, et al. Association of electroconvulsive therapy with psychiatric readmissions in US hospitals. JAMA Psychiatry 2017;74(8):798–804.
[6] Ross EL, Zivin K, Maixner DF. Cost-effectiveness of electroconvulsive therapy vs pharmacotherapy for treatment resistant depression in the United Sates. JAMA Psychiatry 2018;75(7):713–22.
[7] Chan CYW, Abdin E, Seow E, et al. Clinical effectiveness and speed of response of electroconvulsive therapy in treatment-resistant schizophrenia. Psychiatry Clin Neurosci 2019;73(7):416–22.
[8] Sackeim HA. Modern electroconvulsive therapy; vastly improved yet greatly underutilized. JAMA Psychiatry 2017;74(8):779–80.
[9] Bryson EO, Aloysi AS, Farber KG, et al. Individualized anesthetic management. Anesth Analg 2017;124(6):1943–56.
[10] Saoti S. Anesthesia management for electroconvulsive therapy: hemodynamic and respiratory management. J Anesth 2005;19(2):142–9.
[11] Shah AJ, Wadoo O, Latoo J. Electroconvulsive therapy (ECT): important parameters which influence its effectiveness. BJMP 2013;(4):a634.
[12] Aloysi AS, Bryson EO, Kellner CH. Management of prolonged seizures during electroconvulsive therapy. Indian J Psychol Med 2014;36(2):220–1.
[13] Hermida AP, Moshin M, Pinheiro APM, et al. The cardiovascular effects of electroconvulsive therapy and their management. J ECT 2022;38(1):2–9.
[14] Suzuki Y, Miyajima M, Ohta K, et al. A triphasic change of cardiac autonomic activity during electroconvulsive therapy. J ECT 2015;31(3):186–91.
[15] Hartnett S, Rex S, Sienaert. Asystole during electroconvulsive therapy: does electro placement matter? A systematic review. J ECT 2022;00(00):*online ahead of print.*
[16] Burd J, Kettl P. Incidence of asystole in electroconvulsive therapy in elderly patients. Am J Geriatr Psychiatry 1998;6(3):203–11.
[17] Wells DG, Davies GG. Hemodynamic changes associated with ECT. Anesth Analg 1987;66(11):1193–5.
[18] Bryson EO, Popeo D, Briggs M, et al. Electroconvulsive therapy (ECT) in patients with cardiac disease. J ECT 2013;29(1):76–7.
[19] Bhat SK, Acosta D, Schwartz CM. Postictal asystole during ECT. J ECT 2002;18(2):103–6.
[20] Vollmer-Haase J, Folkerts HW, Haase CG, et al. Cerebral hemodynamics during electrically induced seizures. Neuroreport 1998;16(9):407–10.
[21] Saito S, Yoshikawa D, Nishihara F, et al. The cerebral hemodynamic response to electrically induced seizures in man. Brain Res 1995;673(1):93–100.

[22] Tess AV, Smetana GW. Medical evaluation of patients undergoing electroconvulsive therapy. N Engl J Med 2009;360(14):1437–44.
[23] Sunsted KK, Burton MC, Shah R, et al. Preanesthesia medical evaluation for electroconvulsive therapy: a review of the literature. J ECT 2014;30(1):35–42.
[24] Hajak VL, Hajak G, Ziegelmayer C, et al. Risk assessment of electroconvulsive therapy in clinical routine: a 3-year analysis of life-threatening events in more than 3,000 treatment sessions. Front Psychol 2021;23:12767915.
[25] Kaster TL, Vigod SN, Gomes T, et al. Risk of serious medical events in patients with depression treated with electroconvulsive therapy: a propensity score-matched, retrospective cohort study. Lancet Psychiatry 2021;8(8):686–95.
[26] Duma A, Malcecsek M, Panjikara B, et al. Major adverse cardiac events and morality associated with electroconvulsive therapy: a systematic review and meta-analysis. Anesthesiology 2019;130(1):83–91.
[27] Nordenskjöld A, Güney P, Nordenskjöld AM. Major adverse cardiovascular events following electroconvulsive therapy in depression: a register-based nationwide Swedish cohort study with 1-year follow-up. J Affect Disord 2022;296:298–303.
[28] Practice Advisory for the Perioperative Management of Patients with Cardiac Implantable Electronic Devices: Pacemakers and Implantable Cardioverter-Defibrillators 2020: An Updated Report by the American Society of Anesthesiologists Task Force on Perioperative Management of Patients with Cardiac Implantable Electronic Devices. Erratum Anesthesiology 2020;132(2):225–52.
[29] Buday J, Albrecht J, Mares T, et al. Brain tumors and electroconvulsive therapy: a literature overview of the last 80 years. Front Neurol 2020;11:723.
[30] Van Herck E, Sienart P, Hagon A. Electroconvulsive therapy for patients with intracranial aneurysms: a case study and literature review. Tijdschr Psychiatry 2009;51(1):43–51.
[31] Salaris S, Szuba MP, Traber K. ECT and intracranial vascular mass. J ECT 2000;16(2):198–203.
[32] Patkar AA, Hill KP, Weinstein SP, et al. ECT in the presence of brain tumor and increased intracranial pressure: evaluation and reduction of risk. J ECT 2000;16(2):189–97.
[33] Currier MB, Murray GB, Welch CC. Electroconvulsive therapy for post-stroke depressed patients. J Neuropsychiatry Clin Neurosci 1992;4(2):140–4.
[34] Peroski MS, Xhu MM, Doddi SR, et al. The safety of electroconvulsive therapy in patients with implanted deep brain stimulators: a review of the literature and case reports. J ECT 2019;35(2):84–90.
[35] Cochlear. Nucleus cochlear implants important information for Cochlear implant recipients. 2020. Available at: https://www.cochlear.com/a51e3e42-4010-49dc-81d4-e22543f1a5f9/465533_12_01_EN_Rec-IIB_ EMEA_WEB.pdf?MOD=AJPERES&CONVERT_TO=url& CACHEID=ROOTWORKSPACE-a51e3e42-4010-49dc-81d4- e22543f1a5f9-na1WSEc. Accessed June 24 2022.
[36] Albertson LN, Lauridsen JK. A review of electroconvulsive therapy in cochlear implant patients. J ECT 2022;38(1):10–2.
[37] Gahr M, Connemann, Freudenmann RW, et al. Safety of electroconvulsive therapy in the presence of cranial metallic objects. J ECT 2014;30(1):62–8.
[38] Yonkers KA, Wisner KL, Stewart DE, et al. The management of depression during pregnancy: a report from the American Psychiatric Association and the American College of Obstetricians and Gynecologists. Obstet Gyncol 2009;114(3):703–13.
[39] Rose S, Dotters-Katz, kuller JA. Electroconvulsive therapy in pregnancy: safety, best practices, and barriers to care. Obstet Gynecol Surv 2020;75(3):199–203.
[40] Calaway K, Coshal S, Jones KJ, et al. A systematic review of the safety of electroconvulsive therapy use during the first trimester of pregnancy. J ECT 2016;32(4):230–5.
[41] Salzbrenner S, Breeden A, Jarvis S, et al. A 48-year-old woman primigravid via in vitro fertilization with severe bipolar depression and preeclampsia treated successfully with electroconvulsive therapy. J ECT 2011;27(1):e1–3.

[42] Ward HB, Fromson JA, Cooper JJ, et al. Recommendations for the use of ECT in pregnancy; literature review and proposed clinical protocol. Arch Women's Health 2018;21(6): 7145–722.
[43] Mehta V, Mueller PS, Gonzalez-Arriaza HL, et al. Safety of electroconvulsive therapy in patients receiving long-term warfarin therapy. Mayo Clin Proc 2002;79(11):1396–401.
[44] Hirata T, Yasuda K, Uemura T, et al. Electroconvulsive therapy while receiving oral anticoagulation for deep venous thrombosis: report of eight cases and review of the literature. Psychosomatics 2019;60(4):402–9.
[45] Centanni NR, Craig WY, Whitesell DL, et al. Safety of ECT in patients receiving an oral anticoagulant. Ment Health Clin 2021;11(4):254–8.
[46] Pluijms EM, Kamperman AM, Hoogendijk WJ, et al. Influence of adjuvant antidepressant on efficacy of electroconvulsive therapy: a systematic review and meta-analysis. Aust NZ J Psychiatry 2021;55(4):366–80.
[47] Janjua AU, Dhingra AL, Greenberg R, et al. The efficacy and safety of concomitant psychotropic medications and electroconvulsive therapy. CNS Drugs 2020;34(5): 509–20.
[48] Lao KMS, Zhao J, Blais JE. Antipsychotics and risk of neuroleptic malignant syndrome: a population-based cohort and case-crossover study. CNS Drugs 2020;34(11):1165–75.
[49] Murri MB, Guaglianone A, Bugliani M, et al. Second-generation antipsychotics and neuroleptic malignant syndrome: a systematic case review and case report analysis. Drugs RD 2015;15(1):45–62.
[50] Uchinuma N, Yasuda K, Iwata Y, et al. Flumazenil for successful seizure induction with electroconvulsive therapy: case report and literature review. Clin Neuropharmacol 2021;44(1):29–32.
[51] Yi J, Torres J, Azner Y, et al. Flumazenil pretreatment in benzodiazepine-free patients: a novel method for managing declining ECT seizure quality. J ECT 2012;28(3):185–9.
[52] Andrade C, Arumgham SS, Thirthalli J. Adverse effects of electroconvulsive therapy. Psychiatr Clin North Am 2016;39(3):513–30.
[53] Mulder LAC, Grootens KP. The incidence of post-electroconvulsive therapy headache: a systematic review. J ECT 2020;36(3):e22–8.
[54] Bozymski KM, Potter TG, Venkatachalam V, et al. Caffeine sodium benzoate for electroconvulsive therapy augmentation. J ECT 2018;324(4):233–9.
[55] Pinkhasov A, Biglow M, Chandra S, et al. Pretreatment with caffeine citrate to increase seizure duration during electroconvulsive therapy: a case series. J Pharm Pract 2016;29(2):1770180.
[56] Coffey CE, Figiel GS, Weiner RD, et al. Caffeine augmentation of ECT. Am J Psychiatry 1990;147(5):579–85.
[57] Ancill RJ, Carlyle W. Oral caffeine augmentation of ECT. Am J Psychiatry 1992;149(1): 137.
[58] Anastasian ZH, Khan N, Heyer E, et al. Effect of atropine dose on heart rate during electroconvulsive therapy. J ECT 2014;30(4):298–392.
[59] de Arriba-Arnau A, Dalmau A, Soria V, et al. Protocolized hyperventilation enhances electroconvulsive therapy. J Affect Disord 2017;225–32.
[60] Fink M, Johnson L. Monitoring the duration of electroconvulsive therapy seizures: "cuff" and EEG methods. Arch Gen Psychiatry 1982;39(10):1189–91.
[61] Askay SS, Bumb JM, Janke C, et al. New evidence for seizure quality improvement by hyperoxia and mild hypocapnia. J ECT 2014;30(4):287–91.
[62] Gómez-Arnau J, de Arriba-Arnau A, Correas-Lauffer J, et al. Hyperventilation and electroconvulsive therapy: a literature review. Gen Hosp Psychiatry 2018;50:54–62.
[63] McCormick AS, Saunders DS. Oxygen desaturation of patients recovering from electroconvulsive therapy. Anaesthesia 1996;51(7):702–4.

[64] Surve R, Bansal S, Sriganesh K, et al. Incidence and risk factors for oxygen saturation during recovery from modified electroconvulsive therapy: a prospective observational study. J Anesthesiol Clin Pharmacol 2015;31(1):99–103.
[65] Koyama Y, Tzuzaki K, Suzuki T, et al. Prevention of oxygen desaturation in morbidly obese patients during electroconvulsive therapy: a narrative review. J ECT 2020;36(3):161–7.
[66] Kronsell A, Nordenskjold, Bell M, et al. The effect of anaesthetic dose on response and remission in electroconvulsive therapy for major depressive disorder: a nationwide register-based cohort study. BJPsych Open 2021;23(2):e71.
[67] Lihua P, Su M, Ke W, et al. Different regimens of intravenous sedatives or hypnotics for electroconvulsive therapy (ECT) in adult patients with depression. Cochrane Database Syst Rev 2014;2014(4):CD009763.
[68] Kellner CH, Bryson EO. Electroconvulsive therapy anesthesia technique: minimalist versus maximally managed. J ECT 2013;29(2):153–5.
[69] Bryson EO, Aloysi AS, Popeo DM, et al. Methohexital and succinylcholine dosing for electroconvulsive therapy (ECT):actual versus ideal. J ECT 2012;28(3):e29–30.
[70] Fredman B, d'Etienne J, Smith I, et al. Anesthesia for electroconvulsive therapy: effects of propofol and methohexital on seizure activity and recovery. Anesth Analg 1994;79(1): 75–9.
[71] Geretsegger C, Nickel M, Judendorfer B, et al. Propofol and methohexital as anesthetic agents for blind comparison of electroconvulsive therapy seizure quality, therapeutic efficacy, and cognitive performance. J ECT 2007;23(4):239–43.
[72] Vaidya PV, Anderson EL, Bobb A, et al. A within-subject comparison of propofol and methohexital anesthesia for electroconvulsive therapy. J ECT 2021;28(1):14–9.
[73] Tzabazis A, Schmitt HJ, Ihmsen H, et al. Postictal agitation after electroconvulsive therapy: incidence, severity, and propofol as a treatment option. J ECT 2013;189–95.
[74] Janouschek H, Nickl-Jockschat T, Haeck M, et al. Comparison of methohexital and etomidate as anesthetic agents for electroconvulsive therapy in affective and psychotic disorders. J Pyschiatr Res 2013;47(5):686–93.
[75] Singh PM, Arora S, Borle A, et al. Evaluation of etomidate for seizure duration in electroconvulsive therapy: a systematic review. J ECT 2015;31:213–25.
[76] Mehta D, Palta S, Gupta N, et al. Comparison of effect of etomidate with propofol on hemodynamics during modified electroconvulsive therapy. J Anesthesiol Clin Pharmacol 2022;38(1):104–10.
[77] Bryson EO, Ahle GM, Liebman LS, et al. Dosing and effectiveness of ketamine for electroconvulsive therapy (ECT): a case series. Australas Psychiatry 2014;22(5):467–9.
[78] Ainsworth NJ, Sepehry AA, Vila-Rodriguez F. Effects of ketamine anesthesia on efficacy, tolerability, seizure response, and neurocognitive outcome in electroconvulsive therapy: a comprehensive meta-analysis of doubled-blind randomized controlled trials. J ECT 2020;36(2):94–105.
[79] Aoki N, Suwa T, Kawashima H, et al. Sevoflurane in electroconvulsive therapy; a systematic review and meta-analysis of randomized trials. J Psychiatr Res 2012;141:16–25.
[80] Andrade C. Anesthesia for electroconvulsive therapy: a niche role for sevoflurane. J Clin Psychiatry 2021;82(4):21f14173.
[81] Gasteiger L, Heil M, Hörner E, et al. Relationship between anesthesia depth and quality of seizures in patients undergoing electroconvulsive therapy: a prospective observational study. J ECT 2022;38(1):62–7.
[82] Currier G, Gianni MA. Th effectiveness of BIS monitoring during electroconvulsive therapy: a systematic review and meta-analysis. J Clin Anesth 2016;58:100–4.
[83] Mirzakhani H, Guchelaar HJ, Welch CA, et al. Minimum effective doses of succinylcholine and rocuronium during electroconvulsive therapy: a prospective, randomized, crossover trial. Anesth Analg 2016;123(3):587–96.
[84] Bryson EWO, Kellner CH, Li EH, et al. Extreme variability in succinylcholine dose for muscle relaxation in electroconvulsive therapy. Australas Psychiatry 2018;26(4):391–3.

[85] Kadoi Y, Hoshi H, Nishida A, et al. Comparison of recovery times from rocuronium-induced muscle relaxation after reversal with three different doses of sugammadex and succinylcholine during elctroconvulsive therapy. J Anesth 2011;25(6):855–9.
[86] Ittasakul P, Jarernatt P, Tor PC. Prevalence and predictors of postictal confusion after electroconvulsive therapy. Neuropsychiatr Dis Treat 2021;17:283–9.
[87] Allen ND, Allison CL, Goleblowski R, et al. Factors associated with postictal agitation after electroconvulsive therapy. J ECT 2022;38(1):60–1.

Advances in Anesthesia 40 (2022) 223–239

ADVANCES IN ANESTHESIA

ELSEVIER
MOSBY

Advocacy for Anesthesiologists

Richard P. Dutton, MD, MBA[a,*],
Sherif Zaafran, MD[b], Moeed Azam, MD[c]

[a]Department of Anesthesiology, Texas A&M College of Medicine, Baylor University Medical Center, Dallas, TX, USA; [b]Texas Society of Anesthesiologists, Texas Medical Board, Houston, TX, USA; [c]Legislative Committee, Florida Society of Anesthesiologists, Orlando, FL, USA

Keywords

• Advocacy • Practice management • Surprise medical billing • Reimbursement
• Professionalism

Key points

- Every anesthesiologist represents our specialty every day; advocacy is a professional responsibility.
- Anesthesiologists can promote the specialty through membership in specialty and subspecialty societies; through participation in the American Society of Anesthesiologists Political Action Committee; and through active engagement with external stakeholders, such as administrators, regulators, and elected officials.
- Key issues confronting anesthesiology today include workforce supply and demand, reform of reimbursement mechanisms, and management of unexpected insurance coverage gaps.

INTRODUCTION

> America is not governed by the majority, but the majority that participate.
>
> —Thomas Jefferson [1]

We offer this description of advocacy for anesthesiologists, both to improve the reputation of our specialty and in reference to specific issues of today. We offer thoughts on the complexity of modern health care and how anesthesiologists fit within it, and we provide specific recommendations for how every

Note: All authors played a role in the preparation of the article, figures, and boxes. All authors attest to having approved the final manuscript.

*Corresponding author. US Anesthesia Partners, 12222 Merit Drive, Suite 700, Dallas, TX 75251. *E-mail address:* richard.dutton@usap.com

https://doi.org/10.1016/j.aan.2022.07.006
0737-6146/22/

anesthesiologist can get involved. While our presentation is focused on the current US health care system and its unique issues, the need for professional engagement applies to anesthesiologists anywhere in the world.

Advocacy is public support for, or recommendation of, a particular cause or policy. In anesthesiology, it means being a supporter of the profession, representing it to all stakeholders–including patients, surgeons, hospital administrators, regulators, and payers–and speaking out on issues that affect our collective future. We are stronger together, but only if we are pulling in the same direction. Even when consensus is not possible, every anesthesiologist should be motivated to preserve the future of the profession.

WHY GET INVOLVED?

In American politics, "advocacy" conjures an image of political donations, meetings in smoke-filled rooms, and support of candidates for public office. Advocacy is easy to conflate with support for a specific political party or issue, and it is easy to dismiss as unbecoming of a medical professional. In actuality, every anesthesiologist contributes to how our specialty is viewed by patients, fellow clinicians, and administrators. The higher our standing in the eyes of these stakeholders, the better for us all.

Advocacy for anesthesiology means being a proponent of our specialty and the unique value we bring to modern health care. We are leaders of clinical care teams, researchers, teachers, and mentors, and we are respected colleagues by institutional administration, regulators, and health care policymakers. Advocacy means communicating the importance of what we do to patients and administrators, teaching medical students the nature of our work, and pushing for high-quality care today while embracing the scientific progress of evidence-based medicine for the future.

Advocacy, defined as the act of supporting, defending, or arguing for a specific issue, can be used to avoid unintended consequences by regulatory or public policy forces [2]. As professionals, we support these efforts with a contribution of time or money. Time out of the operating room (OR), time to attend a bylaws meeting, time to meet a legislator or interest group, and time to cover for one of your colleagues so they can attend a meeting. Money for a poll, money for a digital letter-writing campaign, money for a governmental relations lobbyist, money for a marketing and educational packet to help educate an elected official or their staff, or money to support a candidate who supports an issue important to our profession. Advocacy is not just lobbying but is the broader act of supporting and promoting a cause or issue in the public or private sector [2]. Lobbying is a specific form of advocacy, with the goal of influencing a decision-maker on a specific piece of legislation or policy. As Joshi states, "Not all advocacy is lobbying, but all lobbying is advocacy." [2] Lobbying activities are regulated at both the state and federal levels, and lobbyists must be registered or licensed by the government. What is permitted or prohibited varies significantly by state, by organization type (political committee, political action committee, tax status, and so on), by membership, contribution sources and limits, and distribution channels.

Health care is a complicated business characterized by multiple intersecting entities. The political process directly impacts how we are reimbursed for services, the regulatory and legal framework in which we provide care, the role of nonphysician providers in our clinical arena, and even who can call themselves an "anesthesiologist." Similarly, seemingly rational actions taken by one group–for example, payers–might have profound effects on other groups. Without constant communication between the stakeholders, it will be impossible to achieve a fair balance of forces and an equitable reward for our work. This communication can only occur if experts in each domain invest the time and energy to educate others. It is not only ethical, but we believe it is our duty to engage in advocacy as a professional responsibility. Public policies and legislation directly affect our patients with respect to access to care, quality standards, and the financial implications of receiving medical care. To remain operational, anesthesiology practices require both reimbursement and supportive economic incentives to provide broad access to care [2]. It would be wonderful if the only thing anesthesiologists had to worry about was providing the best clinical care for the patient in front of them, but in fact, our responsibility is larger than that: we must also care for future patients, promote efficient delivery of population health, and push for wellness and sustainability for the next generation of anesthesiologists. In its broadest sense, advocacy includes our responsibilities as residents of planet Earth; this is illustrated by recent publications on the environmental impact of anesthesia medications and disposables [3,4].

GETTING INVOLVED

Personal participation

We are all passive advocates for anesthesiology, by default. This advocacy begins with professionalism, with how we present ourselves to our patients, our coworkers, and the public. Providing exceptional patient care is a given. We must also strive to be "the grown-up in the room" when managing complex and often emotional interactions between surgeons, OR personnel, administrators, patients, and families. Doing so enhances our collective reputation for being cool under fire, for having strong interpersonal skills, and the ability to prioritize among multiple options with different ratios of risk to benefit. Each of us does this every day as we go about our clinical work, and we should be mindful that we are representing our colleagues and our profession as well as ourselves. This is reflected in American Board of Anesthesiology (ABA) requirements for demonstration of professionalism, and in new residency training activities.

Other components of advocacy require voluntary effort. The simplest is the willingness to show up and participate in relevant nonclinical activities. These include practice or department meetings; hospital committees; state medical or anesthesia society gatherings; or even such things as group charity fundraisers and medical mission trips. Each anesthesiologist should pick the activities that best align with his or her values, whether financial, operational, or humanitarian. The colleague who wants nothing to do with politics or group leadership but who devotes 2 weeks a year to anesthesia service in the developing world is just as much an advocate for anesthesiology as those who run for medical society leadership positions or public office.

Society membership

Participation in "organized medicine" is recommended for every anesthesiologist. At its simplest, this means membership–and payment of dues–in city, state, and national medical societies, and in the American Society of Anesthesiologists (ASA) and the affiliated state society. The ASA is a distinct entity from the ABA, which brings credibility to our profession–a form of advocacy–through certification of the training and professional status of anesthesiologists. It has been said that: the ASA represents the specialty to the public, whereas the ABA ensures the public can trust the specialty.

Even for those who do not attend meetings or speak out on issues, membership is a way of saying "I stand with them." The greater the percentage of eligible physicians who are active members of each society, the greater its credibility when weighing in on important policy issues. Physician anesthesiologists have been in meetings with elected statehouse and Congressional representatives and have been directly asked where the state medical society or the American Medical Association (AMA) stands on that particular issue under discussion. The "opinion" of large medical organizations matters, but it takes active membership to influence positions from within [5].

The AMA represents less than half of all licensed US physicians but is the largest national voice for medicine, and AMA membership is recommended [6]. The fact that AMA membership among anesthesiologists is higher than for other specialties gives us greater influence on the future of American health care; we should seek to continue this advantage.

The ASA currently includes 80% to 85% of all licensed anesthesiologists in the United States, and it is the most influential voice for our profession. Although anesthesiology practice models vary widely from academic departments to government employees to large group practices to independent contractors, we are all providing similar care for similar patients having similar procedures. ASA's ability to deliver educational materials, convene meetings, and create universal standards and guidelines provides value to every anesthesiologist. ASA is large and inclusive enough to serve as the official representative of our specialty to the federal government, other specialty societies, international organizations, and to groups such as the American Hospital Association. For example, ASA's National Anesthesia Clinical Outcomes Registry is one of a small number of Qualified Clinical Data Registries authorized as a conduit for data reporting to the Centers for Medicare and Medicaid Services [7]. National anesthesia organizations in other countries have similar high participation and representation and are equally important for advocacy within their own national health care systems.

ASA membership includes membership in a state or "component" anesthesia society. Participation in the state anesthesia society is an easy approach to

Box 1: An illustration of state-level advocacy

In 2006, the Oklahoma Society of Anesthesiologists conducted a survey of 300 anesthesiologists in the state, demonstrating that over 80% were "totally dissatisfied" with state Medicaid compensation for anesthesia services:

"The final report found that Oklahoma's current methodology for reimbursing anesthesia services is not consistent with current industry standards or with the Medicare methodology. The report also found that the Oklahoma reimbursement rates are on average less than rates paid by third-party payers and in some cases less than the Medicare reimbursement rates."

The OSA worked with state regulators to research anesthesia Medicaid rates in other states and to compare them to existing commercial rates within the state. The result was an increase in Medicaid reimbursement for anesthesia in 2008 to $31.50 per unit, representing an increase in reimbursement of more than $4,000,000 for anesthesia services annually.

From Ref. [8].

involvement at the national level. State anesthesia societies host educational meetings, elect representatives to ASA governance, and engage in local advocacy. Box 1 is an example of how state anesthesia society engagement can produce a benefit for the profession [8].

The big umbrella of anesthesiology includes membership organizations representing a dozen subspecialties and special interests (Box 2). ASA supports and collaborates with most of these societies, and there is often an overlap of leadership positions. These smaller groups provide sounding boards for individual interests, as well as focused meetings, educational materials, and quality improvement initiatives. Membership and active participation in a subspecialty society is a path to engagement for any anesthesiologist with a specialized clinical or educational interest. Many subspecialty societies have meetings in association with ASA meetings, as well as periodic opportunities to contribute to newsletters and guideline development. Participation in a subspecialty society enables connection with like-minded colleagues and networking with academic collaborators.

In addition to subspecialty societies, there are several nonprofit organizations that support our profession. The Anesthesia Patient Safety Foundation is a collaboration of anesthesiologists, safety experts, and industry dedicated to the proposition that "no one shall be harmed by anesthesia care" [9]. The Foundation for Anesthesia Education and Research offers grants to medical students, residents, and early-career researchers with an interest in advancing anesthesia science[10]. The ASA's Wood Library Museum in Schaumburg, Illinois, houses the world's largest collection of anesthesia publications and memorabilia and is a valuable resource for anyone interested in the history of anesthesia [11]. All of these organizations accept charitable contributions from anesthesiologists and practices and offer the opportunity to engage in projects and activities.

Box 2: Subspecialty societies in anesthesiology

- The International Anesthesia Research Society
- The Society for Cardiovascular Anesthesiology
- The Society for Pediatric Anesthesiology
- The Society for Regional Anesthesia and Pain Management
- The Society for Critical Care Medicine
- The Society for Obstetric Anesthesiology and Perinatology
- The Trauma Anesthesiology Society
- The Society of Anesthesiology Academic Associations
- The Society for Technology in Anesthesiology
- The Association of Anesthesia Clinical Directors
- The Society for Education in Anesthesia
- The Society for Neuroscience in Anesthesia and Critical Care

This list is not exhaustive but includes those most likely to have members in the United States; many of these are international organizations, while others have parallel organizations in other countries.

Political action

For those anesthesiologists who wish to participate in the American political process, the easiest starting point is a contribution to ASA's Political Action Committee (ASAPAC). Participation–with a donation of any size–offers the following benefits:

- The ability to educate and inform elected officials on the contributions of our profession to patient safety, quality, and facilitation of procedural care
- The ability to support candidates for office that align with our professional and patient safety interests
- The opportunity to learn from colleagues in anesthesiology advocacy
- Participation in ASAPAC events that include face-to-face meetings with lawmakers and the very important staffers and analysts who craft health care policies
- Access to policy briefs and other educational materials on current issues
- Offsetting the heavily funded advocacy of special interest groups that have diverging agendas from our profession, including payers, hospital systems, and trial lawyers

The ASAPAC is the second largest PAC in health care, trailing only the American Hospital Association [12]. This provides our specialty with a significant influence on health care laws and regulations. ASAPAC contributes to candidates of both parties based purely on their support for the House of Medicine in general and anesthesiologists in particular. The ASAPAC supports a full-time legislative and lobbying team that researches issues and monitors and tracks legislation. For those able and willing to engage more deeply than

Box 3: Active national advocacy issues for US anesthesiologists, 2022

- Payment for anesthesia services
- Supply and demand of anesthesia clinicians
- Physician wellness versus burnout
- Opioid prescribing and opioid use disorder
- Surprise medical billing
- Scope of practice
- Coronavirus disease response

an annual contribution, ASAPAC is a convener of ASA's national legislative conference in Washington, D.C., and is active year-round in organizing fundraisers for political friends of our specialty, as well as one-on-one visits to educate state representatives and Congressional members on the importance of anesthesiology.

Those who truly catch the political bug may wish to leap from the OR to elected office, at either the state or national level. At present, there is only one anesthesiologist in the US Congress, but our profession is represented at the state and civic levels across the country. In the Executive Branch, Dr. Lee Fleisher is Chief Medical Officer and Director of the Center for Clinical Standards and Quality at the Center for Medicare Services and Systems, and Dr. Jerome Adams is the former Surgeon General of the United States. Anesthesiologists serving as statehouse legislators include Dr. Tom Oliverson of Texas; Dr. Suzanne Harrison of Utah; and Dr. Michelle Au of Georgia. Behind these recognized public leaders are numerous anesthesiologists serving at the executive level in large hospitals and medical schools. For those seeking a public role as advocates of the profession, ASA offers training in public speaking, communication, and formal education in executive physician leadership, as well as specific guidance and networking for candidates for public office. Financial support for colleagues running for public office is something that any individual can do. Within one's own practice, facilitating time out of the OR for office-holders and candidates can be a valuable support investment.

What to get involved in—the hot issues of 2022

Anesthesiology is never without issues in the public eye. Some–like payment models and scope of practice–are eternal, while others like surprise medical billing, are intense for a time but will eventually be resolved. Box 3 shows a brief list of the most active issues in 2022. We discuss some of these in detail.

Workforce

The most serious issue confronting most practices today is an overwhelming demand for clinical services and only a limited supply of clinicians. Anesthesiology's ability to facilitate safe and efficient care has led every procedural specialty to request or require our services, leading to an ongoing boom in nonoperating room anesthesia (NORA) [13], such that care outside of the traditional OR suite is approaching 50% of the workload for many anesthesia practices. The demand itself is more than can be met by the existing workforce, and this stress is exacerbated by the inherent inefficiency of NORA sites, both in geographic separation and in time-management challenges.

With every facility requesting more anesthesia services and every anesthesia practice actively seeking more clinicians, intense competition has emerged around recruiting and retaining anesthesiologists, Certified Registered Nurse Anesthetists (CRNAs), and Certified Anesthesiologist Assistants. The rapidly rising cost of labor is a strain on every anesthesia practice, and on every hospital and ASC. Inability to match supply to demand is likely to exacerbate existing inequities in access to care and drive ongoing experimentation with new–and potentially less safe–models of care.

Advocacy around workforce issues is still evolving. Some obvious but likely insufficient solutions will include expanding federal funding for anesthesia residency positions; increasing the number and size of training programs; and providing economic support for hospitals struggling with high anesthesia costs. Future efforts might involve the endorsement of new models of care–assuming they can be proven safe and efficient–fast-tracking newer and safer anesthetic medications, and even direct governmental support for anesthesiologists who work in underserved areas [14].

Opioid prescribing

It is clear in hindsight that the over-emphasis on opioid-based analgesia in the 1990s created an opportunity for manufacturers to influence over-prescription in the hospital, in post-procedural care, and in chronic pain management [15]. This led to the crisis in opioid use today, with large numbers of patients suffering from chronic opioid dependence and follow-on issues including:

- Acute withdrawal syndrome
- The turn to nonprescribed street opioids
- Chronic depression
- Early death, from either intentional suicide or inadvertent overdose

In 2021, the number of Americans dying from opioid overdoses reached a record level, and our health care system will be grappling with this challenge for years to come [16].

Anesthesiologists have played an important role in advocating for these patients and have been at the forefront of identifying, understanding, and mitigating this issue. A recent meta-analysis showed that 7% of patients who are opioid naïve and undergo surgery are still on opioids 12 months later [17]. Our profession has been effective in reducing opioids in the perioperative setting with multimodal analgesia and the use of peripheral nerve blocks. However, on postoperative discharge, many patients continue to be prescribed opioids . As experts in the field of pain control, there are opportunities for us to play a greater role in managing these patients after postoperative discharge and in creating safe and effective means for weaning patients off of opioid medications. This would require a change in our mindset as well as changes in payor payment rules. Anesthesiologist Dr. Sherif Zaafran was one of the lead physicians on the White House Task Force authorized by a congressional directive called the Comprehensive Addiction and Recovery Act. The Pain Management Inter-Agency Task Force Report identified gaps and inconsistencies in pain management and offered recommendations for improving best practices in the management of acute and chronic pain [18].

Anesthesiologists have been instrumental in promoting opioid-free surgery and adopting nonopioid multimodal analgesic regimens (See article "Opioid-Free Anesthesia: The Pros and Cons" by Carcamo-Cavazos in this issue). Anesthesiologists have worked with hospitals on acute pain management protocols that de-emphasize patient-controlled opioid analgesia and have overall contributed to a substantial reduction in perioperative opioid use [19]. Going forward, anesthesiologists must continue to advocate for opioid-sparing perioperative care, for funding of clinical care for chronic opioid users–both medication-facilitated weaning programs and long-term care for those who cannot be weaned–and for basic science and translational research into safer alternatives.

Payment for anesthesia services

Fair payment for anesthesia services is an eternal focus of advocacy for our profession. On the one hand, patients do not intentionally seek out procedural anesthesia and would be surprised if it was not automatically included with a surgical procedure. On the other hand, there are few medical procedures today that are not made safer, more comfortable, or more efficient by the presence of anesthesia professionals. There is an unfortunate tendency on the part of administrators and surgeons to view anesthesia as a commoditized service, to be paid for on a transactional basis just like heat and electricity for the OR. Those with more perspective know better, of course. Significant value is created when a true partnership exists between the facility, the proceduralists, and the anesthesiologists, as illustrated by the rapid adaptation–and proven clinical and economic benefits–of enhanced recovery protocols across multiple surgical specialties [20].

In the United States, professional payment for anesthesia services has followed a relatively simple template for the past 40 years, based on the Current Procedural Terminology (CPT) codes published by the AMA [21]. Every medical procedure has an assigned code, organized by the body region involved. Each procedural code is assigned a corresponding anesthesia code, with a predetermined "base unit" value representing the typical starting costs and complexity of the anesthesia required. Base unit values range from 3 (eg, screening colonoscopy) to 30 (eg, hliver transplant). In addition, one "time unit" is awarded for every 15 minutes of anesthesia care. Reimbursement is based on the total units of care provided for a given case: the base units plus the time units. A 2 hour laparoscopic cholecystectomy (Anesthesia CPT

00790) is thus 6 units (base) plus 8 units (time) for a total of 14 units. Payment is made at a certain dollar value per unit, based on the patient's insurance. Medicare and Medicaid typically pay about $22 per unit, while commercial managed care contracts can pay $80 or more per unit. The gap between government and private sector pay is wider for anesthesia than for any other specialty and has widened steadily since the system was put in place. This issue has distorted the economics of our profession by lending undue importance to the payer mix of a given facility: the ratio of commercially insured to government-insured patients. With a shortage of anesthesiologists nationwide, the inevitable result is a disparity in access to quality anesthesia care. Under-reimbursed anesthesia care from government payors creates disincentives for the provision of anesthesia services in geographies with an unfavorable payor mix. Hospitals and other health care facilities often subsidize the shortfall because they need anesthesia services. Urban and rural hospitals have a doubly difficult task as they operate in environments where it is hard to recruit health care providers due to (1) poor reimbursement and (2) unattractive geography. Today, over 75% of hospitals pay their anesthesiology departments a subsidy, due mainly to the flawed Medicare resource-based relative value unit system for anesthesia services [22]. Box 4 presents an example.

Since early 2000, anesthesiology departments have been increasingly dependent on subsidies from their hosting hospitals to recruit and retain an adequate number of clinicians. Over the past decade, the percentage of hospitals paying anesthesia subsidies has risen from 15% to the current 80%. Reimbursement shifts in commercial anesthesia contracts will directly and quickly impact hospitals. In California, for example, state legislation to address surprise medical bills included the use of a median rate that was highly favorable to payers. This led to decreased rates from commercial payers, which led to an increased need for hospital stipend support. The impact has been most pronounced in nonacademic hospitals and even larger for practices at hospitals serving publicly insured patients. This issue has exacerbated existing health disparities and patient access issues in rural and urban underserved communities. Clinical anesthesia coverage may become commoditized as it becomes impossible to receive an appropriate level of compensation for higher-quality service. In the long run, this is likely to make California less attractive for the best-trained and most capable anesthesiologists, to the detriment of the public. In contrast, the Texas Society of Anesthesiologists was able to work with state officials to craft a state-balanced billing law that accounted for multiple different benchmarks, as well as market variation based on the quality of care delivered [23]. As a result, commercial rates have not been negatively affected.

Anesthesia services are an easy target for cost-cutting efforts by commercial payers, especially given the large and highly visible gap between market rates and government pay. The biggest commercial insurance companies are exponentially larger than even the largest anesthesia practices, allowing them to take a hard line in rate negotiations or ignore smaller practices entirely. The six largest for-profit insurance companies are Anthem, Centene, Cigna, CVS/

Aetna, Humana, and UnitedHealth. They took in a combined total of $1.1 trillion in revenue in 2021. As the discussion later on surprise medical billing illustrates, this economic power has led to physician- and patient-unfriendly behavior. However, surprise medical billing is only one battle in an ongoing war between physicians who would like to receive fair compensation for their efforts and powerful insurers with a strong financial incentive to increase profits by reducing payments for care.

Advocacy around payment for anesthesia occurs at both the micro and the macro level. The necessary links to anesthesia codes are created by the federal Relative Value Scale Update Committee (RUC), which must determine the cost and level of effort required for any given medical procedure, typically by comparison to existing procedures. The RUC must also periodically review existing codes and base unit values to keep the system in balance and in compliance with federal payment laws–the need to maintain zero-sum changes in the system as a whole. Every medical specialty is represented on the RUC; all believe that their services are essential (and undervalued); and the end result is a complex political process. Anesthesiology has been ably represented for years in this arena by ASA's Dr. Stan Stead and the Director of Payment and Practice Management, Sharon Merrick.

On the macro level, ASA is engaged in ongoing efforts to make fundamental changes to the system, with the goal of reducing the public-private payer gap [24]. Ideally, anesthesia payment would be based on diagnostic-related groups and would be synchronized with the work of other medical specialties. Such a major change in something so fundamental will take years to successfully negotiate, and even longer to integrate into practice. In the meantime, the slow but steady increase in prenegotiated flat rates for certain anesthetics, as well as our inclusion in payment bundles offered by hospitals or independent surgeons, indicates a desire for change in the market. Such pilot models are testing alternative approaches, identifying both positive value and unintended consequences, and will help to inform future developments in anesthesia reimbursement [25].

Surprise medical billing

Commercial health insurers create and package health plans to sell to businesses. These health plans have a "network" of doctors and other services and benefits bundled as a product for their customers. An in-network provider is a doctor or health care facility that has signed a contract with an insurance plan, agreeing to accept the insurer's discounted rates. For example, a doctor might charge $160 for an office visit, but they've agreed to accept $120 as payment-in-full when a patient with XYZ insurance receives treatment. If the patient has a $30 copay, the insurer pays $90, the patient pays $30, and the doctor forgoes the remaining $40 since it's above the network negotiated rate. Clinicians trade prices for the volume of patients that can come to them through a network.

An out-of-network (OON) provider, however, does not have any contract or agreement with a specific insurance plan. If they bill $160, they'll expect to

Box 4: The impact of disparate payment rates on access to anesthesia care (Frank Rosemeier, personal communication)

A common example of under-reimbursed anesthesia care is Medicaid payment for labor and delivery. In Florida, anesthesiology services were reimbursed by Medicaid at 14% of commercial rates, only 60 cents to the dollar for the same anesthesia service compared with federally funded Medicare, and less than 20% of the average commercial insurance contract. Further, the state Agency for Healthcare Administration (AHCA) capped the duration of epidural services at 360 minutes, even though approximately half of patients labor more than 6 hours. Medicaid recipients are over-represented in the high-risk obstetric group, of which up to 30% to 40% will undergo an unplanned cesarean section. The AHCA fee schedule reimbursed the anesthesiologist only one additional time unit at $14.50 to care for a Cesarean procedure. The decision to offer obstetric services at a particular facility lies with the hospital facility; as anesthesiologists, we do not choose or restrict the patients we care for, irrespective of insurance status. With the increase in eligible Medicaid recipients in delivery units from 30% to nearly 50%, this under-reimbursement put financial pressure on anesthesia practices, such that many chose not to provide labor analgesia, while those that did required subsidization by the hospital. This reimbursement was so far below market compensation that care was effectively "pro bono," yet unlike hospitals, medical practices and professionals are disallowed from tax credits or exemptions for such community benefit. As market dynamics created inequities in obstetric anesthesia access, it created a risk that policy-makers would allow less-trained personnel to administer labor anesthesia.

Florida anesthesiologists sought better solutions. Dr. Frank Rosemeier, recent past president of the Florida Society of Anesthesiologists, led a committee that advocated to members of the state legislature and the AHCA. Time and money were invested to provide data and evidence, to hire paid lobbyists, and to create summary briefs for agency administrators. Fellow anesthesiologists supported the cause by covering time out of the operating room for the anesthesiologists involved. These efforts resulted in an incremental improvement in the situation. An evergreen reimbursement increase was enacted for Florida Medicaid obstetric anesthesia service codes, ranging between 5% and 58%, resulting in a global increase in anesthesia payments of $1,285,347 across the state in 2021.

collect the full $160. The insurance plan might pay part of the bill if the plan includes out-of-network coverage, but patients are responsible for the full amount if the plan only covers in-network care. This coverage is specified to the patient via the insurance plan's Explanation of Benefits. Some health plans do not reimburse out-of-network providers at all (except in emergency situations), which means that the patient is responsible for the full amount charged by a doctor who is not in the insurer's network. Other health plans offer coverage for out-of-network providers, but the patient responsibility would be higher–sometimes substantially higher–than if seeing an in-network provider.

OON balanced billing, commonly known as "surprise medical billing" but better described as a "surprise gap in health insurance coverage," refers to the specific situation where a patient is treated at a hospital or ASC that has a contract with the payer but one or more clinicians do not–typically an emergency medicine physician, radiologist, anesthesiologist, or surgical assistant administering unanticipated care and not in the health plan's network. The frequent result is a hefty invoice coming directly to the patient from the OON clinician, putting them squarely between the clinicians seeking reimbursement and the payer attempting to deny or reduce it. The fact that the eventually negotiated payment is often in excess of what a prenegotiated contract rate might have been might have led some physician groups to pursue a deliberate "OON" strategy. Needless to say, this practice is a major dissatisfier for the patient who is caught in the middle.

As public unhappiness–and medical debt–has mounted, state and federal governments have taken action to protect patients from surprise medical bills. Although ending surprise medical billing was a patient-centric and noncontroversial initiative, the recent federal legislation was problematic as it threatened to disrupt insurer-physician good-faith negotiations and drive down in-network rates. This became an active issue for anesthesiologists when it became apparent that commercial payers would take advantage of badly written laws (as in the case of California, described earlier) to force anesthesia practices to either accept below-market contracts or minimal–and uncertain–reimbursement through a state or federal arbitration process that does not accurately reflect the free-market cost of recruiting and retaining anesthesia clinicians.

Before the recent surprise medical billing legislation (the No Surprises Act), there was a fair-market mechanism for reimbursement negotiations. However, insurance companies have access to rates across vast geographical regions, whereas physicians do not, implying that there was information asymmetry in the negotiation. By law, independent physician practices cannot exchange rate information with each other. When negotiations failed, both parties had the option of refusing to contract in a network, leaving the patient responsible. In the hard-fought details of the No Surprises Act legislation, the insurance lobby attempted to define a median or benchmark rate (often a percentage of the seriously flawed Medicare rate) as a default. If this benchmark rate is not fairly established, however, clinician practices will lose the ability to negotiate, and there will be an effective floor and ceiling on all reimbursements unrelated to the quality of care. As anesthesiologists, our profession does not typically have the same ability to select whom we care for or which patients and plans we accept; we must care for all patients presenting to the OR. Allowing large insurance companies to set, and then steadily lower, the "median" rates for our services would reduce anesthesia to a commodity and negatively impact the ability to recruit and retain anesthesiologists.

Following mixed experiences with legislation to address surprise medical billing in California, New York, Texas, and other states, advocacy led by the ASAPAC was successful in promoting passage at the federal level of a fair law for arbitrating out-of-network reimbursement [26]. This happened in late 2020, but the insurance industry's efforts to subvert the process continue, through influence on the executive-branch rule-making process required to implement the will of Congress. Final rules are expected in the summer of 2022.

Anesthesiologists have advocated at every level to thwart catastrophic economic consequences for the profession–from grassroots email and letter-writing campaigns to fierce discussion of the legal verbiage in hearings, markups, and extensive negotiations. We have engaged public pressure with battles in the media and press, health economics articles, and influential litigation by state and national societies, including the Texas Medical Association and the AMA.

A final rule that enables commercial payers to unilaterally set rates for anesthesia care will have a chilling effect on reimbursements. Given the workforce issues described earlier, this will in turn require substantial hospital payments to anesthesia groups to recruit and retain the needed supply of clinicians. As such demands for stipends and financial support escalate, hospitals and health systems will look to employ clinicians directly rather than partner with a private practice.

Scope of practice

Every medical specialty has struggled with the question of which medical procedures should be performed only by physicians, which can be performed by nonphysicians under direct supervision, and which can be performed independently by nonphysicians. Anesthesiology is no exception, with conflict extending back many decades over this issue relative to operative care, complex pain management, and specific procedures, such as epidural placement. Federal legislation in the 1990s gave each state the ability to "opt-in" or "opt-out" of a requirement for every anesthetic to be performed or supervised by a physician. To date, 20 states have opted out and allowed CRNAs to practice independently. The reality on the ground, though, is that this status makes little difference in the practice of either profession [27,28]. Almost every large hospital has physician-led anesthesia care, as this is necessary to recruit and retain high-quality surgeons. Independent CRNA practice, however, is common in smaller hospitals and surgery centers, whether the state is opt-out or opt-in; in states where physician supervision is required this requirement is met–on paper at least–through the presence of the attending surgeon or proceduralist.

Given the workload strain on anesthesia services today, one might imagine that scope of practice issues would abate. Involuntary unemployment in either profession is less than 1%. This happy state of affairs–for both professions–has not prevented ongoing provocations. CRNA training programs have added a third year of study to confer a Doctor of Nursing Practice degree on graduates, allowing them to claim the title "Doctor," while their professional organization has renamed itself the American Association of Nurse Anesthesiologists. Advocacy by anesthesiologists in response has led many states and hospital systems to adopt rules preventing title misappropriation, and requiring name badges to distinguish between physicians and nurses. Most anesthesiologists and CRNAs work together every day to deliver high-quality patient care. However, the ongoing war of words fueled by the more outspoken on each side is a threat to the desired culture of safety and cooperation in a high-functioning team and lowers the reputation of both professions in the eyes of the public.

It is debatable how to improve advocacy on the scope of practice. The American College of Obstetrics and Gynecology has been successful in its partnership with the midwife community through deliberate efforts to embrace and endorse the expertise of midwives, as well as collaboration on education, quality improvement, and women's health initiatives, with a consistent emphasis on respectful and inclusive communication [29]. Of note, this occurred in an era of severe workforce stress brought on by the malpractice crisis of the 1980s and 1990s. It is possible that a similar course is open to anesthesiologists, especially in an era when there is more demand for anesthesia services than there are qualified clinicians of any background. There is little doubt that abatement of combative rhetoric by both sides would be welcome to most anesthesiologists and CRNAs, and would improve the reputation of both professions.

SUMMARY

Advocacy is a component of professionalism for anesthesiologists, and every physician should be mindful of how best to represent our specialty to other clinicians, health care facility leaders, surgeons, and the public. Advocacy is obvious in public statements by individuals or professional associations but is also manifest in support for public health initiatives, donations of time and money to charitable organizations, and informed education of our residents and fellows. Anesthesiology is a rewarding career with the opportunity to do good work for patients and society every day. We should do our best to preserve these blessings.

CLINICS CARE POINTS

- Every anesthesiologist is an advocate for the profession.
- Professional success and clinician wellness improve the quality of clinical care.
- Imbalance of the high demand for anesthesia services and a limited supply of clinicians is the largest issue for most practices today.

Disclosure

The authors have nothing to disclose.

References

[1] Available at: file:///C:/Users/Foxri/Downloads/ASA%20Grassroots%20Network%20Advocacy%20Guide%20(1).pdf. Accessed April 17, 2022.
[2] Joshi A, Heller RE 3rd, Acharya PT, et al. Pediatric radiology and advocacy: a professional responsibility. Pediatr Radiol 2022;19:1–8.
[3] McGain F, Muret J, Lawson C, et al. Environmental sustainability in anaesthesia and critical care. Br J Anaesth 2020;125(5):680–92.
[4] Xiao MZX, Abbass SAA, Bahrey L, et al. A Roadmap for Environmental Sustainability of Plastic Use in Anesthesia and the Perioperative Arena. Anesthesiology 2021;135(4):729–37.

[5] Chediak AD, Strollo PJ. The Case for Membership in the AMA. J Clin Sleep Med 2018;14(5):899; https://doi.org/10.5664/jcsm.7140.
[6] Collier R. American Medical Association membership woes continue. CMAJ 2011;183(11):E713–4.
[7] Liau A, Havidich JE, Onega T, et al. The National Anesthesia Clinical Outcomes Registry. Anesth Analg 2015;121(6):1604–10.
[8] Available at: https://oklahoma.gov/ohca/providers/types/physicians/physician-reimbursement-methodology.html. Accessed April 18, 2022.
[9] Theissen A, Capdevila X, Warner MA, et al. A new SFAR/APSF collaboration: Another step towards the common goal of patient safety. Anaesth Crit Care Pain Med 2019;38(6): 671–2.
[10] Speck RM, Ward DS, Fleisher LA. Academic Anesthesiology Career Development: A Mixed-Methods Evaluation of the Role of Foundation for Anesthesiology Education and Research Funding. Anesth Analg 2018;126(6):2116–22.
[11] Bause GS, Vassallo SA, Warner ME, et al. From Park Ridge to Schaumburg to the World Wide Web: the Wood Library-Museum of Anesthesiology. Anesthesiology 2014;121(6): 1135–8.
[12] Available at: https://asapac.asahq.org/home.aspx. Accessed April 18, 2022.
[13] Nagrebetsky A, Gabriel RA, Dutton RP, et al. Growth of Nonoperating Room Anesthesia Care in the United States: A Contemporary Trends Analysis. Anesth Analg 2017;124(4): 1261–7.
[14] Nalley Catlin. Finding Creative Solutions to Workforce Issues in Anesthesia. ASA Monitor 2021;85:20.
[15] Soelberg CD, Brown RE Jr, Du Vivier D, et al. The US Opioid Crisis: Current Federal and State Legal Issues. Anesth Analg 2017;125(5):1675–81.
[16] Available at: https://nida.nih.gov/drug-topics/trends-statistics/overdose-death-rates. Accessed April 23 2022.
[17] Lawal OD, Gold J, Murthy A, et al. Rate and Risk Factors Associated With Prolonged Opioid Use After Surgery: A Systematic Review and Meta-analysis. JAMA Netw Open 2020;3(6): e207367.
[18] Available at: https://www.hhs.gov/sites/default/files/pmtf-final-report-2019-05-23.pdf. Accessed April 18, 2022.
[19] Krauss WE, Habermann EB, Goyal A, et al. Impact of opioid prescribing guidelines on postoperative opioid prescriptions following elective spine surgery: results from an institutional quality improvement initiative. Neurosurgery 2021;89(3):460–70.
[20] Smith TW Jr, Wang X, Singer MA, et al. Enhanced recovery after surgery: A clinical review of implementation across multiple surgical subspecialties. Am J Surg 2020;219(3):530–4.
[21] Available at: https://www.asahq.org/quality-and-practice-management/managing-your-practice/timely-topics-in-payment-and-practice-management/anesthesia-payment-basics-series-codes-and-modifiers?&ct=d95fcf63430094c0bddb49694d7d014d3b144a84ef1e6a2efe74783cba5b9c95b4daf783d5ad197563e2643c5d4-f158a9b4bff47506982683991ca90123745e4. Accessed April 19, 2022.
[22] Available at: https://enhancehc.com/resources/anesthesia-101-anesthesia-subsidy-drivers/. Accessed April 19, 2022.
[23] Available at: https://www.dmagazine.com/healthcare-business/2022/03/texas-physicians-win-battle-against-federal-surprise-billing-rule/. Accessed April 18, 2022.
[24] Nalley Catlin. Payment Progress Series, Part 2: ASA Initiatives to Secure Your Economic Future: The Implications of Health Care Reform. ASA Monitor June 2021;85:19–20.
[25] Merrill DG. Value-Based Payment in Ambulatory Anesthesia: MACRA, MIPS, and More. Anesthesiol Clin 2019;37(2):373–88.
[26] Available at: https://www.asahq.org/advocating-for-you/payment-progress/surprise-medical-billing-solutions. Accessed April 19, 2022.

[27] Feyereisen SL, Puro N, McConnell W. Addressing Provider Shortages in Rural America: The Role of State Opt-Out Policy Adoptions in Promoting Hospital Anesthesia Provision. J Rural Health 2021;37(4):684–91.
[28] Sun EC, Dexter F, Miller TR, et al. Opt Out" and Access to Anesthesia Care for Elective and Urgent Surgeries among U.S. Medicare Beneficiaries. Anesthesiology 2017;126(3): 461–71.
[29] Krolikowski-Ulmer K, Watson TJ, Westhoff EM, et al. The Collaborative Laborist and Midwifery Model: An Accepted and Sustainable Model. S D Med 2018;71(12):534–7.